Challenging Concepts in Obstetrics and Gynaecology

Cases with
Expert Commentary

Edited by

Dr Natasha Hezelgrave
NIHR Clinical Research Fellow in Obstetrics, Women's Health Academic Centre,
King's College London, UK.

Dr Danielle Abbott
Clinical Research Fellow, Women's Health Academic Centre,
King's College London, UK.

Professor Andrew H. Shennan
Professor of Obstetrics, Women's Health Academic Centre,
King's College London, UK

Series editors

Dr Aung Myat BSc (Hons) MBBS MRCP
BHF Clinical Research Training Fellow, King's College London British Heart Foundation Centre of
Research Excellence, Cardiovascular Division, St Thomas' Hospital, London, UK

Dr Shouvik Haldar MBBS MRCP
Electrophysiology Research Fellow & Cardiology SpR, Heart Rhythm Centre, NIHR Cardiovascular
Biomedical Research Unit, Royal Brompton & Harefiled NHS Foundation Trust, Imperial College London,
London, UK

Professor Simon Redwood MD FRCP
Professor of Interventional Cardiology and Honorary Consultant Cardiologist, King's College London
British Heart Foundation Centre of Research Excellence, Cardiovascular Division and Guy's and
St Thomas' NHS Foundation Trust, St Thomas' Hospital, London, UK

OXFORD
UNIVERSITY PRESS

OXFORD
UNIVERSITY PRESS

Great Clarendon Street, Oxford, OX2 6DP,
United Kingdom

Oxford University Press is a department of the University of Oxford.
It furthers the University's objective of excellence in research, scholarship,
and education by publishing worldwide. Oxford is a registered trade mark of
Oxford University Press in the UK and in certain other countries

Published in the United States of America by Oxford University Press
198 Madison Avenue, New York, NY 10016, United States of America

British Library Cataloguing in Publication Data
Data available

Library of Congress Control Number: 2014947259

ISBN 978-0-19-965499-4

Printed in Great Britain by
Ashford Colour Press Ltd, Gosport, Hampshire

Oxford University Press makes no representation, express or implied, that the
drug dosages in this book are correct. Readers must therefore always check
the product information and clinical procedures with the most up-to-date
published product information and data sheets provided by the manufacturers
and the most recent codes of conduct and safety regulations. The authors and
the publishers do not accept responsibility or legal liability for any errors in the
text or for the misuse or misapplication of material in this work. Except where
otherwise stated, drug dosages and recommendations are for the non-pregnant
adult who is not breast-feeding

Links to third party websites are provided by Oxford in good faith and
for information only. Oxford disclaims any responsibility for the materials
contained in any third party website referenced in this work.

FOREWORD

I feel honoured to be asked to write the foreword for this new book *Challenging Concepts in Obstetrics and Gynaecology* as I believe that it offers the reader a new learning experience. It is well recognised in educational circles that each of us learns in different ways and the majority use a plurality of methods to embed knowledge, skills, and attitudes. The use of storytelling in learning is increasingly acknowledged as a powerful part of the teaching armamentarium. This new book combines the stories of women presenting with complex clinical conditions with a holistic exploration of the issues that the obstetrician and gynaecologist needs to consider in order to manage these patients most effectively.

The cases cover all areas of obstetrics and gynaecology without being a reading list ticking off elements of the curriculum. Each case is written by a doctor in postgraduate medical training supported by a local mentor with comments and further emphasis on essential learning points from international experts. It is therefore up to date and relevant to cases that the reader will face in their practice.

The layout makes it easy to read extracts and presents learning points, clinical tips, and identifies the evidence base for further reading. I would recommend this book as a must to all in Obstetrics and Gynaecology as a readily available resource to deliver best care to your patients and as a teaching aid to learn or pass on those clinical gems we all value so much.

Diana Hamilton-Fairley MD, FRCOG,
Consultant Obstetrician and Gynaecologist,
Director for Health Education and Quality,
South London

CONTENTS

EXPERT FACULTY PROFILES

Professor Susan Bewley, Professor of Complex Obstetrics, Women's Health Academic Centre, King's College London, UK

Dr Sarah P Blagden, Consultant Medical Oncologist and Academic Senior Lecturer, West London Cancer Network and Ovarian Cancer Action Research Centre, Imperial College London, London, UK

Dr Fiona Denison, Senior Lecturer and Honorary Consultant in Maternal and Fetal Medicine, MRC Centre for Reproductive Health, Queen's Medical Research Institute, Edinburgh, UK

Dr Ben Fitzwilliams, Consultant Obstetric Anaesthetist, Guy's and St Thomas' NHS Foundation Trust, London, UK

Dr Christina Fotopoulou Consultant and Adjunct Professor in Gynaecological Oncology, West London Gynaecological Cancer Centre and Ovarian Cancer Action Research Centre, Imperial College Healthcare Academic NHS Trust, London UK

Professor Ian Greer, Consultant Obstetrician and Gynaecologist, Faculty of Health & Life Sciences, University of Liverpool, Liverpool, UK

Dr Mohamad Hamady, Consultant and Honorary Senior Lecturer in Clinical and Interventional Radiology, Imperial College Healthcare NHS Trust, London, UK

Dr Judith Hamilton, Consultant Gynaecologist, Early Pregnancy & Acute Gynaecology Unit, Guy's and St Thomas' NHS Foundation Trust, London, UK

Dr Kate Harding, Consultant Obstetrician, Guy's and St Thomas' NHS Foundation Trust

Professor Jenny Higham, Professor and Honorary Consultant Gynaecologist, Imperial College Healthcare NHS Trust, London, UK

Dr Fuad Hussain, Consultant Radiologist, Royal Surrey County Hospital, Guildford, UK

Mr Lawrence W Impey, Consultant Obstetrician, John Radcliffe Hospital, Oxford University, Oxford, UK

Dr Ed Johnstone, Clinical Senior Lecturer in Obstetrics and Fetal Medicine, University of Manchester, UK

Professor Sean Kehoe, Lawson Tait Professor of Gynaecological Cancer, School of Cancer Studies, University of Birmingham, UK

Mr Con Kelleher, Consultant Gynaecologist, Guy's and St Thomas' NHS Foundation Trust, London, UK

Mr Andrew Kent, Consultant Gynaecologist, Royal Surrey County Hospital, Guildford, UK

Professor Henry Kitchener, Professor of Gynaecological Oncology, Institute of Cancer Sciences, University of Manchester, UK.

Professor Sailesh Kumar, Professor of Fetal Medicine, Obstetrics & Gynaecology, Mater Research Institute, University of Queensland, Brisbane, Australia

Professor Pippa Kyle, Professor of Fetal Medicine, Fetal Medicine Unit, Guy's and St Thomas' NHS Foundation Trust, London, UK

Dr Kate Langford, Consultant Obstetrician/Deputy Medical Director Guy's & St Thomas' NHS Foundation Trust, London, UK

Professor William Leigh Ledger, Professor and Head of Discipline of Obstetrics and Gynaecology, University of New South Wales, Royal Hospital for Women, Sydney, Australia

Dr Geraint Lee, Consultant Neonatologist, Guy's and St Thomas' NHS Foundation Trust, London, UK.

Professor David Luesley, Emeritus Professor of Gynaecological Oncology, School of Cancer Sciences, University of Birmingham, UK

Professor Neil Marlow, Professor of Neonatology, Institute for Women's Health, University College London, UK

Professor David R McCance, Consultant Physician/ Honorary Professor of Endocrinology, Regional Centre for Endocrinology and Diabetes, Royal Victoria Hospital, Belfast, UK

Professor Catherine Nelson-Piercy, Professor of Obstetric Medicine, Women's Health Academic Centre, King's Health Partners, Consultant Obstetric Physician, GSTFT and Imperial College Health Care Trust, London, UK

Dr Susan E Robinson, Consultant Haemotologist, Guy's and St Thomas' NHS Foundation Trust, London, UK

Professor Timothy A Rockall, Consultant Surgeon, Director of Minimal Access Therapy Training Unit, Royal Surrey County Hospital, Guildford, UK

Dr Annemiek de Ruiter, Consultant in Genitourinary Medicine and and HIV, Guy's & St Thomas' NHS Foundation Trust, London, UK

Professor Janice Rymer, Professor of Gynaecology, Women's Health Academic Centre, King's College London, UK

Professor Andrew H Shennan, Professor of Obstetrics, Women's Health Academic Centre, King's College London, UK.

Professor Philip J Steer, Emeritus Professor of Obstetrics, Imperial College London, Academic Department of Obstetrics and Gynaecology, Chelsea and Westminster Hospital, London, UK

Dr Lorna Swan, Consultant Cardiologist/Clinical Lead for Adult Congenital Heart Disease, Royal Brompton Hospital, London, UK

Dr Jason Waugh, Consultant in Obstetrics and Maternal Medicine, Newcastle upon Tyne NHS Foundation Trust, Newcastle, UK

External Reviewers

Dr Deborah Bruce, Dr Kate Langford, Dr Lucy Chappell, Mr Geoff Lane, Dr Johanna Trinder, Dr Alex Digesu, Mr James English, Dr Sharmistha Guha, Dr Vik Khullar, Dr Kate Harding, Mr Con Kelleher, Professor Pippa Kyle, Dr Joanna Girling, Dr Melanie Allan, Dr Jane Norman, Professor Andrew Shennan, Professor Scott Nelson, Dr Sonji Clarke, Professor Sailesh Kumar, Mr Kumar Kunde, Miss Diana Hamilton-Fairley

CONTRIBUTORS

Danielle Abbott
Clinical Research Fellow, Women's Health Academic Centre, King's College London, UK

Viren Asher
Subspecialist trainee in Gynaecological Oncology, Department of Gynaecological Oncology, St Mary's Hospital, Manchester, UK

Natalie Atere-Roberts
Specialist Registrar Obstetrics and Gynaecology, John Radcliffe Hospital, Oxford, UK

Helen Bickerstaff
Senior Lecturer and Honorary Consultant Gynaecologist and Obstetrician King's College London and Guy's and St Thomas' NHS Foundation Trust, London, UK

Beth Cartwright
Clinical Research Fellow, Guy's and St Thomas' NHS Foundation Trust, London, UK

Matthew Cauldwell
Specialist Registrar Obstetrics and Gynaecology, South West Thames, London, UK

Manju Chandiramani
Specialist Registrar Obstetrics and Gynaecology, Imperial College Healthcare NHS Trust, London, UK

Jayanta Chatterjee
Subspecialty Fellow in Surgical Gynaecological Oncology, West London Gynaecology Cancer Centre, Imperial College Healthcare Academic NHS Trust, London, UK

Carolyn Chiswick
Clinical Research Fellow, MRC Centre for Reproductive Health, Queen's Medical Research Institute, Edinburgh, UK

Eduard Cortes
Subspecialist Trainee in Urogynaecology, Guy's and St Thomas' NHS Foundation Trust
Louise Webster, Clinical Research Fellow, Women's Health Academic Centre, King's College London, UK

Ruth Curry
Clinical Lecturer/Subspecialist Trainee in Maternal Fetal Medicine, Institute for Women's Health, University College London, UK

Shreelata Datta
Senior Registrar in Obstetrics and Gynaecology, Guy's and St Thomas' NHS Foundation Trust, London, UK

Christina Fotopoulou
Consultant and Adjunct Professor in Gynaecological Oncology, West London Gynaecological Cancer Centre and Ovarian Cancer Action Research Centre, Imperial College Healthcare Academic NHS Trust, London, UK

Gabriella Gray
Senior Registrar in Obstetrics and Gynaecology, Guy's and St Thomas' NHS Foundation Trust, London, UK

Natasha Hezelgrave
NIHR Clinical Research Fellow in Obstetrics, Women's Health Academic Centre, King's College London, UK

Julia Kopeika
Subspecialty Trainee in Reproductive Medicine and Surgery, Guy's and St Thomas' NHS Foundation Trust, London, UK

Sarah Merritt
Clinical Research Fellow, Early Pregnancy & Acute Gynaecology Unit, Guy's and St Thomas' NHS Foundation Trust, London, UK

Shruti Mohan
Senior Registrar in Obstetrics and Gynaecology, St Mary's Hospital, Imperial College Healthcare NHS Trust, London, UK
Jasmine Tay, Specialist Registrar in Obstetrics and Gynaecology, North West Thames, UK

Surabhi Nanda
Subspecialist Trainee in Maternal and Fetal
Medicine, Guy's and St Thomas' NHS Foundation
Trust, London, UK

Muna Noori
Subspecialist Trainee in Maternal and Fetal
Medicine, Queen Charlotte's and Chelsea Hospital,
Imperial College NHS Trust, London, UK

Pubudu Pathiraja
Subspecialist trainee in Gynaecology Oncology,
Nuffield Department of Obstetrics & Gynaecology,
University of Oxford, UK

Srividya Seshadri
Subspecialist Trainee in Reproductive Medicine
& Surgery, Assisted Conception Unit, Guy's and
St Thomas' NHS Foundation Trust, London, UK

Lisa Story
Academic Clinical Fellow, Women's Health Academic
Centre, King's College London, UK

Ai-Wei Tang
Subspecialist Trainee in Maternal and Fetal Medicine,
Liverpool Women's Hospital, Liverpool, UK

Parag K. Thaware
Research Fellow, Regional Centre for Endocrinology
and Diabetes, Royal Victoria Hospital, Belfast, UK

Kavitha Madhuri Thumuluru
Clinical Fellow in Gynaecological Oncology, Royal
Surrey County Hospital, Guildford, UK

Josephine Vivian-Taylor
Clinical Fellow in Obstetrics and Gynaecology, Guy's
and St Thomas' NHS Foundation Trust, London, UK

Sze Jean Wang
Specialist Trainee Obstetrics and Gynaecology,
St Mary's Hospital, Central Manchester Foundation
Trust, Manchester, UK

Natasha Valery Waters
Senior Clinical Fellow in Laparoscopy, Royal Surrey
Hospital NHS Trust, Guildford, UK

ABBREVIATIONS

2D US	two-dimensional ultrasound
3D US	three-dimensional ultrasound
3TC	lamivudine
AA	arterio-arterial
AC	abdominal circumference
ACE	Angiotensin-converting enzyme
ACHOIS	Australian Carbohydrate Intolerance Study in Pregnant Women
ACR	albumin-to-creatinine ratio
ACR	American College of Rheumatologists
ACU	assisted conception unit
A&E	accident and emergency
AFC	Antral follicle count
AFI	amniotic fluid volume
αFP	alpha fetaprotein
AIDS	Acquired Immunodeficiency Syndrome
AFS	American Fertility Society
AMH	anti-Mullarian hormone
anti-dsDNA	anti-double stranded DNA
AP	anterioposterior
aPC	activated protein C
aPCR	activated protein C resistance
APS	antiphospholid syndrome
AR	amnio-reduction
ARB	angiotensin receptor blockers
ART	assisted reproductive techniques
ASFR	age-specific fertility rate
AV	arterio-venous
AVSD	atrioventricular septal defect
AZT	zidovudine
BAC	Birth After Caesarean
βhCG	β human chorionic gonadotrophin
BHIVA	British HIV Association
BMI	body mass index
BPD	biparietal diameter
BPLND	bilateral pelvic lymphadenectomy
BSA	body surface area
BSO	bilateral salpino-oophorectomy
CBAVD	congenital bilateral absence of the vas deferens
CCC	clear cell cancer
CEFM	continuous electronic fetal monitoring
CFTR	cystic fibrosis transmembrane regulator
CHB	congenital heart block
CHIVA	Children's HIV Association
CHOP	Children's Hospital of Philadelphia
CI	confidence interval
CIN	cervical intraepithelial neolasia
CKD	chronic kidney disease
CNS	central nervous system
CNS	clinical nurse specialist
CO	cardiac output
COCP	combined contraceptive pill
CPAP	continuous positive airway pressure
CR	complete response
CRH	crown–rump length
CRP	C-reactive protein
CS	caesarean section
CT	computed tomography
CTEPH	chronic thrombotic and/or embolic disease
CTG	cardiotocograph
CTR	cardiothoracic ratio
CUAVD	congenital unilateral absence of vas deferens
CVP	central venous pressure
D&C	dilatation and curettage
DAU	day assessment unit
DHFR	Di Hydro Folate Reductase
DIC	disseminated intravascular coagulopathy
DOR	duration of response
DV	ductus venosus
DVP	deepest vertical pool
DXA	X-ray densitometry
EBRT	external beam radiotherapy
ECMO	extracorporeal membrane oxygenation
ECOG	Eastern Cooperative Oncology Group
EDF	end-diastolic flow
EFW	estimated fetal weight
EOGBS	early-onset group B streptococcal infection
EPAU	Early Pregnancy Assessment Unit
ERPC	evacuation of retained products of conception
ESHRE	European Society of Human Reproduction and Embryology

ET	endometrial thickness	ICI	International Consultation on Incontinence
EUA	examination under anaesthetic		
FBC	full blood count	ICS	International Urogynaecology & International Continence Society
FDG	fluorodeoxyglucose		
fFN	fetal fibronectin	ICSI	intracytoplasmic sperm injection
FFP	fresh frozen plasma	IOTA	International Ovarian Tumour Analysis
FGM	female genital mutilation	iPH	idiopathic pulmonary hypertension
FGR	fetal growth restriction	IPUV	intra-uterine pregnancy of uncertain viability
FH	fetal heart		
FIGO	International Federation of Gynaecology and Obstetrics	IUP	intra-uterine pregnancy
		IUS	intra-uterine system
FL	femur length	IV	intravenous
FLAP	fetoscopic laser ablation of placental anastomoses	IVF	in vitro fertilization
		IVH	intraventricular haemorrhage
FMRI	fragile X permutation	IVIG	intravenous immunoglobulins
FSH	follicle stimulating hormone	JVP	jugular venous pressure
FVL	factor V Leiden	KCl	potassium chloride
GA	general anaesthetic	KHQ	King's Health questionnaire
GAS	group A sreptococcus	LAVV	left atrioventricular valve
GDM	gestational diabetes mellitus	LB	live birth
GI	glycaemic index	LBC	liquid-based cytology
GM-CSF	granulocyte macrophage colony stimulating factor	LD	longest diameter
		LDA	low-dose aspirin
GNRH	gonadotrophin releasing hormone	LEEP	loop electrosurgical excision procedure
GNRHa	gonadotrophin releasing hormone analogues	LLETZ	large loop excision of the transformation zone
GP	general practitioner	LFT	liver function test
G&S	group and save	LH	luteinizing hormone
GRIT	growth restriction intervention trial	LION	lymphadenectomy in ovarian neoplasms
HAART	highly active retroviral therapy	LLETZ	large loop excision of the transformation zone
HAPO	hyperglycaemia and adverse pregnancy outcome		
		LMP	last menstrual period
HC	head circumference	LMWH	low molecular weight heparin
HELLP	haemolysis, elevated liver enzymes, low platelet count	LND	lymph node dissection
		LNG–IUS	Levornogestrel intra-uterine system
HIV	human immunodeficiency virus	LSCS	low segment caesarean section
HNPCC	hereditary non-polyposis colonic cancer	LUNA	laparoscopic uterine nerve ablation
HPV	human papilloma virus	LUTS	lower urinary tract symptoms
HR HPV	high-risk HPV	LV	left ventricle
HRQoL	health-related quality of life	LVSI	lymphvascular space invasion
HRT	hormone replacement therapy	MAP	mean arterial pressure
HSG	hysterosalpingogram	MCA	middle ceberal artery
HVS	high vaginal swab	MCDA	multiple congenital developmental abnormalities
HyCoSy	hysterocontrast sonography		
IADPSG	International Association of the Diabetes and Pregnancy Study Groups	MEOWS	Modified Early Warning Scoring Systems
		MTCT	mother-to-child transmission
IARC	International Association for Research on Cancer	MEA	microwave endometrial ablation
		MI	Mirena intra-uterine

MIST	miscarriage treatment	POP-Q	Pelvic Organ Prolapse quantification
MPA	main pulmonary artery	PPH	postpartum haemorrhage
MRI	magnetic resonance imaging	PPROM	preterm premature rupture of membranes
MSU	mid-stream urine		
MTX	methotrexate	PPUL	persistent pregnancy of unknown location
MVV	maximum voided volume		
MWT	minute walk test	PPV	positive predictive value
NACT	neoadjuvant chemotherapy	PR	partial response
nCPAP	neonatal continuous positive airways pressure	PRECOG	Pre-eclampsia Community Guideline
		PROM	pre-labour ruptured of membranes
NEC	necrotizing enterocolitis	PROMISE	progesterone in recurrent miscarriages
NICE	National Institute for Clinical Excellence	PROMISE study	Promoting Maternal Infant Survival Everywhere study
NICU	neonatal intensive care unit		
NK	natural killer	pT	primary tumour
NNRTI	non-nucleoside reverse transcriptase inhibitors	PTB	preterm birth
		PTD	preterm delivery
NNT	number needed to treat	PUL	pregnancy of unknown location
NRTI	nucleoside reverse transcriptase inhibitors	PVL	periventricular leukomalacia
		PVR	Post void residual
NSAID	non-steroidal anti-inflammatory drug	PVR	pulmonary vascular resistance
NT	nuchal translucency	qfFN	quantitative fibronectin
NTD	neural tube defect	QOL	quality of life
NYHA	New York Heart Association	RAC	rapid access clinic
PAMG-1	placental α-microglobulin-1	RART	robotic abdominal radical trachelectomy
PAP	pulmonary arterial pressure	RAVV	right atrioventricular valve
PAPP-A	plasma-associated plasma protein A	RBS	random blood sugar
PCOS	polycystic ovarian syndrome	RCT	randomized controlled trial
PCP	pneumocystis carinii pneumonia	RECIST	Response Evaluation Criteria in Solid Tumours
PD	progressive disease		
PEP	post-exposure prophylaxis	RFA	radiofrequency ablation
PESA	percutaneous epididymal sperm aspiration	RI	resistance index
		RM	recurrent miscarriage
PET	positron emission tomography	RMI	risk of malginancy
PFMT	Pelvic floor muscle training	ROMA	risk ovarian malignancy algorithm
PFS	progression-free survival	RPOC	retained products of conception
PGD	pre-implantation genetic diagnosis	RR	relative risk
PGD	prenatal genetic diagnosis	RV	right ventricle
PGP	pelvic girdle pain	RVSP	right ventricular systolic pressure
PGS	pre-implantation genetic screening	SBAR	situation— background—assessment—recommendation
PH	pulmonary hypertension		
PI	protease inhibitors	SCC	squamous cell carcinoma
PI	pulsatility index	SD	stable disease
PIH	pregnancy-induced hypertension	SFA	seminal fluid analysis
PKA	protein kinase A	SGO	Society of Gynaecological Oncology
PLGF	free placental growth factor	SIGN	Scottish Intercollegiate Guideline Network
pNK	peripheral		
POD	Pouch of Douglas	SLE	systemic lupus erythematous
POF	premature ovarian failure	sPTB	spontaneous preterm birth

SSR	surgical sperm removal	TVT-O	Tension-free Vaginal Tape–Obturator
STAN	ST Analysis	TVUS	transvaginal ultrasound scan
STI	sexually transmitted infection	TWR	two-week rule
SVR	systemic vascular resistance	UAE	uterine artery embolization
TAH	total abdominal hysterectomy	UFH	unfractionated heparin
TAPS	twin anaemia polycythaemia sequence	UI	urinary incontinence
TCRE	transcervical resection of endometrium	uNK	uterine
TCRF	transcervical resection of fibroids	US	ultrasound
TESA	testicular sperm aspiration	UTI	urinary tract infection
TESE	testicular sperm extraction	UVJ	urethrovesical junction
TOE	trans-oesophageal echocardiography	VB	vaginal brachytherapy
TRAP	twin reversed arterial perfusion	VBAC	vaginal birth after caesarean section
TRUST	the randomized uterine septum trans-section trial	VL	viral load
		VTE	venous thromboembolic disease
TTTS	twin-to-twin transfusion	VV	veno-venous
TV	transvaginal	WHI	Women's Health Initiative
TVT	tension-free vaginal tapes		

MRCOG SYLLABUS: CURRICULUM MAPS

IT, Clinical Governance and Research	Core Surgical Skills, Postoperative Care And Surgical Procedures	Antenatal Care	Maternal Medicine	Management of labour and delivery	Gynaecological Problems	Subfertility	Early Pregnancy Care	Gynaecological Oncology	Urogynaecology and Pelvic floor
Case 17	Case 2	Case 6	Case 11	Case 17	Case 1	Case 4	Case 3	Case 22	Case 21
	Case 21	Case 7	Case 12	Case 18	Case 2	Case 20	Case 5	Case 23	
		Case 8	Case 13	Case 19	Case 20			Case 24	
		Case 9	Case 14						
		Case 10	Case 16						
		Case 15							

ATSM CURRICULUM GUIDE

A 'classic' case of heavy menstrual bleeding?

Shruti Mohan and Jasmine Tay

Expert Commentary Jenny Higham
Guest Expert Mohamad Hamady

Case history

A 41-year-old Para 3 woman was referred to the general gynaecology clinic by her general practitioner (GP). She presented with increasingly heavy periods over the past year. She continued to have a regular 28-day cycle, but was now bleeding for six days each month, four of which she felt were excessively heavy, such that her daily activities were interrupted. She was not experiencing any inter-menstrual or post-coital bleeding, but did describe a feeling of 'pressure' in the pelvis. She was otherwise fit and well. Her smear tests were up to date and had always been normal.

Having had three caesarean sections (CS) in the past, she expressed a desire to retain her fertility, although she had no immediate plans to conceive. For the previous four months the patient had been using tranexamic acid as prescribed by her GP, but had not noted any significant improvement in her symptoms.

A pelvic examination was performed. The patient was noted to have a slightly bulky uterus, of approximately 10/40 size. The cervix was normal and there were no adnexal masses. The patient was referred for a full blood count and pelvic ultrasound scan. A menstrual calendar was provided in order for the patient to record the duration and severity of her bleeding prior to her subsequent review. In the meantime she was advised to continue taking the tranexemic acid.

⊗ Learning point Assessment and quantification of menstrual blood loss

Menstrual blood loss can be assessed both subjectively (by the patient) and objectively. Based on population studies a monthly blood loss of over 80 ml has been taken as the objective definition of menorrhagia. Approximately 10% of women experience a loss of over this level and it carries an association with anaemia [1].

Numerous methods for the objective measurement of blood loss have been described, including recording numbers of sanitary products used, weighing of sanitary products, use of a menses cup to collect blood passed, and chemical analysis of blood content of used sanitary products. Assessment of the number of sanitary products used can serve as a guide to lifestyle impact, but has been shown to be as related to a patient's hygiene practices as it is to the volume of blood lost. Many of the other documented methods have significant practical limitations, and some have been used solely as research tools.

In practice, any blood loss which a woman finds to be significantly detrimental to her quality of life should prompt treatment, and use of such subjective definitions is now encouraged. However, pictorial blood loss charts [2] and menstrual calendars remain useful, both for a patient's understanding of her symptoms as well as to monitor response to treatment.

⊕ Clinical tip Examination of women with menorrhagia

Symptoms such as unscheduled (post-coital or inter-menstrual) bleeding, pelvic pain, or pressure symptoms raise the possibility of structural abnormalities and other pathology. In practice, all women presenting to secondary care with heavy menstrual bleeding should be examined in order to assess the size and mobility of the uterus and for the presence of any cervical polyp. Where indicated outpatient endometrial biopsy may be performed simultaneously.

✪ **Learning point** Causes of menorrhagia

The causes of menorrhagia are varied **(Table 1.1)**. History, examination, and investigations should be directed towards the identification of the likely common causes, in order to plan appropriate management.

Table 1.1 Causes of menorrhagia

Pelvic	Uterine fibroids
	Adenomyosis
	Endometrial polyps
	Pelvic infection
	Endometrial hyperplasia
	Endometrial adenocarcinoma
	Presence of copper containing intra-uterine contraceptive device
	Uterine vascular malformations
	Myometrial hypertrophy
Systemic	Coagulation disorders, e.g. thrombocytopenia, Von Willebrand's disease
	Hypothyroidism
	Systemic lupus erythematosus
	Chronic liver failure
Functional	Dysfunctional uterine bleeding

✪ **Learning point** Investigation of menorrhagia

Blood tests—Full blood count is indicated in all women presenting with menorrhagia. In certain cases (relevant personal/family history, presence since menarche), testing for coagulation disorder may be appropriate. Thyroid function tests are only indicated if other signs and symptoms of thyroid disease are present. Routine hormone profile testing is of no benefit if the menses are regular.

Ultrasound is the first-line imaging modality. Imaging is indicated in the vast majority of women presenting to secondary care with menorrhagia and certainly it should be undertaken where the uterus is palpable per abdomen, a pelvic mass is found on bi-manual examination or where previous pharmaceutical treatment has failed. Both trans-vaginal and trans-abdominal scanning have a role, depending on the size of the uterus and patient acceptability.

MRI has no advantage over ultrasound as an investigation tool in most cases. However, where ultrasound is inconclusive it may provide valuable additional information (Figure 1.1). An example is the differentiation of adenomyosis from the presence of multiple small fibroids. It is also used to map position and size of fibroids prior to uterine artery embolization, and other developing treatment modalities such as MRI-guided focused ultrasound.

Endometrial biopsy: Although post-menopausal bleeding is the hallmark symptom which necessitates exclusion of endometrial pathology, up to 25% of women with endometrial cancer will present prior to the menopause [3]. In pre-menopausal women suspicious symptoms (eg inter-menstrual or continuous bleeding), suspicious scan findings or failure of pharmacological treatments, particularly in a patient over 45 years of age, should prompt endometrial biopsy. Blind, outpatient biopsy is convenient but is known to miss significant pathology in a proportion of cases.

Hysteroscopy (and directed biopsy) is indicated where there are inconclusive scan findings or a high index of suspicion regarding endometrial pathology. Occasionally it is performed because sampling is required but has not been possible in the outpatient setting. It is generally considered the gold-standard investigation due to high sensitivity and specificity for detecting atypical hyperplasia and endometrial cancer [4].

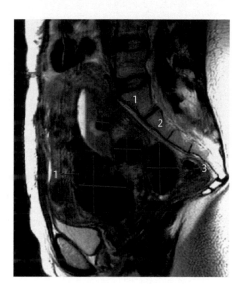

Figure 1.1 MRI picture demonstrating uterus enlarged with multiple fibroids. Note that the uterine cavity is obstructed by an additional large submucous fibroid (arrowed) to the left.

1. Submucous fibroid
2. Intramural fibroid
3. Subserous fibroid

⊛ **Learning point** Pharmacological treatments for heavy menstrual bleeding

Historically, pharmacological methods have been offered to women as the first line of treatment, and they continue to be the only treatments available in primary care **(Table 1.2)**. The following have all been shown to cause clinically significant reductions in blood loss in some women, and a variable amount of comparative data is available. However, the choice of treatment will depend upon the patient's preference in terms of hormonal or non-hormonal methods, contraception requirements and mode of administration.

The success of many of these treatments is often limited by their side-effect profiles and need for continued, regular usage. Patients will frequently seek more definitive solutions. The Levornogestrel IUS has, however, transformed the management of menorrhagia.

Table 1.2 Pharmacological treatments for HMB

Treatment	Administration	Hormonal	Contraceptive
Tranexamic acid	Oral tablets, to be taken whilst bleeding	No	No
NSAIDs	Oral tablets, to be taken whilst bleeding	No	No
Levornogestrel containing IUS	Intra-uterine device	Yes	Yes
Combined oral contraceptive pill	Oral tablet taken for 21-days of 28-day cycle	Yes	Yes
Oral progestagens	Oral tablets to be taken from day 5 to day 26 of each cycle	Yes	Yes
Injected/ Implanted progestagens	12 weekly intramuscular injection or 3-yearly subdermal implant	Yes	Yes
GNRH analogues	Monthly injection	Yes	No

She was reviewed in gynaecology clinic one month later. Her Hb was 10.2 g/dl (normal range 12.0-15.5 g/dl) and pelvic ultrasound demonstrated an enlarged fibroid uterus; one subserosal fibroid of 4 cm, one intramural of 3 cm, and one submucous fibroid of 3 cm diameter. No endometrial or adnexal abnormality was noted (Figure 1.2).

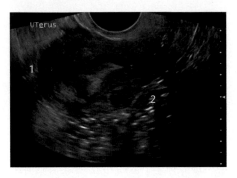

Figure 1.2 Transvaginal ultrasound picture demonstrating uterus in sagittal section:

1. Submucous fibroid indenting uterine cavity
2. Subserous fibroid

> ✔ **Evidence base** Levonogestrel intrauterine system (LNG–IUS)
>
> The LNG–IUS was first marketed in Scandinavia in the early 1990s as a contraceptive device. It quickly became apparent that it caused a reduction in menstrual blood flow, and, although not licensed for use in menorrhagia until 2001, it has dramatically altered the treatment of heavy menstrual bleeding in the past 15 years.
>
> An early investigation of its potential in the setting of menorrhagia [7] found an 86% reduction in menstrual loss after three months and 97% reduction after 12 months of use. 37% of women were amenorrhhoeic at one year. A Cochrane review [8] of RCTs compared the LNG–IUS with medical and surgical treatments. Compared with cyclical norethisterone the IUS was more effective and women were more likely to continue treatment. The IUS led to a smaller reduction in blood flow when compared to endometrial ablation; however, satisfaction scores were the same in both groups. When compared with hysterectomy, quality of life scores were not significantly different with the IUS, but the IUS was more cost effective. However, this was based on a single trial with follow-up of up to five years only.
>
> By its continuous release of 20 mcg of levonorgestrel every 24 hours, the IUS prevents endometrial proliferation and goes on to cause endometrial suppression. The hormone is largely absorbed by the endometrium itself, with little reaching the systemic circulation. Therefore progestagenic side-effects, although experienced by some women, are relatively infrequent and generally minor. However, patients should be warned about the possibility of irregular bleeding which is common for 3–6 months post insertion.
>
> The LNG–IUS holds a number of advantages over other treatments for menorrhagia including ease of insertion, no requirement for anaesthetic, excellent reversible contraception, and avoidance of risks of surgery. However, it is not suitable or effective for every woman, and there is evidence that a significant proportion of patients with an IUS will go on to request hysterectomy in the future.

The management options were presented as follows, with written information provided on each.

a. Hysteroscopy with trans-cervical resection of fibroid as appropriate, +/– insertion of Levornogestrel intra-uterine system (LNG–IUS)
b. Insertion of LNG–IUS without resection of fibroid
c. Uterine artery embolization

The patient opted for hysteroscopy and transcervical resection of fibroids (TCRF). In view of the anticipated resection, and patient preference, this was arranged under general anaesthetic, as a day case. A moderate sized Grade 1 submucous fibroid was noted and resected (Figure 1.4). Due to fluid overload and risk of hyponatraemia, the procedure was abandoned prior to complete resection.

> 🔓 **Expert comment**
>
> A fluid deficit equal to or greater than 1000 ml glycine should warn the surgeon to the possibility of hyponatraemia and hypo-osmolality. However, modern bipolar resectoscopes allow resection in saline and virtual elimination of the risks of fluid overload.

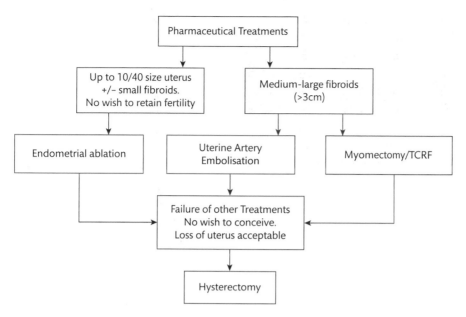

Figure 1.3 Treatment ladder in menorrhagia.

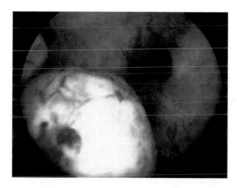

Figure 1.4 Hysteroscopic view of a sub-mucosal fibroid

Image courtesy of Ms Deborah Holloway.

> ⭐ **Learning Point** Treatment ladder in menorrhagia
>
> Treatments for menorrhagia may be considered in Figure 1.3. The patient's wishes will ultimately determine which treatments are given, and in which sequence.

> ➕ **Clinical tip** GA vs outpatient hysteroscopy
>
> Traditionally hysteroscopy has been performed under general anaesthetic (GA) in an operating theatre. Outpatient hysteroscopy is usually performed without anaesthetic or with a cervical block, ideally in a dedicated treatment room. This holds a number of advantages including greater convenience, faster recovery, avoidance of risks of general anaesthetic, and reduced risk of uterine perforation. In addition it is significantly more cost-effective, both for the patient and for healthcare providers.

An LNG–IUS was inserted although she was counselled on the possible need to remove the IUS and repeat the procedure if her symptoms were not adequately controlled. She was warned regarding the risk of irregular bleeding in the short term (up to six months) after IUS insertion. She was discharged on the same day with a normal blood sodium level.

> ❝ **Expert comment**
>
> First-line treatments for menorrhagia associated with fibroids may differ from those in a woman with a structurally normal uterus. Pharmaceutical treatments are likely to be less effective, including the Mirena IUS, which may also be more difficult to site in the presence of fibroids. However, alternative treatments are more limited in women with fibroids of a significant size. In addition they are generally more invasive, associated with significant risks, and have implications for fertility. Therefore finding an effective and agreeable treatment for these women poses a particular challenge and is the focus of considerable ongoing research. Currently UK national guidelines state that in the presence of symptomatic fibroids of 3 cm or over, myomectomy, uterine artery embolization, and hysterectomy should be offered [6].

> ❝ **Expert comment**
>
> Increasingly operative hysteroscopy such as the removal of small polyps, resection of small fibroids, endometrial ablation, and trans-cervical sterilization are also performed in the outpatient setting, dependent upon facilities available and operator experience. For women in whom the anticipated procedure does not necessitate general anaesthetic, outpatient hysteroscopy should be offered.

⭐ **Learning point** Fibroids and menorrhagia

- Fibroids are common, affecting 20–40% of women of reproductive years, with a higher prevalence in Afro-Caribbean populations.
- Although fibroids are often asymptomatic, their association with heavy menstrual bleeding is well established [5].
- Symptoms are likely to be related to the number, size and location of fibroids.
- Submucous fibroids, which may disrupt and expand the endometrium, are particularly implicated.

❝ Expert comment

The choice of treatment will depend upon the pattern of fibroids, the patient's desires regarding retention of the uterus and fertility and their preferences regarding undergoing surgery. Overall myomectomy is associated with greater blood loss than hysterectomy and patients should be warned of the small risk of proceeding to hysterectomy should catastrophic bleeding ensue.

⭐ **Learning point** Myomectomy

This is the excision of fibroid tissue from the uterus. It may take the form of trans-cervical resection of fibroid (TCRF), open myomectomy, or laparoscopic myomectomy.

- TCRF is a hysteroscopic procedure in which the uterine cavity is distended by fluid and an electrocautery loop used to excise the fibroid. This technique is suitable for submucous fibroids extending more than 50% into the endometrial cavity (grade 0 or grade 1 fibroids) whilst resection of fibroids which extend < 50% into the myometrium (grade 2 fibroids) may carry an increased risk of treatment failure and uterine perforation.
- Open myomectomy is the excision of fibroids via laparotomy. This is the traditional method but carries with it the operative risks and longer recovery period of open surgery.
- Laparoscopic myomectomy is offered increasingly widely and is suitable for subserous and intramural fibroids, depending on their size, number, and distribution.

The patient returned for review 6 months following surgery. Unfortunately she felt her symptoms had deteriorated over time and were becoming increasingly disruptive. She was offered further pelvic imaging and the treatment options were discussed once more:

a) Further hysteroscopy with TCRF or endometrial ablation as appropriate
b) Uterine artery embolization
c) Myomectomy
d) Hysterectomy

The procedures, risks, recovery, and likely success of each treatment modality were explained in detail, and she was counselled that having undergone three caesarean sections, she may have formed significant intra-abdominal adhesions and a thin anterior uterine scar. These would increase the risks of endometrial ablation and of any further surgery. In addition the patient was undecided as to whether her family was complete and expressed a preference for treatments which would allow her the option of conceiving in future.

✔ **Evidence base** Endometrial ablation

This is the destruction or removal of the endometrium. It should be considered in women with a uterus under 10–12 week-size (depending on technique) or fibroids measuring < 3 cm in diameter, who do not wish to conceive in the future. Overall, the average rate of amenorrhoea at 12 months is around 40%. A Cochrane review in 2013 showed that overall 90% of patients reported satisfactory reduction in menstrual loss at one-year follow-up. It further demonstrated that 20–30% patients required secondary treatment at two-year follow-up (9).

First-generation techniques

- These involve resection or ablation of the endometrium under direct hysteroscopic vision using electro-cautery (monopolar or bipolar) and include TCRE (transcervical resection of endometrium), rollerball, and laser.
- The MISTLETOE study (10) found rollerball ablation to be safer than loop resection and a 4.4% rate of significant complications including two deaths in just over 10 000 women.
- Potential complications are associated with dilutional hyponatraemia (cerebral oedema, seizures, and death) if excessive absorption of 1.5% glycine which is used as a distention medium occurs.
- These techniques require a considerable amount of training and experience in order to be performed safely. However, where hysteroscopic myomectomy is to be performed concurrently, the use of first-generation technique is appropriate.

(continued)

Second-generation techniques

- These are newer techniques which do not require hysteroscopic guidance, and are generally quicker. Some can be performed in the outpatient setting.
- Examples include microwave endometrial ablation (MEA), fluid-filled thermal balloon endometrial ablation and impedance-controlled bipolar radiofrequency ablation.
- They should be used as first line where no structural or histological abnormality is present.
- The overall success rates and complication profile are reported to be favourable when compared to first generation techniques [11].
- The long-term hysterectomy rate post second-generation technique treatment is low at 16% [12].
- Randomized controlled trials (RCT) comparing various second-generation ablation techniques show no significant differences in complication rates, amenorrhoea rates, or quality of life post procedure [13]. Therefore, choice of instrument will depend on operator experience and local availability of equipment.

✪ Learning point Uterine artery embolization

This is a minimally invasive procedure performed under moderate sedation and local anaesthesia by interventional radiologists. It has been increasingly used since the late 1990s. The femoral artery is canulated using 5F vascular sheath. The uterine arteries are then catheterized using micro catheters (2.7F) and micro embolic particles (350–900 micron) are injected in order to partially occlude the uterine arteries. Fibroid necrosis and shrinkage then follows. Patients are usually discharged within 24 hours with a relatively swift return to normal activities. Short-term symptoms including pain and fever are normal. Serious complications are uncommon although systemic infection due to septic fibroid degeneration is a recognized consequence and reported to be less than 1%.

Uterine artery embolization (UAE) is an alternative treatment for women with menorrhagia secondary to fibroids. It is less invasive and recovery time is faster when compared to myomectomy and hysterectomy and therefore it is an attractive option for women who wish to avoid surgery.

Trials have demonstrated that UAE alleviates symptoms in 60–90% of women, and that the effects last for an average of 5 years [14,15]. There is a mean uterine volume reduction of 40% post procedure. [16]. The HOPEFUL study, a retrospective cohort study comparing UAE and hysterectomy, found that 20% of patients required further intervention at 4–5-year follow-up [17]. Serious complications are rare and there are no major safety concerns associated with UAE. However, in most centres, prophylactic antibiotics are given at the time of the procedure to reduce infective complication rates. The effects on fertility and pregnancy following UAE are unclear; therefore patients should be counselled appropriately prior to undertaking this procedure.

✔ Evidence base Myomectomy vs uterine artery embolization

Both myomectomy and UAE are suitable for women with fibroids who wish to retain their uterus. Women in this situation will naturally wish to understand the relative risks and efficacy of these interventions. Only one small RCT, involving 63 women, has been published directly comparing the two procedures [18]. UAE was associated with shorter hospital stay (mean difference 1.6 days) and shorter time to resumption of normal activities (mean difference 16 days) as compared to myomectomy. Despite a suggestion of increased minor complications in the UAE group, there was no significant difference between the groups for need for antibiotics, need for blood transfusion, re-admission to hospital, or major complications. Relief from fibroid-related symptoms at 6-months follow-up was also comparable. However, the proportion of women requiring further intervention for their fibroids was markedly higher (odds ratio 8.97) in the UAE group as compared to the myomectomy group. In addition a number of cohort and observational studies have reported on this subject. Some have found lower transfusion and complication rates with UAE.

Overall the results support the conclusion that avoidance of surgery with UAE has benefits in terms of shorter hospital stay and reduced impact on lifestyle. However, as we might expect with a treatment which gives a variable degree of fibroid shrinkage, the proportion of patients requiring

(continued)

> **❝ Guest expert comment (radiology)**
>
> A recent randomized trial (FEMME) comparing UAE and myomectomy, funded by NIHR, has started in UK and the first report is expected in 2014.

> **❝ Guest expert comment (radiology)**
>
> Current evidence is conflicting regarding the use of GnRHa prior to uterine artery embolization. Despite the lack of clear evidence, almost all interventionists prefer to do UAE at least 4–6 weeks post GnRHa due to concerns that this hormone could lead to vasospasm and prevents injection of adequate embolic material.

further treatment (usually surgical) is higher with UAE. Evidence regarding complication rates remains conflicting, but the less invasive procedure (UAE) is also associated with re-admissions and occasionally significant adverse effects.

✔ Evidence base   Pre-treatment preparation with GnRH analogues

Administration of gonadotrophin releasing hormone analogues (GNRHa) leads to a down regulation of the hypothalamic–pituitary–ovarian axis. The reduction in gonadotrophins and ovarian sex steroid production can also lead to thinning of the endometrium and fibroid shrinkage. Long-term treatment is not recommended due to the effective induction of the menopause in patients. However, clinicians have often utilized short courses prior to surgery for menorrhagia, with the rationale that this may increase the effectiveness and reduce complications of treatment. A systematic review of over 20 RCTs considering GnRHa treatment prior to myomectomy was published in 2001 [19].

- Women treated with GnRHa had a significant reduction in uterine volume and a significant rise in haemoglobin concentration prior to surgery.
- As expected, they did experience more menopausal symptoms than those not treated or given placebo.
- Intra-operatively, women pre-treated with GnRHa required fewer vertical incisions, and there was some evidence of reduced blood loss.
- There was no difference in rates of blood transfusions or operating time (it has been postulated that administration of GnRHa can increase the difficulty of finding surgical planes and therefore increase surgical time).
- There was conflicting evidence regarding an increased rate of fibroid recurrence in women who were pre-treated, and insufficient evidence to assess implications for fertility.

In view of this, routine GnRHa treatment prior to myomectomy is not recommended. However, 3–4 month courses should be considered in patients with a greatly enlarged uterus or significant anaemia.

A new drug, Ullipristal, is now available and can be used as a substitute for GnRH analogues to reduce the size of fibroids [20].

★ Learning point   Fertility and treatment of menorrhagia

The majority of treatments for menorrhagia have an influence on fertility. Many pharmacological treatments are contraceptive, including the Mirena IUS. However, these are reversible methods of contraception, providing the patient with the option of pregnancy in the future.

Other treatments may have more permanent effects:

Endometrial ablation Ablation is unsuitable for women who wish to conceive in the future. Destruction of the endometrium impairs implantation and therefore reduces fertility. In addition the literature suggests that those pregnancies which do follow ablation are associated with high rates of miscarriage, fetal loss, and other complications such as retained placenta [21]. For this reason, the requirement for contraception post ablation must be discussed with patients considering this treatment.

Uterine artery embolization In some cases embolization will directly affect fertility by inducing ovarian failure. Reduction of collateral ovarian blood supply has been documented to lead to amenorrhoea in between 0.5% and 15% of patients in different series. Although this is more likely in women aged over 45, amenorrhoea has also been reported in far younger women.

Data regarding pregnancies which do occur after this relatively new procedure are now beginning to accrue. A 2009 review of over 200 pregnancies following UAE found a miscarriage rate of 35%, pre-term delivery of 14%, Caesarean section 66%, and postpartum haemorrhage rate of 14% overall [22]. The rates of pre-term delivery and malpresentation were similar in post UAE delivery and control pregnancy with fibroids. Although it is acknowledged that women who have undergone UAE are in a poor prognostic group in terms of pregnancy (often with significant residual fibroids and generally older), these results are alarming for women considering the procedure with a view to future pregnancy.

(continued)

Myomectomy This is the traditional treatment for women with bulky, symptomatic fibroids who wish to conceive. Risks include haemorrhage (rarely necessitating hysterectomy), infection, and adhesion formation, all of which will potentially reduce fertility.

Two studies have compared pregnancy outcomes following UAE and myomectomy:

- A retrospective review of 53 pregnancies occurring after UAE, compared with 139 pregnancies occurring after laparoscopic myomectomy [23], demonstrated a significantly higher risk of pre-term delivery (odds ratio [OR] 6.2; CI 1.4–27.7) and malpresentation (OR 4.3; CI 1.0–20.5) after UAE. There was also a trend towards higher rates of miscarriage, postpartum haemorrhage and caesarean delivery, although these did not reach significance.
- An RCT comparing pregnancy outcomes post UAE ($n = 17$) with outcome following open and laparoscopic myomectomy ($n = 25$) [24] demonstrated lower pregnancy rates post UAE than myomectomy (50% versus 77.5%, $p < 0.05$) as well as significantly higher rates of miscarriage (64% versus 24%, $p < 0.05$) and lower rates of live birth (36% versus 76%, $p < 0.05$) after UAE compared with myomectomy.

✪ Learning point Treatment of menorrhagia after previous CS

In a patient who has undergone previous caesarean section, certain treatments may be contra-indicated and others will carry increased risk of complications. The risks after multiple previous caesareans will be further increased.

Endometrial ablation The risk of uterine perforation and subsequent damage to the abdominal viscera is increased in the presence of a thin lower segment caesarean scar. The myometrium may be deficient at the site of the previous surgical incision and any scar tissue is a point of weakness. Therefore ultrasound assessment of the scar is recommended prior to first- or second-generation ablation. A scar thickness of under 8–10 mm (depending on the particular technique) is considered a contra-indication to treatment.

Myomectomy/Hysterectomy The presence of significant adhesions following caesarean will increase the risks of laparotomy, laparoscopy, and vaginal surgery. Bowel adhesions may be present and the bladder may be high and adherent to the uterine incision, particularly after multiple previous caesareans. Any patient in this situation considering surgical management of her menorrhagia should be warned regarding the increased risk of heavy blood loss, bowel and bladder injury, and likely longer length of surgery and recovery. Therefore these patients may have a higher threshold for considering surgical management and preferentially pursue treatments such as pharmacological methods and uterine artery embolization.

Uterine artery embolization Previous surgical history does not affect the success rate of UAE.

❝ Expert comment

UAE should be performed in women wishing to conceive in future only after careful counselling and explanation of potentially poor reproductive outcome compared with myomectomy.

❝ Guest expert comment (radiology)

Repeat UAE following initial successful results has gained growing interest. Recent studies have shown that recanalization of the uterine arteries post embolization is not uncommon. Also, alternative blood supply, for example from ovarian arteries, can be blamed for the regrowth. Therefore, repeating UAE can be considered in these cases. In a study of 39 patients who underwent a repeat UAE, 94% reported significant symptomatic relief [25].

In view of her surgical history and wish to maintain the option of a further pregnancy, the patient opted for uterine artery embolization. She was referred to a consultant interventional radiologist and the procedure was uneventful. She was reviewed six months later. She continued to have regular periods but these had become significantly less heavy. The patient was satisfied with the result and was therefore discharged.

Two years later she returned to the clinic. Her periods had become excessively heavy once again. Now aged 44, the patient felt certain that her family was complete and she requested hysterectomy. She had sought further information regarding the procedure through a number of health-related websites and in particular was keen to discuss the option of a subtotal hysterectomy.

She was counselled extensively regarding the risks of surgery, the recovery period, and potential psychological and psychosexual sequelae. The risks and benefits of total versus subtotal hysterectomy and of oophorectomy were discussed.

✪ **Learning point** Route and complications of hysterectomy

Hysterectomy may be performed by laparotomy, vaginally, or laparoscopically. The route of hysterectomy will be determined by:

- Uterine size
- Size and location of any fibroids
- Uterine descent
- History of previous pelvic surgery
- Surgical expertise

A systematic review of 27 RCTs comparing routes of hysterectomy (28) concluded that the route of hysterectomy should be considered preferentially in the following order: vaginal, laparoscopic, abdominal.

Vaginal hysterectomy is associated with a quicker recovery time and reduced post-operative complications. It is also the preferred route when a pelvic floor repair is indicated. Evidence is now building regarding the benefits of laparoscopic hysterectomy. Although associated with longer operating times and possibly higher rates of urinary tract injury, this is offset by shorter recovery, reduced blood loss, and reduced infective complications. Where oophorectomy is required in addition to vaginal hysterectomy, it can have a specific role. The advantages are likely to be even greater in the obese patient, but clearly specific expertise is required to perform these procedures.

Before opting for a total abdominal hysterectomy, patients should be counselled regarding the risks associated with major surgery (infection, bleeding, damage to visceral organs, venous thromboembolism, and anaesthetic risk) The RCOG quotes an overall risk of serious complications from abdominal hysterectomy as 4 in 100 (common).

❝ **Expert comment**

Hysterectomy remains the definitive treatment for menorrhagia, essentially guaranteeing amenorrhoea. A significant proportion of women will continue to require and request hysterectomy, usually where other treatments have failed. Potential benefits of retaining the cervix (subtotal hysterectomy) have been debated for decades. Only rarely, technical difficulties such as poor access or adhesions may prevent removal of the cervix and necessitate subtotal hysterectomy. It has been suggested that the reduced requirement for bladder dissection in subtotal hysterectomy is associated with a lower rate of urinary tract injury and urinary dysfunction as compared with total hysterectomy. However, this is not borne out by the three RCTs comparing the two procedures, with some evidence suggesting less urinary incontinence in women who had the cervix removed [26]. It is the concept that sexual function is less disrupted by retention of the cervix which leads many women to request subtotal hysterectomy. In fact, an improvement in sexual satisfaction has often been demonstrated with hysterectomy for clinical indications such as menorrhagia, likely to be related to relief from the underlying symptoms. The RCT evidence suggests no difference between the two operations in terms of sexual function [27]. Women considering subtotal hysterectomy must be counselled that this will necessitate continued smear tests and carries the small risks of continued bleeding from the cervical stump and cervical prolapse. Despite this, particularly in the highly subjective and sensitive area of sexual function, women who feel they will be better served by subtotal hysterectomy should be given due consideration.

✪ **Learning point** Oophorectomy

Bilateral oophorectomy was previously performed regularly at the time of hysterectomy for menorrhagia. It was felt that the reduction in risk of ovarian cancer, and the potential increased difficulty of performing oophorectomy after hysterectomy should it become necessary in future, justified the procedure.

In keeping with a general trend towards more conservative treatment and away from the removal of healthy organs, routine oophorectomy is no longer advised. The effects of inducing menopause

(continued)

including increased risk of osteoporosis, loss of the cardio-protective effects of oestrogen and menopausal symptoms should be explained. It is known that a high proportion of women who intend to use hormone replacement therapy following surgery will discontinue treatment within one year. In individual cases, for example in a patient with a strong family history of breast or ovarian cancer, there may be greater indication to perform the procedure. The risks and benefits of oophorectomy should be discussed in advance of any hysterectomy.

✪ **Learning point** Emerging treatments for mennorhagia

Novel treatments for menorrhagia, in particular in association with fibroids, continue to be developed. The following appear to be safe in initial studies, although most require a greater evidence base before being introduced into more widespread practice.

Laparoscopic myolysis This technique involves laparoscopic use of an energy source (laser, cryoprobe, or diathermy) to coagulate and shrink fibroids. Fibroids of up to 8 cm size have been treated in this manner, but subsequent pregnancy is not advised due to collateral devascularization of the myometrium.

MRI-guided high-intensity focused ultrasound An ultrasound beam is delivered directly to the target fibroid(s) percutaneously under ultrasound guidance. Reports suggest that due to the targeted effect of the ultrasound energy, adverse effects are reduced. However, the procedure is less suitable for women with multiple fibroids or previous abdominal surgery (burns can occur in association with scar tissue).

MRI-guided percutaneous laser ablation In this procedure, four needles are inserted into each target fibroid and laser wires are threaded through under MRI guidance. Once the tips reach the fibroid core thermal ablation is performed. Again, this procedure carries the advantages of using accurately directed energy, but may be less applicable where numerous fibroids are present.

Interstitial laser photocoagulation This procedure also employs laser fibres passing through needles directly into fibroids for treatment. However, in this case the needles are sited laparoscopically. Therefore MRI is not required and this procedure can be performed by gynaecologists.

In view of the patient's enlarged uterus and history of three previous caesarean sections, abdominal hysterectomy was advised. She opted for total hysterectomy but was advised of the small possibility that it may be necessary to retain the cervix and perform a subtotal procedure, should there be significant bladder adhesions or distortion of the pelvic anatomy related to the previous surgery. The operation was uneventful and a total abdominal hysterectomy was performed. The patient made a good recovery and was discharged from the hospital on day 3.

Discussion

Menorrhagia is a major cause of ill health in women. In addition, it is an important issue for gynaecology services, accounting for approximately 20 % of all new outpatient referrals. Despite this, until relatively recent times hysterectomy has been the only effective long-term treatment.

In the UK the number of hysterectomies for menorrhagia declined by 64 % between 1990 and 2002 [29]. There are a number of factors accounting for this dramatic change with the proliferation of effective, safer, alternative treatments such as the Mirena IUS and ablation probably the most significant. In addition there has been a shift in attitude and a recognition that some women experience physical, psychological, and psychosexual difficulties following hysterectomy. Women are now more likely to find a solution which suits their lifestyle and wishes regarding future pregnancy.

However, challenges still exist. Clinicians are increasingly faced with women who are delaying pregnancy until later in life, yet may have severe heavy menstrual bleeding symptoms resistant to medical treatment. The options remain limited for women seeking treatment which has no impact on reproductive outcomes.

In addition, as the caesarean section rate rises, we will continue to see more patients who have previously undergone considerable pelvic surgery. This has an enormous influence on the technical difficulty and risks of surgical treatments such as myomectomy and hysterectomy. Hysterectomy continues to be a life-altering operation for many women who have suffered debilitating menstrual symptoms. At a time when falling numbers of hysterectomies mean that surgical trainees are struggling to acquire and maintain appropriate skills, the greater complexity of the operations which are performed is a major concern. The search continues for an effective, non-surgical treatment, without impact on fertility and pregnancy.

A Final Word from the Expert

Heavy menstrual bleeding remains the commonest symptom leading women to seek the advice of a gynaecologist, hence effective and sensitive handling of this complaint is central to the specialty.

The trend towards more minimally invasive, outpatient-based therapies in all aspects of medicine is also reflected here and recent advances in both medical and surgical options mean that women now have a wide range of treatments from which to choose. Despite this, hysterectomy will ultimately be the chosen treatment for many women.

Hysterectomy is an operation which carries significant cultural and social implications. Enormous variation in attitudes towards the operation exist between cultures and individuals. For some, the loss of the uterus is viewed as loss of femininity and womanhood. The high rates of hysterectomy in years gone by has also been seen an indicator of male dominance in the political and medical establishments. Although evidence regarding sexual function post hysterectomy is conflicting, it is true that proper counselling and discussion regarding psychosexual issues prior to the procedure is associated with better outcomes. The paradox for the doctor is to reassure those women with severe, intractable symptoms who are likely to be best served by hysterectomy that their overall quality of life, including sexual function, is likely to be improved following surgery, whilst explaining to those women who attend convinced that they require hysterectomy having not fully explored other options, that their symptoms may well be relieved with more conservative measures.

Hysterectomy should only be considered in women who have completed their families and where other treatments have failed or are inappropriate. In practice, this means that those hysterectomies which are performed for menorrhagia are likely to be surgically more challenging; for example, for the enlarged fibroid uterus. The increasingly surgical nature of obstetrics is also having an impact, with a large proportion of women in their 40s and 50s having undergone multiple previous caesarean sections.

As the number of hysterectomies performed dwindles, providing adequate surgical training to enable gynaecologists to meet these challenges is proving difficult. Simulation will have a greater role and is particularly employed in training for laparoscopic surgery [30]. As technology develops effective virtual reality simulators for open surgery are likely to become more common, although their usefulness may also be limited by expense and availability.

For the foreseeable future, there is unlikely to be a replacement for the experience of operating on patients and therefore we now see a small proportion of trainees focusing on obtaining the skills required to perform more complex surgery. This trend is likely to become more pronounced, necessitating increasing specialization within gynaecology, with the majority of surgeons performing outpatient and minor procedures only. This in turn has implications for recruitment into obstetrics and gynaecology, and for the structure of services, which will need to accommodate greater referral between specialists. The priority is to maintain a system in which women have access to high calibre, appropriately trained doctors who can offer the breadth of treatments they need.

References

1. Hallberg L, Högdahl AM, Nilsson L, Rybo G. Menstrual blood loss: a population study. Variation at different ages and attempts to define normality. *Acta Obstet Gynecol Scand* 1966;45:320–5.

2. Higham JM, O'Brien PM, Shaw RW. Assessment of menstrual blood loss using a pictorial chart. *Br J Obstet Gynaecol* 1990; 97:734–9.

3. Rose, PG. Endometrial Cancer. *N Engl J Med* 1996;335:640–9.

4. Ceci O, Bettocchi S, Pellegrino A, Impedovo L, Di Venere R, Pansini N. Comparison of hysteroscopic and hysterectomy findings for assessing the diagnostic accuracy of office hysteroscopy. *Fertil Steril* 2002;8(3):677–84.

5. Wegienka G, Baird DD, Hertz-Picciotto I, Harlow SD, Steege JF, Hill MC, *et al.* Self-reported heavy bleeding associated with uterine leiomyomata. *Obstet Gynecol* 2003;101(3):431–7.

6. NICE Guideline, Heavy Menstrual Bleeding. January 2007. <http://www.nice.org.uk/nicemedia/live/11002/30404/30404.pdf>

7. Andersson JK, Rybo, G. Levonorgestrel-releasing intrauterine device in the treatment of menorrhagia. *BJOG* 1990:97:690–4.

8. Lethaby A, Cooke I, Rees M. Progesterone or progestogen-releasing intrauterine systems for heavy menstrual bleeding. *Cochrane Database of Sys Rev* 2005, Issue 4.

9. Fergusson RJ, Lethaby A, Shepperd S, Farquhar C. Endometrial resection and ablation versus hysterectomy for heavy menstrual bleeding. *Cochrane Database of Syst Rev* 2013, Issue 2.

10. Overton C, Hargreaves J, Maresh M. A national survey of the complications of endometrial destruction for menstrual disorders: the MISTLETOE study. *BJOG* 1997;104:1351–9.

11. Lethaby AM. Endometrial destruction techniques for heavy menstrual bleeding. (Cochrane Review). In: *Cochrane Database of Syst Rev*, Issue Oxford, 2005.

12. Cooper KG, Bain C, Lawrie L, Parkin DE. A randomised comparison of microwave endometrial ablation with transcervical resection of the endometrium; follow up at a minimum of five years. *BJOG* 2005;112:470–75.

13. Abbott J, Hawe J, Hunter D, Garry R. A double-blind randomized trial comparing the Cavaterm™ and the NovaSure™ endometrial ablation systems for the treatment of dysfunctional uterine bleeding. *Fertil Steril*, July 2003;80(1):203–8.

14. Walker W, Pelage JP. Uterine artery embolisation for symptomatic fibroids: clinical results in 400 women with imaging follow up. *BJOG* 2002;109:1262–72.

15. Moss J, Cooper KG, Khaund A, Murray LS, Murray GD, Wu O, et al. Randomised comparison of uterine artery embolisation (UAE) with surgical treatment in patients with symptomatic uterine fibroids (REST trial): 5-year results. BJOG 2011;118:936–44.
16. Coleman P. Review body for interventional procedures, Sheffield: Commissioned by the National Institute for Clinical Excellence. National Institute for Clinical Excellence 2004.
17. Dutton S, Hirst A, McPherson K, Nicholson T, Maresh M. A UK multicentre retrospective cohort study comparing hysterectomy and uterine artery embolisation for the treatment of symptomatic uterine fibroids (HOPEFUL study): main results on medium-term safety and efficacy. *BJOG* 2007;114:1340–51.
18. Mara M, Fucikova Z, Maskova J, Kuzel D, Haakova L. Uterine fibroid embolization versus myomectomy in women wishing to preserve fertility: Preliminary results of a randomized controlled trial. *Eur J Obstet Gyn R B* 2006;126(2):226–33.
19. Lethaby A, Vollenhoven B, Sowter M. Pre-operative GnRH analogue therapy before hysterectomy or myomectomy for uterine fibroids. *Cochrane Database of Syst Rev* 2001;Issue 2.
20. Hare AA. Pregnancy following endometrial ablation: a review article. *J Obstet Gynaecol* 2005;25(2):108–14.
21. Homer H, Saridogan E. Pregnancy outcomes after uterine artery embolisation for fibroids. *Obstet Gynaecol* 2009;11:265–70.
22. Goldberg J, Pereira L, Berghella V, Diamond J, Daraï E, Seinera P, et al. Pregnancy outcomes after treatment for fibromyomata: uterine artery embolization versus laparoscopic myomectomy. *Am J Obstet Gynecol* 2004;191:18–21.
23. Mara M, Maskova J, Fucikova Z, Kuzel D, Belsan T, Sosna O. Midterm clinical and first reproductive results of a randomized controlled trial comparing uterine fibroid embolization and myomectomy. *Cardiovasc Intervent Radiol* 2008;31:73–85.
24. Lucas B, Reed RA. Repeat uterine artery embolization following poor results. *Minim Invasive Ther Allied Technol* 2009;18(2):82–6.
25. Gimbel H, Zobbe V, Andersen BM, Filtenborg T, Gluud C, Tabor A. Randomised controlled trial of total compared with subtotal hysterectomy with one-year follow up results. *BJOG* 2003;110(12):1088–98.
26. Learman LA, Summitt RL Jr, Varner RE, McNeeley SG, Goodman-Gruen D, Richter HE, et al.; Total or Supracervical Hysterectomy (TOSH) Research Group. A randomized comparison of total or supracervical hysterectomy: surgical complications and clinical outcomes. *Obstet Gynecol* 2003;102I (3):453–62.
27. Johnson N, Barlow D, Lethaby A, Tavender E, Curr L, Garry R. Methods of hysterectomy: systematic review and meta-analysis of randomised controlled trials. *BMJ* 2005;330:1478.
28. Reid P, Mukri F. Trends in number of hysterectomies performed in England for menorrhagia: examination of health episode statistics, 1989 to 2002. *BMJ* 2005;330:938.
29. Coleman RL, Muller CY. Effects of laboratory-based skills curriculum on laparoscopic proficiency: a randomized trial. *Am J Obstet Gynecol* 2002;186:836–42.

Severe endometriosis in a young woman with unexpected end-organ failure

Natasha Valery Waters

ⓘ **Expert Commentary** Andrew Kent
ⓘ **Guest Experts** Timothy Rockall and Fuad Hussain

A 24-year-old nulliparous woman presented to a gynaecologist with 1-year history of worsening period pain radiating to her rectum with extremely painful defecation (dyskezia). Her menses started at the age of 14 and she had been taking the combined contraceptive pill (COCP) since the age of 16. Her pain had been manageable until one year earlier, when it failed to be relieved with simple analgesia. She complained of severe deep dyspareunia and had one recent admission to an accident and emergency (A&E) department with severe dysmenorrhoea, which was managed with simple analgesia.

Prior to this presentation she had been reviewed in clinic on two occasions by gynaecologists, who had both concluded that her pain was not 'typical' of endometriosis and was unlikely to be of gynaecological origin. There was no documented pelvic examination, but they recommended that she continue taking the COCP. However, her daily severe dyskezia was significantly affecting her quality of life and so a decision was made by the current gynaecologist to perform a laparoscopy.

✪ **Learning point** Pathogenesis and diagnosis of endometriosis

Endometriosis is a common and frequently debilitating condition, characterized by the presence of ectopic endometrial tissue outside the uterine cavity. It can present as a local disorder as well as complex, chronic systemic disease. Commonly associated with pelvic pain and infertility, its diagnosis and management can be extremely challenging for the clinician.

Whilst the exact aetiology is unknown, one of the most widely accepted theories—'retrograde menstruation'—proposes that the passage of menstrual blood containing endometrial fragments through the fallopian tubes into the pelvic cavity in a retrograde direction results in the formation and persistence of endometrial deposits. The retrograde menstruation theory, however, does not explain rectovaginal endometriosis and why endometriosis develops in some but not most women. Recently, ectopic endometriotic tissue was found in fetuses; empirical evidence supporting the new embryological theory [1] that postulates abnormal migration and differentiation of endometriotic cells during embryonic formation of female genital tract. Moreover, various environmental and genetic factors may cause gene abnormality in progenitor cells, predisposing the adult woman to

(continued)

❝ Expert comment

When determining the best treatment for endometriosis it becomes much more difficult to argue the case for radical surgery in case of retrograde menstruation theory as the disease will inevitably be recurrent in a woman who retains her uterus. The embryological theory is the only mechanism which readily explains the nature of the disease, but more importantly, when the conclusion is that one is dealing with a congenital disease, then a genuine cure may be obtained by means of radical surgery.

❝ Expert comment

It is not unusual for young women who present with these symptoms to experience resistance from the medical profession (primary and secondary care) with regards to referral or operative investigation. This often reflects a lack of understanding of the ramifications of endometriosis and pelvic pain. Vaginal examination is a key part of a gynaecological assessment and should always be performed at the first visit unless there is a good reason not to. In this case, it would have prompted the diagnosis of a rectovaginal nodule.

endometriosis [2]. These ectopic endometriotic tissues may be activated during menarche and have abnormally high levels of oestrogen and aromatase, and some are resistant to progesterone.

Endometriosis usually affects young women, with the highest prevalence in the 25–35 age group [3, 4]. It can progress like a cancer involving surrounding tissues distorting anatomy, and destroying surgical planes, yet the extent of disease is very variable, and correlates poorly with symptoms and sequalae, even in advanced stages.

On average, there is a lag between first presentation with symptoms and diagnosis of endometriosis of eight years. The three clinically distinct forms of endometriosis are implants on peritoneum and ovaries, endometriotic cysts within ovaries, and a complex mass containing endometriotic glands with adipose and fibromuscular tissue situated in the space between vagina and rectum and referred as rectovaginal endometriosis or deep infiltrating endometriosis. The symptoms of endometriosis vary. The most consistent are dysmenorrhoea (painful menstruation, affecting about 60 % of sufferers), and dyspareunia (pain with intercourse, affecting 60 % of sufferers). Other symptoms include chronic pelvic pain, menorrhagia, intermenstrual spotting, fatigue, dyskezia, and infertility [5].

Bowel involvement is the most challenging in terms of management and in endometriosis is rare (around 5 %), but may signify severe deep infiltrating endometriosis. Painful defecation and rectal bleeding especially during a period (signifies transmucosal involvement) and worsening constipation should alert clinician to suspect bowel involvement [6, 7].

The prevalence of endometriosis in women with pelvic pain who are seen GP surgeries is as low as 2 % [8]; however, it is higher in specialist gynaecology clinics, and amongst women presenting to specialist gynaecology clinics with infertility and chronic pelvic pain, it could be as high as one in three [9].

Laparoscopy is considered and remains a 'gold standard' for diagnosing, staging, and histological confirmation of endometriosis, unless disease is visible in the vagina or elsewhere [8].

✪ Learning point   Clinical assessment of endometriosis

Abdominal and pelvic examinations are usually unremarkable. However, in severe disease vaginal examination is invaluable and with experience can be as useful as MRI and transvaginal ultrasound to define the management strategy. 'Blue nodules' (retro-cervical endometriotic nodules), although rare, can be seen during speculum examination; a 'frozen pelvis' can be found on vaginal examination, and nodules can be palpated. If there are bowel symptoms, a 'per rectum' examination may reveal nodules in the rectovaginal septum and strictures in the rectum, if the lesion is low enough. The uterus is typically retroverted and immobile with severe disease. Abdominal palpation may reveal a mass (e.g. endometrioma).

It is very helpful if there is a transvaginal scanner available in the gynaecology clinic but a high-resolution, dedicated transvaginal or transrectal ultrasound in the radiology department is also useful. An MRI examination can help to determine if there is bowel involvement but it is expensive and must be interpreted by a radiologist familiar with how to detect endometriosis, as there is no specific marker.

Ultrasound and MRI have high specificity and sensitivity for deep infiltrating endometriosis only in experienced hands in dedicated radiology services, but still have low correlation with operative findings, especially in mild disease [6]. They are used to plan surgery, counsel pre-operatively, and they involve appropriate members of the multidisciplinary team (e.g. a colorectal surgeon or urologist).

Ultrasound, however, might be very useful for the assessment of urological disease, which is rare and often silent. Ureteric involvement is capable of producing significant morbidity as it can lead to hydronephrosis and ultimately to renal failure. A high index of suspicion is necessary to obtain an early diagnosis [10]. For some surgeons once deep infiltrating endometriosis is diagnosed, it is a routine practice to obtain a pre-operative renal ultrasound as many will be found to have significant hydronephrosis, ureteric obstruction, or reduced renal cortex in which case a MAG3 (Mercaptoacetyltriglycine) or DMSA (dimercaptosuccinic acid) can be performed.

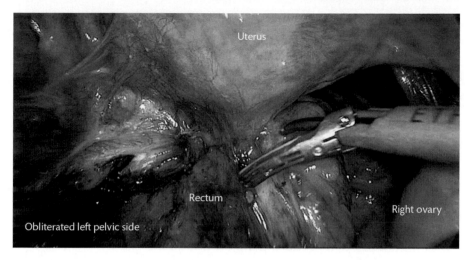

Uterus

Rectum

Right ovary

Obliterated left pelvic side

Figure 2.1 Left pelvic sidewall and adnexae obstructed by adhesions: view at laparoscopy.

A laparoscopy was performed 12 weeks later. This revealed extensive sigmoid adhesions to the pelvic sidewall. The left side of the pelvis was obstructed to view and assessment of adnexae and Pouch of Douglas was not possible due to bowel adhesions overlying pelvic structures. However, the right side of the pelvis appeared normal (Figure 2.1).

Two possible diagnoses were proposed: tubo-ovarian abscess or endometriosis. Post procedure, the patient was advised to take GNRH (gonadotropin releasing hormone) analogues for six months and was referred to a colorectal colleague specializing in endometriosis, and a gynaecologist specializing in severe endometriosis, for the planning of a future joint procedure. The patient declined the GNRH analogue, due to reluctance to accept the side effects, and continued to take the COCP.

> **❝ Guest expert comment (Colorectal)**
>
> In my experience, pre-operative imaging seems to add very little to the surgical management of this disease. A careful clinical examination together with a laparoscopy gives the best information regarding the likely stage and site of the disease and any bowel involvement. Even this, however, cannot entirely predict what type of bowel surgery might be required to radically excise the disease. The ability to separate or shave superficial deposits off the anterior rectum, to perform a disc resection with primary suture, and to perform a segmental resection with primary anastomosis all need to be within the ability of the operating team, so this necessitates the regular involvement of a colorectal surgeon.

> **✪ Learning point** Classification of endometriosis
>
> The current classification of endometriosis with the revised American Fertility Society (AFS) endometriosis classification system (last modified in 1985) is accepted worldwide as the international standard for endometriosis and is well known to both patients and clinicians (Figure 2.2). It describes four stages of endometriosis: minimal, mild, moderate, and severe, depending on the extent of lesions and associated adhesions (visualized at laparoscopy). However, it does not have any correlation with symptoms nor does it have prognostic value to predict the outcome of treatment [11–13]. Moreover, it has serious limitations in rectovaginal endometriosis involving the rectovaginal septum (Figure 2.3).)
>
> To overcome these limitations, several scores have been proposed including fertility assessment [14], and for the surgical strategy to assess vertical and horizontal spread [15] (ENZIAN score; See Figure 2.4). However, there is still no common 'language' that enables surgeons to standardize and compare surgery, facilitate research, and specify diagnosis.

THE AMERICAN FERTILITY SOCIETY
REVISED CLASSIFICATION OF ENDOMETRIOSIS

Patient's Name _____ Date _____

Stage I (Minimal) - 1-5
Stage II (Mild) - 6-15
Stage III (Moderate) - 16-40
Stage IV (Severe) - >40
Total _____

Laparoscopy _____ Laparotomy _____ Photography _____
Recommended Treatment _____
_____
Prognosis _____

PERITONEUM	ENDOMETRIOSIS	<1cm	1-3cm	>3cm
	Superficial	1	2	4
	Deep	2	4	6
OVARY	R Superficial	1	2	4
	Deep	4	16	20
	L Superficial	1	2	4
	Deep	4	16	20

	POSTERIOR CULDESAC OBLITERATION	Partial		Complete	
		4		40	

	ADHESIONS	<1/3 Enclosure	1/3-2/3 Enclosure	>2/3 Enclosure
OVARY	R Filmy	1	2	4
	Dense	4	8	16
	L Filmy	1	2	4
	Dense	4	8	16
TUBE	R Filmy	1	2	4
	Dense	4*	8*	16
	L Filmy	1	2	4
	Dense	4*	8*	16

*If the fimbriated end of the fallopian tube is completely enclosed, change the point assignment to 16.

Additional Endometriosis: _____

Associated Pathology: _____

To Be Used with Normal Tubes and Ovaries

L   R

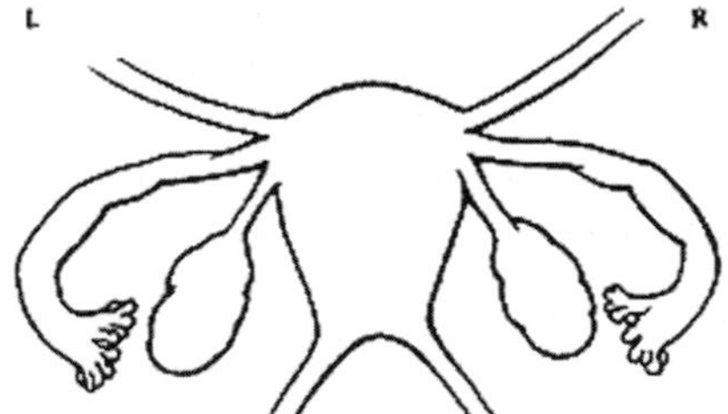

To Be Used with Abnormal Tubes and/or Ovaries

L   R

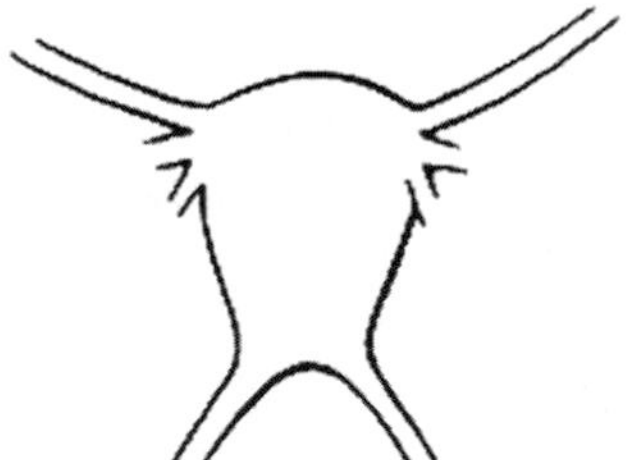

Figure 2.2 American Fertility Society revised classification of endometriosis.

Reprinted from *Fertil Steril* 67, 5, Robert S Schenken, David S Guzick, Revised endometriosis classification, 815–16, Copyright 1997, with permission from Elsevier.

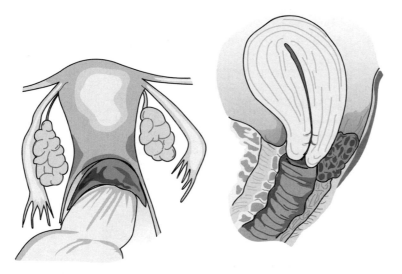

Figure 2.3 Discrepancy in severity assessment of rectovaginal endometriosis. Minimal disease (stage I) according to AFS classification, E3c according to ENZIAN score (infiltration of the rectum).

---

⑥ Expert comment

GnRH analogues are not a treatment for endometriosis in their own right; they just suppress symptoms. They are a useful adjunct to surgery, particularly with two-stage procedures. There is no evidence to suggest benefit once surgery is completed. Consequently the patient probably was wise not to take the GnRH analogues, but I would have stopped her combined pill to reduce the levels of circulating oestrogen which may drive the endometriosis.

✪ Learning point ESHRE (European Society of Human Reproduction and Embryology) guideline for diagnosis and treatment of endometriosis [16] (2005)

For women presenting with symptoms suggestive of endometriosis, a definitive diagnosis of most forms of endometriosis requires visual inspection of the pelvis at laparoscopy as the 'gold standard' investigation. However, pain symptoms suggestive of the disease can be treated without a definitive diagnosis using a therapeutic trial of a hormonal drug to reduce menstrual flow.

In women with laparoscopically confirmed disease, suppression of ovarian function for six months reduces endometriosis-associated pain; all hormonal drugs studied are equally effective although their side-effects and cost profiles differ. Ablation of endometriotic lesions reduces endometriosis-associated pain and the smallest effect is seen in patients with minimal disease; there is no evidence that also performing laparoscopic uterine nerve ablation (LUNA) is necessary.

In minimal to mild endometriosis, suppression of ovarian function in order to improve fertility is not effective, but ablation of endometriotic lesions plus adhesiolysis is effective compared to diagnostic laparoscopy alone. There is insufficient evidence available to determine whether surgical excision of moderate to severe endometriosis enhances pregnancy rates. IVF is appropriate treatment especially if there are coexisting causes of infertility and/or other treatments have failed, but IVF pregnancy rates are lower in women with endometriosis than in those with tubal infertility.

The management of severe/deeply infiltrating endometriosis is complex and referral to a centre with the necessary expertise is strongly recommended. Patient self-help groups can provide invaluable counselling, support and advice.

Enzian Score

a • Cul-de-sac • Vagina	b • Uterosacral ligament • Cardinal ligament	C Bowel, rectum Rectosigmoid

E1a = isolated nodule the pouch of Douglas

E1b = isolated nodule <1 cm from the uterine sacral ligament (USL)

E1bb = bilateral infiltration of the USL

E1c = isolated nodule in the rectovaginal space

E2a = infiltration of the upper third of vagina

E2b = infiltration of the USL >1 cm

E2bb = bilateral

E2c = infiltration of rectum <1 cm

E3a = Infiltration of the middle part of the vagina

E3b = Infiltration of the cardinal ligament (without ureterohydronephrosis)

E3bb = Bilateral

E3c = Infiltration of the rectum 1–3 cm without stenosis

E4a = Infiltration of uterus and/or lower third of the vagina and/or lower third of the vagina

E4b = Infiltration of the cardinal ligament to pelvic side wall and/or ureterohydronephrosis cardinal ligament to pelvic side and/or ureterohydronephrosis

E4bb = Bilateral

E4c = Infiltration of the rectum >1 cm and/or rectal stenosis Infiltration of the rectum >3 cm and/or rectal stenosis

FA = Adenomyosis uteri

FB= Deep infiltration of the bladder

FU = Ureteral infiltration (intrinsic)

FI = Intestinal infiltration (other side than rectum or sigmoid)

FO = Other locations

Figure 2.4 ENZIAN score for staging endometriosis, assessing vertical and horizontal spread

✚ Clinical tip How to prevent laparoscopic entry-related injuries [17]. The following information taken from the RCOG guidelines describes ways to reduce entry-related complications.

Serious complications during laparoscopy occur in about one in 1000 cases and the majority take place during the blind insertion of needles, trocars, and cannulae through the abdominal wall, hence the period of greatest risk is from the start of the procedure until visualization within the peritoneal cavity has been established. This guideline aims to highlight strategies to reduce these complications. Gynaecologists favour the closed or Veress needle entry technique.

The risk of bowel damage is 0.4/1000 and of major vessel injuries is 0.2/1000.13. It might be anticipated that the open (Hasson) technique would be less likely to cause major vessel injury than the closed method.

The primary incision for laparoscopy should be vertical from the base of the umbilicus. Care should be taken not to incise so deeply as to enter the peritoneal cavity.

The Veress needle should be sharp, with a good and tested spring action. A disposable needle is recommended, as it will fulfil these criteria.

The operating table should be horizontal (not in the Trendelenburg tilt) at the start of the procedure.

The abdomen should be palpated to check for any masses and for the position of the aorta before insertion of the Veress needle.

The lower abdominal wall should be stabilized in such a way that the Veress needle can be inserted at right angles to the skin and should be pushed in just sufficiently to penetrate the fascia and the peritoneum. Two audible clicks are usually heard as these layers are penetrated.

The test of most value that the Veres is in the peritoneal cavity is to check that the initial insufflation pressure is relatively low (less than 8 mmHg) and is flowing freely.

An intra-abdominal pressure of 20–25 mmHg should be used for gas insufflation before inserting the primary trocar.

The distension pressure should be reduced to 12–15 mmHg once the insertion of the trocars is complete.

Once the laparoscope has been introduced through the primary cannula, it should be rotated through 360 degrees to check visually for any adherent bowel. If this is present, it should be closely inspected for any evidence of haemorrhage, damage, or retroperitoneal haematoma.

If there is concern that the bowel may be adherent under the umbilicus, the primary trocar site should be visualized from a secondary port site, preferably with a 5 mm laparoscope.

Secondary ports must be inserted under direct vision perpendicular to the skin, while maintaining the pneumoperitoneum at 20–25 mmHg.

During insertion of secondary ports, the inferior epigastric vessels should be visualized laparoscopically to ensure the entry point is away from the vessels.

(Reproduced from Royal College of Obstetricians and Gynaecologists. Preventing Laparoscopic Injury Green-top Guideline No. 49. London: RCOG, 2008, with the permission of the Royal College of Obstetricians and Gynaecologists)

✪ Learning point Medical treatment of endometriosis

Endometriosis is a 'surgical' disease, with the goal of treatment to remove all areas of endometriosis and divide adhesions, thus restoring normal anatomy. Currently, the only place for medical treatment of endometriosis is pain management (usually by ovarian suppression) and control of the bleeding.

● Combined oral contraceptive pill (COCP)

Although the combined oral contraceptive pill (COCP) has been used to 'treat' endometriosis for many years, it is mainly used to suppress ovulation, providing a bleed-free time, and reduce dysmenorrhoea when used in bi- and tricycling fashion. There is no evidence that it reduces endometriotic deposits

(continued)

and from a surgical prospective, the oestrogen in the COCP makes tissues more vascular and friable. It is sensible to change to progesterone-only preparations when a diagnosis is confirmed on laparoscopy.

- Intra-uterine system (IUS)

Recent evidence regarding the Mirena® progesterone-releasing intra-uterine coil demonstrates its equal effectiveness with GNRH analogues in reducing pain and achieving reduction in ultrasonographic size of rectovaginal nodules [18–20]. It may have a direct effect on deposits through peritoneal fluid and reduces the volume of retrograde menstruation [18,21–24]. A Mirena® can be used for long-term symptom control in surgically proven endometriosis.

- Gonadotrophin-releasing hormone (GNRH) analogues

GNRH analogues can be used for short-term pain relief and preparation for surgery, via ovarian suppression. If used for longer than 6 months an addition of oestrogen hormone replacement therapy known as 'add-back' therapy is recommended to prevent bone loss and counteract side effects, without interfering with the efficacy of the treatment.

- Aromatase inhibitors

Based on the observation that endometriotic tissue over-expressed aromatase, an aromatase inhibitor may be added in cases of severe endometriosis. Aromatase inhibitors suppress biosynthesis of estradiol in all tissues, including ovary, fat, skin, and endometriotic deposits, and is therapeutic in endometriosis [25]. These medications are used used before surgery only due to side effects (largely related to increased risk of osteoporosis), and are used off-licence [26, 27].

'Old' preparations like Danazol, an anti-oestrogen, have no place in modern management of endometriosis should not be used in this group of young women. It is ineffective and causes unacceptable side effects, including male-pattern baldness and deepening of the voice.

Six months later a second laparoscopy was performed by a joint team which included a colorectal surgeon and a gynaecologist. An examination under anaesthetic revealed a large nodule on the left side of pelvis involving pelvic sidewall protruding into the vagina. A blue nodule in the vagina could be seen. On rectal examination the nodule did not extend to the rectal lumen, but the rectum was deviated. The aim of the surgery was to remove all the visible disease and to conserve reproductive organs as much as possible. The surgical strategy during procedure was as follows:

1. Restoration of normal anatomy. For this, the sigmoid adhesions to pelvic sidewall, left uterosacral ligament, and to the uterus were divided. The bowel was shaved off the pelvic sidewall without the disruption of serosal layer.
2. Understanding the extent of the disease, i.e. the endometriotic nodule. It became obvious that the nodule encircled the distal ureter down to the bladder insertion (Figure 2.4). This was unexpected and only evident once overlying adhesions were removed. An attempt to insert a ureteric stent failed due to complete obstruction of the ureteric lumen and 5 mm of distal ureter close to bladder insertion had to be removed. The nodule extended to the bladder and a small part of the bladder wall was also removed. A guide wire was inserted through the bladder in a retrograde manner with simultaneous laparoscopic and cystoscopic control and the ureter was re-anastomosed laparoscopically. A 6 French JJ ureteric stent was inserted to complete the procedure and was left for 6 weeks. During this process a small part of the vagina with endometriotic nodule had to be removed and the defect was closed laparoscopically with interrupted sutures.
3. Prevention of a post-operative urinary fistula by providing urine drainage and allowing spontaneous healing of the ureter. Post-operatively, an indwelling urinary catheter was inserted to prevent a ureteric reflux until there was no leak on imaging.

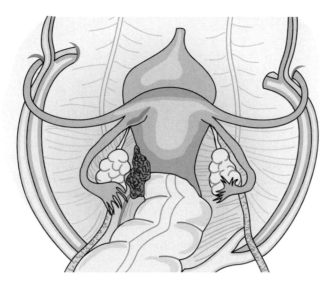

Figure 2.5 Endometriotic nodule involving left uterosacral ligament, distal ureter, vaginal vault, and bladder.

✪ Learning point Laparoscopic approach versus open surgery versus robotic surgery

The advantages of laparoscopy in this case are:

- The ability to use magnification and present areas with abnormal anatomy closer for the surgeon to view, to use exposure techniques to improve visibility in the pelvis, and to allow microsurgical techniques of dissection.
- Creation of a pneumoperitoneum allows the surgeon to open up planes; the cavitation effect of vapour and steam from energy sources provides further advantage.
- Laparoscopic technique enables careful dissection and sparing of reproductive and pelvic organs and their function (fertility, voiding, defecation, sexual function) and enhances ability to diagnose even small iatrogenic injuries to pelvic organs.
- The tactile feedback is not lost as compared with robotic surgery [29].
- The fact that the entire procedure is displayed on the screen makes every member of surgical team an active participant in the surgery, relevant when acute complications occur and invaluable in teaching, both at the site and during 'live' transmission (in laparoscopic training centres).
- Minimally invasive techniques offer faster recovery and reduction of post-operative adhesion formation. In the future, it may be possible to develop nerve-sparing techniques, which will reduce 'functional' complications after surgery. These include reduced bladder sensitivity, urine retention, bowel frequency and urgency, which can last up to a year after surgery.

✪ Learning point To operate or not to operate?

Surgical strategy must be tailored to a patient's symptoms; an expectant management approach is sensible in an asymptomatic patient. Once surgery is contemplated, the approach depends on the location and size of the endometriotic lesions, as well as the patient's future fertility requirements.

(continued)

Unlike cancer, the surgical treatment of endometriosis does not necessitate maximal debulking. There is evidence to suggest that the complete laparoscopic excision of endometriosis offers good long-term symptomatic relief, especially for those with severe or debilitating symptoms [13,29]. Thus, a pelvic clearance with removal of the ovaries might be an option for women who have completed their family. However, given that patients are frequently young and that they require fertility-preserving procedures, conservation of reproductive organs is often a priority. On occasions, it might be preferable to leave residual disease rather than perform major resective surgery resulting in, for example, a colostomy, which will greatly affect the social life of a young woman.

To confirm the integrity of the ureter, a contrast study for the renal system was performed 2 days after the procedure. It revealed very small flow through the left ureter but no evidence of obstruction. A nuclear magnetic renogramm (MAG3) of renal function revealed an essentially non-functioning small left kidney with 9 % remaining function (see Figure 2.6). The biochemical tests of renal function showed normal creatinine and urea. Surgery is the treatment of choice to relieve ureteral obstruction which was achieved. The kidney was still functional, albeit less than 25 %, and the renal function tests were normal, therefore an expectant management without nephrectomy was considered to be more appropriate by urological colleagues.

On day 10 post-operatively, the patient noted clear fluid leaking from the vagina. A vesico-vaginal fistula was confirmed on speculum examination. The mechanism of injury in this instance was devascularisation of the ureter during extensive dissection and therefore manifested only on day 10, which is typical for this type of injury. The best way to manage a vesicovaginal fistula is drainage of urine with a ureteric stent insertion and a bladder catheter to prevent vesicoureteric reflux. The patient underwent ureteric stent insertion and went home the same day with antibiotic cover to prevent urinary-tract ascending infection due to presence of foreign bodies (stent and indwelling catheter).

The vesico-vaginal fistula healed spontaneously in three weeks, while the ureteric stent and indwelling catheter remained in situ. The patient continued on GNRH analogues, antibiotics, and barrier cream to prevent skin maceration from the urine leak. She recovered fully and her renal function was normal six weeks after operation. After a consultation with a urologist a decision for a conservative management of non-functioning kidney was made.

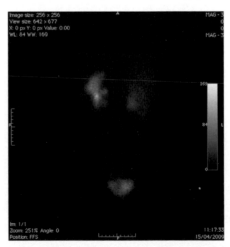

Figure 2.6 MAG-3 renogramm showing 9 % of function of the left kidney.

✪ **Learning point** Post-operative vesico-vaginal fistula

The risk of vesico-vaginal and ureteric fistula after endometriosis surgery is less than 1% [30] and is related to the severity of the disease and segmental blood supply to the ureter. It is a late complication (usually occurs 10–14 days post-operatively), and occurs as a result of poor healing and devascularization, rather than direct injury. Surgical correction is difficult due to inflammation. It is mostly treated conservatively with drainage by insertion of ureteric stents or nephrostomy if stent insertion is not possible.

It is not possible to predict who will develop a urinary tract fistula, but careful ureterolysis with respect of segmental blood supply to the ureter, and insertion of ureteric stent at the start of procedure if extensive dissection is planned are both beneficial [30].

In severe endometriosis there is high chance of ureteric involvement; some experts recommend performing a pre-operative renal contrast study if a rectovaginal nodule > 3 cm is detected [30–32].

❝ **Guest expert comment (Colorectal)**

The juxtaposition of vaginal and rectal incisions/anastomosis clearly represents a risk for fistula formation. In these circumstances, mobilization and interposition of the greater omentum is recommended to reduce this risk. From a urinary point of view, stents and a bladder catheter effectively drain the urinary system in case of fistula formation. For a rectovaginal fistula a colostomy or ileostomy would be required for defunctioning.

✪ **Learning point** Rectovaginal endometriosis

Rectovaginal endometriosis presents a particular surgical challenge, due to access difficulties and risk of bowel injury. A sub-peritoneal disease, it has been compared to the tip of an iceberg. In practical terms this means that the peritoneum must be opened and the retroperitoneal space is entered and explored.

Rectovaginal disease is different from ovarian endometriosis. It resembles adenomyosis with glands invading smooth muscle, which results in distortion of tissue planes, and therefore requires sharp dissection during surgery. The active fibrosis causes retraction of surrounding tissues which can then affect other closely related pelvic organs.

Experienced gynaecologists treating severe endometriosis know that this surgery can involve ureterolysis, adhesiolysis, decisions regarding radicality towards the approach to the bowel, and the possibility of stoma formation. Risks of post-operative fistulae should be openly discussed with the patient and clearly documented in the notes and consent form.

The patient recovered well and became pregnant 8 months after the operation. However, she developed severe pre-eclampsia at 35 weeks' gestation with deranged urea and creatinine, high uric acid, and severe proteinuria, and she underwent a caesarean section after failed induction. The caesarean section and recovery was uneventful. The patient's renal function post pregnancy remained normal.

🕙 **Landmark trial** Laparoscopic surgery in infertile women with minimal or mild endometriosis. Canadian Collaborative group on endometriosis [33].

Background A randomized controlled trial to determine whether laparoscopic surgery enhanced fecundity in infertile women with minimal or mild endometriosis.

Results Among the 172 women who had resection or ablation of endometriosis, 50 became pregnant and had pregnancies that continued for 20 weeks or longer, compared with 29 of the 169 women in the diagnostic–laparoscopy group (cumulative probabilities, 30.7% and 17.7%, respectively; $p = 0.006$ by the log-rank test). The corresponding rates of fecundity were 4.7 and 2.4 per 100 person–months (rate ratio, 1.9; 95% confidence interval, 1.2: to 3.1). Fetal losses occurred in 20.6% of all the recognized pregnancies in the laparoscopic–surgery group and in 21.6% of all those in the

(continued)

diagnostic–laparoscopy group (*p* = 0.91). Four minor operative complications (intestinal contusion, slight tear of the tubal serosa, difficult pneumoperitoneum, and vascular trauma) were reported (three in the surgery group, and one in the control group).

Conclusion Laparoscopic resection or ablation of minimal and mild endometriosis enhances fecundity in infertile women.

Discussion

Endometriosis is a chronic, often disabling condition characterized by the presence of endometrial tissue outside of the uterine cavity, most commonly in the pelvic cavity, typically on the utero-sacral ligaments and ovaries. It can also affect the vagina, umbilicus, bladder, rectum, abdominal wound scars, and rarely, the lungs. It should be suspected in any women of reproductive age presenting with chronic pelvic pain or dysmennorhoea. However, the clinical presentation is varied, with poor correlation between symptoms and signs and the extent of disease. Whilst the theory of retrograde menstruation predominates, embryological and immunogical processes have been proposed. Given that retrograde menstruation has been demonstrated to be near universal in women, it is unlikely to explain all cases of endometriosis.

Endometriosis involving the renal tract is a particular challenge. Less than 50 % of involving endometriosis of the renal tract are symptomatic and a negative physical examination cannot exclude bladder and ureteric endometriosis [4,5,29]. In cases of complete ureteric stenosis associated with endometriosis, there is approximately 30 % association with 'silent' renal atrophy. The mainstay of treatment in these cases is surgery, although accurate data about location and size of urinary tract endometriosis cannot be obtained pre-operatively. Therefore a surgeon contemplating operating for severe endometriosis should have skills to perform cystoscopy, ureteric stent insertion, ureterolysis, and ureteric repair, and he or she requires the support of an interventional radiologist.

The majority of endometriotic lesions involving the urinary tract are associated with rectovaginal adenomyosis or ovarian endometriosis, therefore the range of skills should extend to the ability to deal with bowel disease. In this particular case, the formation of a post-operative vesico-vaginal fistula may have been a consequence of devascularization and extensive dissection from the ureter being encircled by the disease. In cases like these, expectant management with effective urine drainage (stents, nephrostomy, an indwelling catheter) is feasible and should be the first line of management. The recurrence rate of urinary tract endometriosis depends on ability to resect maximal disease, and ranges from 5–30 %. The Mirena® progesterone releasing intrauterine system may reduce endometriosis symptoms recurrence post-operatively.

In infertile patients, there is clear evidence of fertility benefit after surgery for disease at any stage [33]. It is clear that if there are endometriomas and distortion of pelvic anatomy by adhesions, surgery improves implantation rate and pregnancy rate in both spontaneous and IVF pregnancies. However, there is no evidence that resection of rectovaginal nodules and bowel resection improves fertility, so the decision for these operations should be made with care and tailored to patient's symptoms.

In a young patient with loss of kidney function, a conservation of the kidney is a feasible option, but pre-pregnancy counselling and careful monitoring during pregnancy for hypertensive disorders should be a mainstay. The mode of delivery is based on obstetric indications. However in women who have undergone segmental resection, most colorectal surgeons would recommend an elective caesarean due to the fact that in case of dehiscence of rectosigmoid anastomosis, the subsequent management is difficult, and healing is impaired.

Despite scientific advances, endometriosis remains a 'mysterious disease' of unknown aetiology, with no 'silver bullet' for cure or symptom management. However, with current advances in minimal access surgery, a new specialty of a 'pelvic' surgeon is emerging. Together with the help of allied surgical specialties and radiologists, advances in surgical techniques may improve management of the disease and quality of life for endometriosis sufferers.

A Final Word from the Expert

This lady had a very severe form of endometriosis. Only 1–2% of endometriotic nodules infiltrate the ureter and in this case the resulting ureteric obstruction had severely compromised the kidney. All the signs and symptoms of severe disease were there from the outset. Vaginal examination would have confirmed the presence of a rectovaginal nodule and laparoscopy is the gold standard for the diagnosis and establishing the extent of disease. Early referral to an endometriosis centre is preferable. Extensive endometriosis is best removed surgically, ideally laparoscopically, by a multidisciplinary team specializing in the treatment of endometriosis.

References

1. Signorile PG, Baldi F, Bussani R, D'Armiento M, De Falco M, Baldi A. Ectopic endometrium in human foetuses is a common event and sustains the theory of müllerianosis in the pathogenesis of endometriosis, a disease that predisposes to cancer. *J Exp Clin Cancer Res* 2009;28:49–53.
2. Bulun SE. Mechanism of disease. Endometriosis. *N Engl J Med* 2009;360:268–79.
3. Kennedy S, Hadfield R, Mardon H, Barlow D. Age of onset of pain symptoms in non-twin sisters concordant for endometriosis. *Hum Reprod* 1996;11(2):403–5.
4. Hadfield R, Mardon H, Barlow D, Kennedy S. Delay in the diagnosis of endometriosis: a survey of women from the USA and the UK. *Hum Reprod* 1996;11(4):878–80.
5. Sinaii N, Cleary SD, Younes N, Ballweg ML, Stratton P. Treatment utilization for endometriosis symptoms: a cross-sectional survey study of lifetime experience. *Fertil Steril* 2007;87(6):1277–86.
6. Kinkel K, Chapron C, Balleyguier C, Fritel X, Dubuisson JB, Moreau JF. Magnetic resonance imaging characteristics of deep endometriosis. *Hum Reprod* 1999;14(4):1080–6.
7. Fauconnier A, Chapron C, Dubuisson JB, Vieira M, Dousset B, Breart G. Relation between pain symptoms and the anatomic location of deep infiltrating endometriosis. *Fertil Steril* 2002;78(4):719–26.
8. Pugsley Z, Ballard K. Management of endometriosis in general practice: the pathway to diagnosis. *Br J Gen Pract* 2007;57(539):470–6.
9. Balasch J, Creus M, Fabregues F, Carmona F, Ordi J, Martinez-Roman S, et al. Visible and non-visible endometriosis at laparoscopy in fertile and infertile women and in patients with chronic pelvic pain: a prospective study. *Hum Reprod* 1996;11(2):387–91.

10. Arrieta Bretón S, López Carrasco A, Hernández Gutiérrez A, Rodríguez González R, de Santiago García J. Complete loss of unilateral renal function secondary to endometriosis: a report of three cases, *Eur J Obstet Gynecol Reprod Biol* 2013 171:132–7.

11. Porpora MG, Koninckx PR, Piazze J, Natili M, Colagrande S, Cosmi EV. Correlation between endometriosis and pelvic pain. *J Am Assoc Gynecol Laparosc* 1999;6(4):429–34.

12. Guzick DS, Bross DS, Rock JA. Assessing the efficacy of The American Fertility Society's classification of endometriosis: application of a dose-response methodology. *Fertil Steril* 1982;38(2):171–6.

13. Chopin N, Vieira M, Borghese B, Foulot H, Dousset B, Coste J, et al. Operative management of deeply infiltrating endometriosis: results on pelvic pain symptoms according to a surgical classification. *J Minim Invasive Gynecol* 2005;12(2):106–12.

14. Adamson GD, Pasta DJ. Endometriosis fertility index: the new, validated endometriosis staging system. *Fertil Steril* 2010 94(5):1609–15.

15. Tuttlies F, Keckstein J, Ulrich U, Possover M, Schweppe KW, Wustlich M, et al. ENZIAN-score, a classification of deep infiltrating endometriosis. *Zentralbl Gynakol* 2005;127(5):275–81.

16. Kennedy S, Bergqvist A, Chapron C, D'Hooghe T, Dunselman G, Greb R et al. ESHRE guideline for the diagnosis and treatment of endometriosis. *Hum Reprod* 2005;20(10):2698–704.

17. RCOG Green-top Guidelines No. 49. Preventing entry related gynaecological laparsocpic injuries. http://www.bsge.org.uk/guidelines.php

18. Panay N. Advances in the medical management of endometriosis. BJOG 2008;115(7):814–17.

19. Lockhat FB, Emembolu JO, Konje JC. The evaluation of the effectiveness of an intrauterine-administered progestogen (levonorgestrel) in the symptomatic treatment of endometriosis and in the staging of the disease. *Hum Reprod* 2004;19(1):179–84.

20. Lockhat FB, Emembolu JO, Konje JC. The efficacy, side-effects and continuation rates in women with symptomatic endometriosis undergoing treatment with an intra-uterine administered progestogen (levonorgestrel): A 3-year follow-up. *Hum Reprod* 2005;20(3):789–93.

21. Vercellini P, Fedele L, Pietropaolo G, Frontino G, Somigliana E, Crosignani PG. Progestogens for endometriosis: forward to the past. *Hum Reprod Update* 2003;9(4):387–96.

22. Vercellini P, Frontino G, De Giorgi O, Pietropaolo G, Pasin R, Crosignani PG. Endometriosis: preoperative and postoperative medical treatment. *Obstet Gynecol Clin North Am* 2003;30(1):163–80.

23. Vercellini P, Trespidi L, Zaina B, Vicentini S, Stellato G, Crosignani PG. Gonadotropin-releasing hormone agonist treatment before abdominal myomectomy: a controlled trial. *Fertil Steril* 2003;79(6):1390–5.

24. Petta CA, Ferriani RA, Abrao MS, Hassan D, Rosa ESJC, Podgaec S, et al. Randomized clinical trial of a levonorgestrel-releasing intrauterine system and a depot GnRH analogue for the treatment of chronic pelvic pain in women with endometriosis. *Hum Reprod* 2005;20(7):1993–8.

25. Bulun SE. Mechanism of disease. Endometriosis. *N Engl J Med* 2009;360:268–79.

26. Ailawadi RK, Jobanputra S, Kataria M, Gurates B, Bulun SE. Treatment of endometriosis and chronic pelvic pain with letrozole and norethindrone acetate: a pilot study. *Fertil Steril* 2004;81(2):290–6.

27. Takayama K, Zeitoun K, Gunby RT, Sasano H, Carr BR, Bulun SE. Treatment of severe postmenopausal endometriosis with an aromatase inhibitor. *Fertil Steril* 1998;69(4):709–13.

28. Cho JE, Shamshirsaz AH, Nezhat C, Nezhat F. New technologies for reproductive medicine: laparoscopy, endoscopy, robotic surgery and gynecology. *A review of the literature. Minerva Ginecol* 2010 62(2):137–67.

29. Abbott JA, Hawe J, Clayton RD, Garry R. The effects and effectiveness of laparoscopic excision of endometriosis: a prospective study with 2–5 year follow-up. *Hum Reprod* 2003;18(9):1922–7.

30. Frenna V, Santos L, Ohana E, Bailey C, Wattiez A. Laparoscopic management of ureteral endometriosis: our experience. *J Minim Invasive Gynecol* 2007;14(2):169–71.

31. Jadoul P, Feyaerts A, Squifflet J, Donnez J. Combined laparoscopic and vaginal approach for nephrectomy, ureterectomy, and removal of a large rectovaginal endometriotic nodule causing loss of renal function. *J Minim Invasive Gynecol* 2007;14(2):256–9.

32. Donnez J, Squifflet J. Laparoscopic excision of deep endometriosis. *Obstet Gynecol Clin North Am* 2004;31(3):567–80, ix.

33. Marcoux S, Maheux R, Berube S. Laparoscopic surgery in infertile women with minimal or mild endometriosis. Canadian Collaborative Group on Endometriosis. *N Engl J Med* 1997;337(4):217–22.

3 Pregnancy of unknown location: a diagnostic and management dilemma

Sarah Merritt

❝ Expert Commentary Judith Hamilton

Case history

A 38-year-old woman (Gravida 2 Para 0) presented to the early pregnancy assessment unit (EPAU) at four weeks and six days' gestation by her last menstrual period (LMP). She gave a three-day history of mild, intermittent, generalized, lower abdominal pain. The pain was described as 'crampy', spreading across the lower abdomen and there were no exacerbating or relieving factors. There was no vaginal bleeding, no feeling of faintness or shoulder-tip pain.

Eight years previously, she had undergone a laparoscopic salpingectomy for a right tubal ectopic pregnancy. She had a regular, uneventful, 28-day menstrual cycle. Cervical screening was up to date and had always been normal. Her current pregnancy was spontaneously conceived with her husband of seven years. The couple had suffered from five years of unexplained subfertility prior to the natural conception of their first pregnancy. There was no history of pelvic infection or surgery and her past medical history was unremarkable. The patient was taking folic acid but no other medication.

Observations (temperature, pulse, and blood pressure) were normal. Abdominal examination found a soft, non-tender abdomen with no palpable masses. Bimanual pelvic examination revealed a normal sized, anteverted uterus with no palpable adnexal masses, cervical excitation, or tenderness. Speculum examination showed an apparently healthy, closed cervix, and no blood in the vagina.

> **❝ Expert comment**
>
> Non-specific lower abdominal pain is a common symptom in early pregnancy. In the recently published National Institute for Health and Care Excellence (NICE) Guideline on Ectopic Pregnancy and miscarriage [1], women under six weeks' gestation with vaginal bleeding but no pain are to be managed expectantly, in the community. The risk factors for an ectopic pregnancy in this patient are the previous ectopic pregnancy and the history of subfertility. The 24-month cumulative rate of recurrence of ectopic pregnancy is 18.5% after surgical treatment (salpingectomy or salpingostomy), and 25.5% after medical treatment. Recurrence is less likely if there is a history of subfertility (as is conception rate) or previous live birth. Voluntary termination of a previous pregnancy also appears to be a risk factor for recurrence [2].

> ✪ **Learning point** Early pregnancy assessment units [1, 3, 4]
>
> - Dedicated area, easily accessible for referrals and advice from general practitioners and other departments (most commonly emergency and genito-urinary medicine).
> - Led by health care professionals specializing in the management of early pregnancy problems to facilitate preferably 'one stop' diagnosis and to provide (for the majority) outpatient care with continuity of the healthcare professionals involved.
> - Must have access to transvaginal ultrasound scanning, laboratory investigations, inpatient facilities, an emergency operating theatre, and 24-hour, 7-days-a-week direct patient access to emergency medical support.
> - All (including non-clinical) staff should have training in breaking bad news.

A transvaginal ultrasound scan (TVUS) was performed (Figure 3.1). The uterus was anteverted and the endometrial thickness (ET) was 14.9 mm. There was no evidence of an intra-uterine pregnancy (IUP) or retained products of conception (RPOC).

> ✪ **Learning point** Scanning in early pregnancy
>
> - TVUS is the first-line investigation for early pregnancy problems. [1] It should complement the history and clinical examination.
> - TVUS determines location and viability, and detects multiple pregnancies at much earlier gestations and with greater accuracy than the transabdominal route [5, 6].
> - An intra-uterine gestation sac (for which well-established description criteria now exist) can be detected from as early as four weeks and three days' gestation using TVUS in a woman with a regular, 28-day cycle.
> - Serum βhCG levels should **not** be used to determine who should have a scan.
> - TVUS should be available to all **symptomatic** women presenting in early pregnancy and it should not be deferred due to an early gestation based on estimated LMP.
> - Confirmation of viability or non-viability is related to gestational age. In **asymptomatic,** low-risk women, waiting until 49 days' gestation to perform an ultrasound scan has been shown to reduce the number of pregnancies of unknown location (PULs) and IUPs of uncertain viability (IPUV) scans [7].
> - In 90% of cases of suspected early pregnancy complications, a single scan can provide all the information required for further management [8].
> - TVUS can detect 75–80% of clinically significant ectopic pregnancies at initial examination (Figure 3.2) [9].

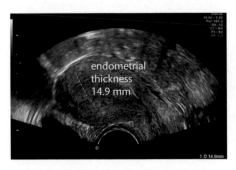

Figure 3.1 Endometrial thickness measured in AP in a longitudinal image of an anteverted uterus. The midline is represented by the bright echogenic line.

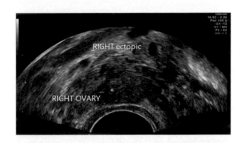

Figure 3.2 Right tubal ectopic pregnancy. The ectopic pregnancy is separate to the ovary.

➕ **Clinical tip** Systematic technique for transvaginal scanning

- Explain why the transvaginal route is required, reassure patient it will not harm the pregnancy, and obtain verbal consent.
- Ensure probe has been adequately cleaned.
- Gently insert probe into vagina and move it vertically (remembering that the majority of uteri are anteverted) until the uterus is seen in longitudinal section.
- Locate the cervix, in longitudinal section.
- Follow the cervical canal to the endometrium and visualize the endometrial cavity up to its fundal end.
- Sweep through the uterus from side to side in longitudinal section.
- Rotate the probe 90° to see the uterus in transverse section.
- Scan through from cervix to the fundus; ensure that the interstitial section of each tube is seen.
- From the interstitial area, follow the path of the tube, denoted by the hypoechogenic structures passing laterally within the broad ligament to the pelvic sidewall and iliac vessels. The ovary should lie at the distal end just medial to the iliac vessels. Scan through the ovary in transverse section noting the areas above and below it, and then turn the probe 90° and scan through the ovary in longitudinal section passing out laterally and then medially towards the uterus.
- Repeat with the contralateral side.
- Measurement of the endometrium occurs in longitudinal section where the endometrium is at its thickest from anterior to posterior. The ovaries are measured in three perpendicular planes.

⭐ **Learning point** The endometrium on ultrasound scan

- Description of the endometrial appearance on TVUS should include whether the midline echo is intact or disrupted.
- An intact, trilaminar appearance consists of the hyperechoic anterior and posterior margins of the endometrium with the midline echo separating the two (Figures 3.3 and 3.4).
- Identification of the midline echo is an essential diagnostic criterion for confirming the presence of an early intra-uterine pregnancy.
- During the fourth week of gestation the gestational sac is typically visualized as a regular spherical structure surrounded by a ring of hyperechoic tissue, which represents the echogenic trophoblast (Figure 3.5). The gestational sac is eccentrically placed to one side of the intact midline echo of the endometrium [8]. This is crucial in distinguishing a small gestational sac from a so-called 'pseudosac' (Figures 3.6 and 3.7) which represents a collection of fluid within the midline, which follows the contour of the endometrial cavity. This is possibly secondary to bleeding and there is no surrounding echogenic ring. The shape and size of this fluid may change during scanning and/or secondary to pressure from the scanning probe.

Both ovaries and adnexae could be assessed and no extra-uterine pregnancy was seen. There was a single corpus luteum on the left ovary and no fluid was visible in the Pouch Of Douglas (POD). No pain was elicited by pressure from the scanning probe. An ultrasound conclusion of pregnancy of unknown location (PUL) was made.

❝ **Expert comment**

It is of note that the corpus luteum was on the same side as the remaining tube, as 71.2% of ectopic pregnancies are ipsilateral to the site of ovulation in women with a previous salpingectomy [10].

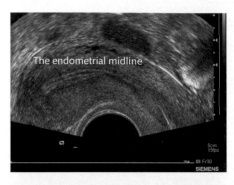

Figure 3.3 An anteverted uterus in longitudinal section showing the typical trilaminar appearance of an intact endometrium.

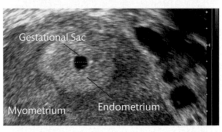

Figure 3.4 The same uterus in transverse section showing the trilaminar appearance.

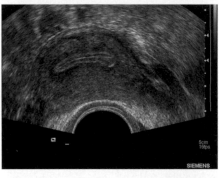

Figure 3.5 A single gestational sac situated within the endometrium.

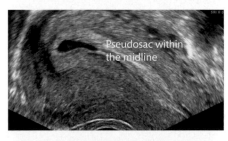

Figure 3.6 Pseudosac present within a longitudinal image of an anteverted uterus. Note that the fluid is within the midline.

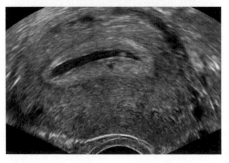

Figure 3.7 The same pseudosac seen within the midline in transverse section of the uterus.

☼ Learning point Pregnancy of unknown location (PUL)

- A PUL is concluded if a TVUS cannot identify an intra- or extra-uterine pregnancy or retained products of conception (RPOC) in a woman with a positive pregnancy test.
- PUL replaces the terms 'pregnancy of undetermined location' [11] and 'pregnancy of uncertain site' [12].
- The European Society of Human Reproduction and Embryology (ESHRE) Special Interest Group in early pregnancy recognized the term PUL as the absence of an identifiable pregnancy on ultrasound examination with a positive urine or serum hCG pregnancy test [13].
- PUL is a descriptive term and not a final diagnosis, and follow-up is mandatory from a safety perspective [14].
- The prevalence of PUL varies from 8–31 % [15–17], depending on the gestation at which scanning is commenced, the technical skills of the individual performing the scan, and the resolution of the scanning machine.
- EPAUs should aim to maintain PUL rates of below 15 % [18].
- The possible outcomes of a PUL are [15, 16, 19, 20–22]:
  1. An intra-uterine pregnancy too early to be seen on scan (22–46.5 %)
  2. A failing pregnancy whose location is never established (45–69 %).
  3. An ectopic pregnancy, too early to be seen or missed on scan (7–14 %).
  4. A persistent pregnancy of unknown location (PPUL).

⊕ Clinical tip Endometrial thickness and PUL

- ET is thinner in PULs where the final diagnosis is an ectopic pregnancy [23].
- As ET increases so too does the likelihood that a PUL is an IUP [24–26].
- The range of ET is wide and there is overlap between different outcome groups, preventing it from being reliable on its own as a predictor of outcome [15, 25, 16].
- Despite promising initial results [16] endometrial diameter or appearance has not been found to increase the power of mathematical models to predict the outcome of PUL [20, 27].

⊕ Clinical tip The danger of diagnosing 'complete miscarriage' on ultrasound scan

- Complete miscarriage is a possible outcome of PUL but the diagnosis can only be made if the woman has had a previous scan confirming an IUP.
- Up to 5.9 % of women with an apparent complete miscarriage defined by an ET of less than 15 mm and a history of heavy vaginal bleeding will have an ectopic pregnancy [28].
- There was a single maternal death in the 2000–2002 triennium of a woman given a diagnosis of a 'complete miscarriage' on a single ultrasound scan and who had no biochemical follow-up [29]. Death was secondary to a ruptured, undiagnosed ectopic pregnancy.
- Even when complete miscarriage is suspected, a woman should be managed as a PUL and followed up biochemically until this diagnosis is confirmed.

The patient's serum βhCG and progesterone levels were checked. The scan findings were explained fully and the possible outcomes discussed. The patient was clinically well so she went home and was called later with her blood test results and management plan. She was asked to return 48 hours later for a repeat hCG blood test. The βhCG level had increased by 41 % over this time period (Table 3.1). The patient remained well with minimal discomfort and no bleeding.

Table 3.1 Serum BhCG, progesterone and Hb results on presentation and day 2

	βhCG (IU/l)	Progesterone (nmol/l)	Haemoglobin (g/dl)
Day 0	580	11	12
Day 2	818	-	-

✚ **Clinical tip** Exert caution when interpreting βHCg

- 15% of viable IUPs will have a slowly rising βhCG [32].
- 10–13% of ectopic pregnancies will have a normal rate of increase in serial serum βhCG [8, 32].
- Slowly rising βhCG levels **cannot** differentiate between an ectopic pregnancy and a failing intra-uterine pregnancy [8].

✪ **Learning point** Free β human chorionic gonadotrophin (βhCG) measurements

Serum βhCG should be checked:

- To aid in predicting the outcome/managing women with a PUL [2, 30].
- To help decide the appropriate management of women with a confirmed ultrasound diagnosis of ectopic pregnancy.
- As part of ongoing surveillance in women with ectopic pregnancy having expectant or medical management.

In women with a PUL, βhCG should not be used to determine location of the pregnancy but instead to assess trophoblastic proliferation [1].

βhCG can be detected in the urine by most commercially available monoclonal antibody-based kits at a level which equates to a serum measurement of 25 IU/l and above. In a regular 28-day cycle, this corresponds to day 23 or nine days after conception [31].

In early pregnancy, a serum βhCG increase of ≥ 66% of the baseline value over a 48-hour interval is usually associated with a viable intra-uterine pregnancy (VIUP).

A prolonged βhCG doubling time is usually associated with an abnormal pregnancy.

Serum hCG ratios have a better performance than an absolute single hCG level in predicting an outcome of ectopic pregnancy in a PUL [30].

✪ **Learning point** The discriminatory zone

This term refers to the level of βhCG above which a normal IUP is usually visible on ultrasound scan. Using high-resolution transvaginal ultrasound scanning this level is estimated to be around 1000 IU/l [33,34], and on transabdominal scanning, 6500 IU/l.

- Over 50% of ectopic pregnancies visualized on TVUS have βhCG levels **under** 1000 IU/l [16].
- PULs with βhCG levels greater than 1000 IU/l can reflect complete or early delayed miscarriages, where the βhCG initially remains high due to its half life of 24–36 hours [8].
- Multiple intra-uterine pregnancies have higher hCG levels and are not always seen at initial scan despite the βhCG being > 1000 IU/l.
- The diagnostic accuracy of varying discriminatory zones (1000 IU/l, 1500 IU/l, and 2000 IU/l) has been evaluated. There was no significant improvement in the detection of ectopic pregnancies in women with PUL between each of these threshold levels [34].
- βhCG levels are affected by gestational age, maternal weight, racial origin, parity, smoking, and mode of conception [35, 36].

❝ **Expert comment**

The discriminatory zone is a historical concept which does not take into account that so-called 'doubling times' for serum βhCG levels do not apply to the majority of ectopic pregnancies. Many ectopic pregnancies which can be seen on TVUS will never reach an hCG level above the cut-off for the discriminatory zone. An ultrasound policy which will not allow women to be scanned until this hCG level is exceeded will delay diagnosis of ectopic pregnancies. These women may become clinically unwell, despite low hCG levels. If scanning is not offered until such symptoms develop, management by non-surgical means may no longer be safe.

One cannot be reassured that the pregnancy site has not been visualized on TVUS just because the hCG level is less than 1000 IU/l unless all efforts have been made to exclude an extra-uterine pregnancy.

If the gestation, initial scan findings of a PUL and serum biochemistry suggest that there is an early IUP, there is no benefit, in rescanning a patient who is clinically well before the hCG can be estimated to exceed 1000 IU/l.

(continued)

Use of serum βhCG in second-trimester screening tests has recognized that levels can be affected by other factors, including race. Afro-Caribbean women have higher hCG levels at the same gestation and recent work has confirmed that this also applies in the first trimester [35, 36]. Mathematical models have been proposed, based largely on serial hCG levels, but these are complex and have been found to have variable reproducibility in differing centres [37, 38].

✪ **Learning point** The use of serum progesterone levels in management of PUL

Progesterone levels of less than 20 nmol/L are associated with falling βhCG levels and have been found to identify failing pregnancies with a sensitivity of 94% and a specificity of 91% [16]. Levels of over 60 nmol/L are associated with a doubling βhCG and usually indicate viable IUPs. Levels between 20–60 nmol/L are associated with abnormal pregnancies. Single-visit protocols for management of PULs using, most recently, a progesterone 'cut-off' level of ≤ 10 nmol/l, have been proposed as triage for women who can be safely discharged after their initial visit, thereby reducing the number of follow-up visits [15, 16, 39].

Caution:

- Progesterone levels cannot predict the location of a pregnancy.
- Viable IUPs can occur with a progesterone level below 60 nmol/L and EPs can have a level above this cut-off.
- Progesterone levels may be increased in women taking progestagen suppositories.

A recent meta-analysis found (from 5 studies with 1998 participants) that a single progesterone measurement in symptomatic women with inconclusive ultrasound findings predicted a non-viable pregnancy with a pooled sensitivity of 74.5% and specificity of 98.4% [40].

❝ **Expert comment**

The serum progesterone level does not alter in an ongoing IUP. Estimation should only be repeated to support a likely diagnosis of a failing pregnancy. There is considerable overlap between progesterone levels secondary to failing corpora lutea in delayed miscarriages and ectopic pregnancies. Both these diagnoses are likely to have a progesterone level between 20–60 nmol/L. A low progesterone level in a woman taking progestagen supplementation is reassuring with regard to the likelihood of a failing pregnancy, if the ultrasound diagnosis is of a PUL, so it is still worth checking in these patients. The efficacy and safety of 'single-visit' protocols based on a low progesterone level have only been validated in a tertiary referral setting with dedicated, specialist expertise in transvaginal scanning. Of note, progesterone levels are not available on the same day in all hospitals.

The patient was asked to return for a scan five days later (day 7). The endometrium remained thickened at 11 mm but no intra- or extra-uterine pregnancy was visualized. There was no evidence of internal bleeding and scanning did not provoke any tenderness.

As this was a persistent PUL (PPUL), serum βhCG was rechecked and was 1831 IU/l.

✪ **Learning point** Management of PUL

Aims

- To determine the location of the pregnancy.
- To assess the likelihood of the need for intervention.
- To minimize the anxiety caused by investigation and diagnosis.

(continued)

This should be achieved through:

- A minimum number of follow-up visits.
- No unnecessary interventions.
- Keeping the patient safe.

Expectant management in a clinically stable patient is safe and important in order to differentiate between women who have a resolving pregnancy and those with a potentially significant ectopic pregnancy requiring intervention [16, 17]. NICE recommends checking two serum βhCG measurements 48 hours apart but does not include measuring an initial progesterone level [1]. Rescan/review can be arranged guided by these levels.

ⓕ Expert comment

A minority (7–14%) of women with a PUL will have an ectopic pregnancy [7, 15, 16, 20–22]. As this is potentially the most dangerous outcome, there is a tendency for health professionals without specialist early pregnancy knowledge to over-monitor women with PULs. EPAUs are often run by specialist nurses or midwives without the support of a dedicated consultant with specific training in ultrasound scanning and/or early pregnancy problems. Decisions on hCG levels are too often made by junior doctors who do not have continuity of care for the patient or the experience required to make any decision other than to repeat the hCG level in another 48 hours. Returning for repeated blood tests and being continually warned you may have an ectopic pregnancy is extremely disruptive for the function and well-being of any patient. Compliance with follow-up of these patients is essential from a safety perspective [14] but this must be appropriate, at a time and in a form that is likely to help finalize the diagnosis and inform the patient's management. Whatever the planned follow-up, the patient must be able to access emergency medical care at any time, on any day, if she has concerns.

✚ Clinical tip Are we missing ectopic pregnancies at initial scan?

- Diagnosis of an ectopic pregnancy should be **based on visualizing an ectopic mass** and **should not be based on the failure to identify an intra-uterine pregnancy** [41, 42].
- TVUS has the ability to detect the location of a pregnancy in 91.3% of women on initial scan and it has a high sensitivity for detecting ectopic pregnancies of 73% and specificity of 99.9% [43].
- Small, non-viable ectopic pregnancies will not develop to a stage where they can be seen on scan or at laparoscopy. These will be classified as failing PULs where the pregnancy site is never visualized but the serum βhCG steadily declines. The majority of failing PULs will be IUPs which also failed before becoming visible on scan.
- Growing ectopic pregnancies may become visible on a follow-up TVUS. These ectopic pregnancies are associated with a lower serum βhCG, higher progesterone levels, and significantly lower mean gestational age at initial presentation than those visualized on first scan. Ectopic pregnancies initially classified as a PUL are probably merely too small and early to be seen on the first scan [44].

✪ Learning point Ectopic pregnancies

Traditionally ectopic pregnancies have been managed surgically, most recently by laparoscopy and salpingectomy. Medical and expectant management are increasingly recognized as safe options [3, 45, 46]. Clinical presentation, ultrasound scanning, and biochemical markers can help to identify women suitable for these management options. Many ectopic pregnancies resolve spontaneously, just as an intra-uterine pregnancy can miscarry, and these women are often suitable for expectant management.

ⓕ Expert comment

Women know about pregnancies earlier in their gestation than they once did. EPAUs facilitate access to TVUS, which in itself is of a higher resolution and often now performed by health professionals with more specialist expertise in this area. Small ectopic pregnancies (which would previously have failed on their own and were not diagnosed) are increasingly being found. These ultrasonographically diagnosed ectopic pregnancies do not behave in the same manner and do not pose the same threat to safety as the typical, traditional ectopic pregnancy, which made itself known through clinical symptoms [45, 46]. It is worth explaining to women being followed up for a PUL that even if we could visualize an ectopic pregnancy, the management (monitoring of symptoms, repeat scanning, and/or serum biochemistry) would not differ.

✪ Learning point Methotrexate in the management of ectopic pregnancies/PPULs

- Folate antagonist [reversibly inhibits Di Hydro Folate Reductase (DHFR)].
- Effective on rapidly dividing trophoblast.
- Safety data and potential teratogenicity for future pregnancies based on long established use in gestational trophoblastic disease.

Table 3.2 Criteria for methotrexate use [1, 47, 48]

Criteria	Inclusion	Exclusion
Clinical	• Clinically stable, normal heart rate, blood pressure • Minimal or no pain • Soft abdomen and no/ little tenderness on bimanual pelvic examination • Willing and able to comply with several weeks of follow-up	• Haemodynamically unstable • Significant pain, after exclusion of other causes • Falling Hb levels • Breast feeding • Unwilling to undergo medical management • Unable to comply with follow-up
Ultrasound	• No haemoperitoneum • Absence of fetal cardiac activity • Adnexal mass diameter of less than 3 cm • No evidence of an intra-uterine pregnancy	• Haemoperitoneum • Fetal cardiac activity • Co-existing intra-uterine pregnancy (heterotopic)
Biochemistry	• Initial serum βhCG < 5000 IU/l • 3500 – 5000 IU/l: discuss with consultant	• Declining βhCG • βhCG > 5000 IU/l (discuss with consultant)
Medical History	• No contraindications to use of MTX	• Acute infection • Moderate to severe anaemia • Renal/liver impairment • Active peptic ulcer disease • Colitis • Active pulmonary disease • Immunodeficiency • Leucopenia • Thombocytopenia

Table 3.3 Regimen for single dose systemic methotrexate (MTX)

Day	Action	Information to patient
1	• Written consent • Baseline serum βhCG • Liver function tests (LFTs), renal function (U&Es), full blood count (FBC), group and save (G&S) • Height and weight to calculate body surface area (BSA) • Intramuscular injection of MTX based on the BSA and dosage of 50 mg/m^2	• Counsel patient • Explain expected symptoms • Avoid sunlight, vitamins, NSAIDs, until treatment is complete • Keep well hydrated • Abstain from alcohol • Avoid sexual intercourse until treatment is complete • Use adequate contraception for three months after treatment is completed
4	• Serum βHcg.	
7	• Serum βhCG, FBC, LFTs, U&Es, enquire regarding symptoms. • If βhCG falls by > 15% between days 4 and 7 and clinically well, repeat levels weekly until hCG level is undetectable. • Give second dose of MTX if the βhCG level falls by < 15% between days 4 and 7, followed by 30 mg of folinic acid orally 24-hours later and repeat βhCG weekly, if declining, provided the patient remains clinically well. • Specialist clinical review is required if the βhCG level has increased. The patient's symptoms and the examination, including ultrasound findings, will guide whether it is appropriate to give a second dose. It is normal for the βhCG level to increase between days 1 and 4. • If βhCG levels do not fall by > 15% after the second injection, surgical management is required.	

⊕ Clinical tip Side effects of methotrexate

- 75% will have increased abdominal pain usually 2–6 days after treatment, secondary to separation of the trophoblast.
- Tiredness.
- Nausea.
- Vaginal bleeding due to shedding of the endometrium.
- Stomatitis, conjunctivitis, gastritis, photosensitivity, bone marrow suppression, and impaired liver function are quoted but rarely seen with this low-dose single or two-dose regime.
- Avoid pregnancy for three months after last administration of methotrexate due to the risk of miscarriage and potential teratogenicity in a subsequent pregnancy.

The patient was symptom-free, her observations stable, and clinical examination was unremarkable. She was very keen to avoid intervention. She was told that although it was not yet clear on scanning where the pregnancy was situated, the βhCG level was increasing sub-optimally (i.e. at a rate lower than that expected for an ongoing IUP). She was informed that although an ectopic pregnancy had not been seen, as the patient had only one tube remaining, intervention could be considered at this stage because of the rising hCG and the reasonably high absolute level. This intervention would be with methotrexate treatment (Tables 3.2 and 3.3).

❂ Learning point Methotrexate and persistent pregnancy of unknown location (PPUL)

- The incidence of PPUL is low, 1.3–2.5% [20, 22, 49, 50], although there is no agreed definition of when a PUL becomes a PPUL.
- PPULs biochemically mimic ectopic pregnancies or failing IUPs with slowly rising or plateauing βhCG levels. The location of the pregnancy cannot be identified on scan or at laparoscopy and there is no evidence of gestational trophoblastic disease.
- Small numbers of asymptomatic women with PPUL have been successfully treated with systemic methotrexate [32, 49].
- Methotrexate should only be used when there is a persistently increasing or plateauing hCG level in an asymptomatic woman where the pregnancy cannot be visualized after expert review, and an ultrasound scan performed by an operator experienced in early pregnancy scanning [49, 51].
- Early intervention with methotrexate, in the absence of a diagnosis and as a precaution against the minority of PULs which will turn out to be ectopic pregnancies, runs the risk of inadvertent administration to a woman with an intra-uterine pregnancy which is too early/small to detect on initial scan. The methotrexate is unlikely to work in such a situation so the clinician and patient will be faced with management of an ongoing pregnancy which has been exposed to a teratogenic drug. The number of reported cases like this in America (and the attendant lawsuits) is such that caution is being urged against early, over-treatment with methotrexate [52].
- All women receiving methotrexate should have their serum hCGs monitored until resolution to ensure that treatment has succeeded and that other causes of persistent βhCG are not present.

To ensure that the patient's serum βhCG level had not peaked between days 2 and 7 and was now declining, its level was rechecked on day 10 (72 hours, not 48 hours, later, at the patient's request). A repeat TVUS showed a PPUL with an unchanged ET and no worrying features to suggest an extra-uterine pregnancy. The patient was asymptomatic

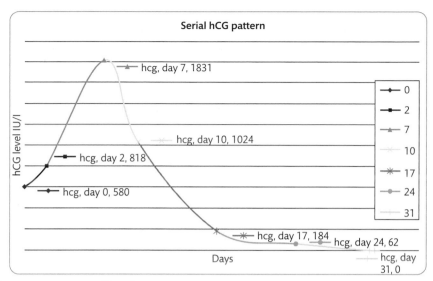

Figure 3.8 Serial serum βhCG from initial visit until resolution

and not tender on examination or scanning. Serum βhCG, a full blood count, renal and liver function were assessed in preparation for methotrexate administration.

The βhCG level had decreased by 44.1 % to 1024 IU/l. Expectant management of the now-resolving PPUL was advised, with the patient's agreement. Four days later she began to bleed heavily with the passage of small clots vaginally, associated with central lower abdominal cramping pains. One and two weeks later the serum βhCG levels were 184 and 62 IU/l respectively (Figure 3.8). Her bleeding by this time was minimal and the cramping had stopped. One week after the last βhCG, her urinary pregnancy test was negative when she was discharged back to her GP.

Although this was not the ongoing pregnancy that the patient wanted, she was pleased to avoid intervention, which could effect or delay her fertility, and had no concerns over her follow-up.

> **❝ Expert comment**
>
> The clinical and biochemical behaviour of this pregnancy are in keeping with an early, delayed, intra-uterine miscarriage which did not develop to an extent where it was visible on TVUS. The patient was Afro-Caribbean which contributed to the fact that her absolute hCG level was higher than might have been expected from the scan findings. The case illustrates the advantages of judicious monitoring but no unnecessary intervention in a clinically stable patient. There was additional pressure and potentially a lower threshold to intervene in this case, as we wanted to preserve her single, remaining tube. There is no evidence that methotrexate speeds up the rate of hCG decline once the trophoblast is in regression. Intervention on day 7 would have ensured this patient did not have an accurate diagnosis and would have presumed that she had had a second ectopic pregnancy in her remaining tube, with the associated implications for future fertility.

> ✪ **Learning point** Surgical management (laparoscopy and endometrial curettage) in PPUL
>
> Surgical intervention, by means of an evacuation of retained products of conception (ERPC) or laparoscopy, is required (for an increasing βhCG or worsening symptoms) in 9–29% of women with a PUL [16, 17].
>
> **Laparoscopy**
> - Diagnostic laparoscopy was regarded as the gold standard for detecting ectopic pregnancy [56].
> - If diagnostic laparoscopy was used in the management of all PULs, this would give a more accurate figure of the prevalence of ectopic pregnancies within this population [57].
> - Laparoscopy does not detect all ectopic pregnancies [58]. False negative laparoscopies occur if there is an early ongoing ectopic pregnancy, too small to see, or a failing ectopic pregnancy which never becomes big enough to be visualized [41, 58].
> - Laparoscopy has surgical complications and anaesthetic risks and it is difficult to support this course of management in women with a PUL who are clinically well when the majority of PULs either fail and/or are IUPs.
> - Laparoscopy should be reserved for treatment and not used to make a diagnosis. Women with a PUL who are clinically unwell, haemodynamically unstable, have a significant haemoperitoneum at the time of ultrasound scan, are tender on scanning or examination, or who develop worsening symptoms during expectant management will need surgical intervention.
>
> **Uterine/'diagnostic' curettage**
> - Uterine curettage is most commonly used in America, [59] in PULs where ectopic pregnancy is thought to be a possibility.
> - Dilatation and curettage (D&C) has been assessed in clinically stable women with a PUL and a single βhCG level of > 2000 IU/l or an initial level of < 2000 IU/l and an abnormal rise/fall in serial βhCG levels. D&C was concluded to be a useful diagnostic tool in differentiating ectopic pregnancies from non-viable IUPs and in preventing administration of methotrexate (MTX) to women with a failing IUP [60–62].
> - 50% [16] and 81% [63] of women with spontaneously failing pregnancies would undergo an unnecessary invasive procedure based on βhCG or progesterone results, respectively, based on the inclusion criteria.
> - The risk of inadvertent termination of an early, viable IUP is estimated to be 0.5–12.3% [63].
> - Chorionic villi can be absent if the diagnosis is complete miscarriage as well as ectopic pregnancy.
> - Curettage has no place in the investigation of women with PUL in the UK, outside the context of research trials.
> - ERPC may be required to treat women with plateauing hCG levels and minimal vaginal bleeding where all the evidence points to an IUP, despite lack of definitive diagnosis on TVUS [16].

Discussion

There was a single maternal death in the last reported triennium in a patient initially described as having a PUL [14]. This led to the report concluding that the term should be abandoned and 'active steps to exclude an ectopic pregnancy' should be taken in any patient who fulfilled the criteria for this diagnosis. This conclusion was widely criticized by the early pregnancy community from those involved in research and those involved in direct patient care [64, 65]. It ignores the fact that a PUL is a relatively common finding (5–31% of women attending with early pregnancy problems [65]), it is not a final diagnosis, and follow-up is mandatory. After review of the case, follow-up was reported as substandard and the important issues of inappropriate delegation of management to junior members of staff, poor quality and poorly supervised scanning, and a lack of specialist knowledge about early pregnancy management were highlighted. Investment in and recognition of the fundamental importance of specialist training in early pregnancy scanning is the single most important initiative which is likely to reduce PUL rates. This, in combination with all EPAUs having a dedicated lead clinician with expert early pregnancy and scanning knowledge, will best help keep potential mothers safe in the first trimester. Regressing to the days when women who had a positive pregnancy test and a pregnancy which could not be seen on scan were presumed to have an ectopic pregnancy until proven otherwise will not.

The NICE guideline on PUL gives initial guidance on management based on the percentage change in hCG levels over 48 hours [1]. Absolute hCG levels are only mentioned in the management of women in whom the hCG level increases by more than 63 % over this time, with review by a senior gynaecologist recommended in women with an hCG level greater than 1500 IU/l in whom a pregnancy has not been visualized on ultrasound scanning. It does not include progesterone in its algorithm but stresses that this cannot be used to ascertain pregnancy location. The algorithm does not address PPUL or specify subsequent management if the diagnosis is not clear after the 48-hour review. This is the first national guidance on the management of early pregnancy problems and it has not been received without controversy [65]. Important points that it does make with regard to PUL are as follows:

- Do not use serum hCG measurements to determine the location of the pregnancy.
- Place more importance on clinical symptoms than hCG results and review the patient if her symptoms change, regardless of previous results and assessments.
- Use hCG measurements only for assessing trophoblastic proliferation to help determine subsequent management.
- Take two serum hCG measurements as near as possible to 48 hours apart. Take further measurements only after review by a senior healthcare professional.

The NICE guidelines would not have given us specific advice on how to manage the patient described in this chapter. After the initial 41 % rise in her hCG level, their recommendation would be that she was reviewed in the EPAU within 24 hours. No further detail is given, unless a specific diagnosis is made at that stage. Unless there is uncertainty about the quality of the initial scan, there is nothing to be gained from review so soon. The majority of outcomes of PULs need time to manifest themselves and follow-up should be timed and involve tests which are most likely to give a diagnosis. It is not just the absolute length of time for which a woman is followed up with a PUL that needs to be considered but the number of occasions she has to attend hospital within this period.

Appropriate counselling of the patient is essential. Whilst stressing the importance of seeking medical care if their symptoms change, women should overall be reassured that the least likely outcome is an ectopic pregnancy. Even if it is the latter, this will tend to be early and potentially non-viable, requiring no more intervention than the monitoring and follow-up which is already occurring.

The ultimate rationalization of PUL management is to discharge women after a single or two visits if there is evidence that, regardless of site, their pregnancy is failing [39, 67]. Tertiary referral centres with specialist expertise in early pregnancy scanning and management have demonstrated that, in their hands, this practice is safe. It leaves the unresolved question for the patient as to the location of her pregnancy.

Patients may have a poor understanding of the term PUL. Once the possibility of an ectopic pregnancy is mentioned they tend to remember little else. There is no published literature on the future fertility of PULs managed expectantly and, specifically, no data on recurrent ectopic pregnancy rates. Whether early, failing ectopic pregnancies have any implications for tubal function either before or after occurrence can be debated. If a patient presents to a different hospital in her next pregnancy and tells them her last pregnancy was a possible ectopic pregnancy, this may distort her risk assessment. It is important that all health professionals are familiar with the term PUL and understands that the most likely cause of a resolved PUL is an IUP too underdeveloped to ever be visualized on ultrasound scanning.

A Final Word from the Expert

The evolution of specialist EPAUs over the last 20 years, in conjunction with advances in transvaginal scan technology and the training and expertise of those using it, has led to the development of the concept of PULs. The term was introduced to standardize nomenclature and allow consistency amongst published research [19, 64]. Even though a minority of women with an initial diagnosis of PUL will ultimately have an ectopic pregnancy, there has been a tendency to counsel and manage all of these cases as if this were the most likely outcome. This leads to significant anxiety and social disruption to the woman and an unnecessarily heavy and expensive workload on the EPAU managing the case. Specialist expertise in early pregnancy scanning should now be available in all EPAUs and health professionals managing cases of PULs should understand that modern transvaginal scanning can identify ectopic pregnancies that may not be visible at laparoscopy. The focus inevitably has to move on to how to rationalize the follow-up of these cases. Any such strategy will always have to achieve a balance between being safe and effective in units with less specialist ultrasound scanning skills and expert support, and those who strive to achieve a 'one-stop' strategy for the majority. The only way to bring these two extremes closer together and raise the overall standard of early pregnancy care is to invest in ultrasound training and ensure all EPAUs have a dedicated consultant with the requisite skills for modern early pregnancy management.

References

1. NICE guideline on ectopic pregnancy and miscarriage. 2012.
2. De Bennetot M, Rabischong B, Aublet-Cuvelier B, Belard F, Fernandez H, Bouyer J, Canis M, Pouly JL. Fertility after tubal ectopic pregnancy: results of a population based study. *Fertil Steril* 2012;98:1271–6.
3. Royal College of Obstetricians and Gynaecologists. 2006. <http://www.rcog.org.uk/files/rcog-corp/uploaded-files/GT25ManagementofEarlyPregnancyLoss2006.pdf>
4. Sawyer E, Jurkovic D. Ultrasonography in the Diagnosis and Management of Abnormal Early Pregnancy. *Clin Obstetr Gynaecol* 2007;50(1):31–54.
5. Gurel S, Sarikaya B, Gurel K, Akata D. Role of sonography in the diagnosis of ectopic pregnancy. *J Clin Ultrasound* 2007;35:509–17.
6. Jain KA, Hamper UM, Sanders RC. Comparison of transvaginal and transabdominal sonography in the detection of early pregnancy and its complications. *Am J Roentgenol* 1988;151:1139–43.
7. Bottomley C, Van Belles V, Mukri F, Kirk E, Van Huffel S, Timmerman D, Bourne T. The optimal timing of an ultrasound scan to assess the location and viability of an early pregnancy. *Hum Reprod* 2009;24:1811–17.
8. Jurkovic D, Valentin L, and Vyas S. *Gynaecological ultrasound in practice.* London: RCOG Press, 2009; 1–5.
9. Condous G, Okaro E, Khalid A, Lu CVan Huffel S, Timmerman D. The accuracy of transvaginal sonography for the diagnosis of ectopic pregnancy prior to surgery. *Hum Reprod* 2005;20:1404–9.

10. Ross JA, Davison AZ, Sana Y, Appiah A, Johns J, Lees CT. Ovum transmigrationafter salpingectomy for ectopic pregnancy. *Hum Reprod* 2013;28(4):937–41.

11. Brumstead J, Gibson M. Unusual chorionic gonadotrophic patterns in pregnancies of undetermined location. *Int J Fert* 1989;34(5):333–6.

12. Hahlin M, Thorburn J, Bryman I. The expectant management of early pregnancies of uncertain site. *Hum Reprod* 1995;10:1223–7.

13. Farquharson RG, Jauniaux E, Exalto N on behalf of the ESHRE Special Interest Grup for Early Pregnancy (SIGEP). Updated and revised nomenclature for description of early pregnancy events. *Hum Reprod* 2005;20:3008–11.

14. Saving Mothers' Lives: Reviewing Maternal deaths to make motherhood safer: 2006-2008. The eighth report of the Confidential Enquiries into Maternal Deaths in the United Kingdom. *Br J Obstet Gynecol* 2011;118:Suppl; 1–203: 81–4.

15. Banerjee S, Aslam N, Zosmer N, Woefer B, Jurovic D. The expectant management of women with pregnancy of unknown location. *Ultrasound Obstet Gynecol* 1999;14:231–6.

16. Banerjee S, Aslam N, Woefer B, Lawrence A, Elson J, Jurovic D. Expectant management of early pregnancies of unknown location: a prospective evaluation of methods to predict spontaneous resolution of pregnancy. *BJOG* 2001;108:158–63.

17. Hahlin M, Thorburn J, Bryman I. The expectant management of early pregnancies of uncertain site. *Hum Reprod* 1995;10:1223–7.

18. Condous G, Timmerman D, Goldstein S, Valentin L, Jurkovic D, Bourne T. Pregnancies of unknown location: consensus statement *Ultrasound Obstet Gynecol* 2006;28:121–2.

19. Barnhart K, Norah M, Bourne T, Kirk E, Van Calster B, Bottomley C, Chung K, Condous G, Goldstein S, Hajenius P, Mol BW, Molinaro T, O'Brien KL, Husicka R, Sammel M, Timmerman D. Pregnancy of unknown location: A consensus statement of nomenclature, definitions and outcome. *Fertil Steril* 2011;95:857–66.

20. Gevaert O, De Smet F, Kirk E, Van Calster B, Bourne T, Van Huffel S, Moreau Y, Timmerman D, De Moor B, Condous G. Predicting the outcome of pregnancies of unknown location: Bayesian networks with expert prior information compared to logistic regression. *Hum Reprod* 2006;21(7):1824–31.

21. Kirk E, Condous G, Haider Z, Lu C, Van Huffel S, Timmerman D, Bourne T. The practical application of a mathematical model to predict the outcome of pregnancies of unknown location. *Ultrasound Obstetr Gynecol* 2006;27:311–15.

22. Kirk E, Condous G, Van Calster B, Van Huffel S, Timmerman D, Bourne T. Rationalizing the follow-up of pregnancies of unknown location. *Hum Reprod* 2007;22(7):1744–50.

23. Spandorfer S, Barnhart K. Endometrial stripe thickness as a predictor of ectopic pregnancy. *Fertil Steril* 1996; 66;3;474–7.

24. Moschos E, Twickler DM. Endometrial thickness predicts intrauterine pregnancy of unknown location. *Ultrasound Obstetr Gynecol* 2008;32;929–34.

25. Levgur M, Tsai T, Kang K, Feldman J, Kory L. Endometrial Stripe thickness in tubal and intrauterine pregnancies. *Fertil Steril* 2000;5:889–91.

26. Hammoud AO, Hammoud I, Bujold E, Gonik B, Diamond MP, Johnson SC. *Am J Obset Gynecol* 2005;192:1370–5.

27. Condous G, Van Calster B, Kirk E, Halder Z, Timmerman D, Van Huffel S, Bourne T. Clinical information does not improve the performance of mathematical models in predicting the outcome of pregnancies of unknown location. *Fertil Steril* 2007;88(3);572–80.

28. Condous G, Okaro E, Khalid A, Bourne T. Do we need to follow up complete miscarriages with serum human chorionic gonadotrophin levels? *BJOG* 2005;112:827–9.

29. CEMACH. *Why Mothers Die 2000–2002. The Sixth Report of the Confidential Enquiries into Maternal Deaths in the United Kingdom*. London: RCOG Press, 2004.

30. Van Mello NM, Mol F, Opmeer BC, Ankum WM, Barnhart K, Coomarasamy A, Mol BW, van der Veen F, Hajenius PJ. Diagnostic value of serum hCG on the outcome of pregnancy of unknown location: a systematic review and meta-analysis. *Hum Reprod Update* 2012;18:603–17.

31. Braunstein GD, Rasor J, Adler D, Danzer H, Wade ME. Serum human chorionic gonadotrophin levels throughout normal pregnancy. *Am J Obstet Gynecol* 1976;126:678–81.
32. Condous G, Okaro E, Bourne T. The conservative management of early pregnancy complications: a review of the literature. *Ultrasound in Obstet Gynecol* 2003;22:420–30.
33. Cacciatore B, Stenman U-H., Pekka Y. Diagnosis of ectopic pregnancy by vaginal ultrasonography in combination with a discriminatory serum hCG of 1000 iu/l (IRP). *BJOG* 1990;97:904–8.
34. Condous G, Kirk E, Lu C, Van Huffel S, Gevaert O, De Moor B, De Smelt F, Timmerman D, Bourne T. Diagnostic accuracy of varying discriminatory zones for the prediction of ectopic pregnancy in women with a pregnancy of unknown location. *Ultrasound Obstet Gynecol* 2005;26:770–5.
35. Ball S, Ekelund C, Wright D, Kikegaard P, Norgaard P, Peterson OB, Tabor A. Temporal effects of maternal and pregnancy characteristics on serum pregnancy-associated plasma protein-A and free β-human chorionic gonadotrophin at 7-14 weeks' gestation. *Ultrasound Obstet Gynecol* 2013;41:33–9.
36. Dillon KE, Sioulas VD, Sammel MD, Chung K, Takacs P, Shaunik A, Barnhart KT. How and when human chorionic gonadotrophin curves in women with an ectopic pregnancy mimic other outcomes: differences by race and ethnicity. *Fertil Steril* 2012;98:911–16.
37. Barnhart KT, Sammel MD, Appleby D, Rausch M, Molinaro T, Van Calster B, Kirk E, Condous G, Van Huffel S, Timmerman D, Bourne T. Does a prediction model for pregnancy of unknown location developed in the UK validate on a US population? *Hum Reprod* 2010;25:2434–40.
38. Van Calster B, Abdallah Y, Guha S, Kirk E, Van Hoorde K, Condous G, Preisler J, Hoo W, Stalder C, Bottomley C, Timmerman D, Bourne T. Rationalizing the management of pregnancies of unknown location: temporal and external validation of a risk prediction model on 1962 pregnancies. *Hum Reprod* 2013;28:609–16.
39. Cordina M, Schramm-Gajraj K, Ross JA, Lautman K, Jurkovic D. Introduction of a single visit protocol in the management of selected patients with pregnancy of unknown location: a prospective study. *BJOG* 2011:118(6):693–7.
40. Verhaegen J, Gallos ID, van Mello NM, Abdel-Aziz M, Takwoingi Y, Harb H, Deeks JJ, Mol BW, Coomarasamy A. Accuracy of single progesterone test to predict early pregnancy outcome in women with pain or bleeding: meta-analysis of cohort studies. *BMJ* 2012;345:e6077.
41. Sagili H, Mohamed K. Review Pregnancy of Unknown Location: an evidence-based approach to management. *The Obstetrician and Gynaecologist*. 2008:10:224–30.
42. Jurkovic D, Farquharson R. *Acute Gynaecology and Early Pregnancy*. RCOG Press, 121–31.
43. Kirk E, Papageorghiou AT, Condous G, Tan L, Bora S, Bourne T. The diagnostic effectiveness of an initial transvaginal scan in detecting ectopic pregnancy. *Hum Reprod* 2007;22:2824–8.
44. Kirk E, Daemen A, Papageorghiou AT, Bottomley C, Condous G, De Moor B, Timmerman D, Bourne T. Why are some ectopic pregnancies characterized as pregnancies of unknown location at the initial transvaginal ultrasound examination? *Acta Obstetrcia et Gynecologica* 2008;87:1150–4.
45. Jurkovic D. hCG as a patient. *Ultrasound Obstet Gynecol* 2010;36:395–9.
46. Van Mello NM, Mol F, Ankum WM, Mol BW, van der Veen F, Hajenius PJ. Ectopic pregnancy: how the diagnostic and therapeutic management has changed. *Fertil Steril* 2012;98:1066–73.
47. Lloyd ME, Carr M, Mcelhatton P, Hall GM, Hugues RA. The effects of Methotrexate on pregnancy, fertility and lactation. *QJM* 1999;92:551–63.
48. Royal College of Obstetricians and Gynaecologists. 2004. < http://www.rcog.org.uk/womens-health/clinical-guidance/management-tubal-pregnancy-21-may-2004>

49. Tan L, Kirk E, Papageorghiou AT, Condous G, Mukri F, Bora S, Bourne T. Persisting pregnancies of unknown location: challenges in diagnosis and management. *Ultrasound in Obstetrics and Gynecology* 2007;30:387–8.

50. Condous G, Okaro E, Khalid A, Timmerman D, Lu C, Zhou Y, Van Huffel S, Bourne T. The use of a new logistic regression model for predicting the outcome of pregnancies of unknown location. *Hum Reprod* 2004;19(8):1900–10.

51. Van Mello NB, Mol F, Verhoeve HR, van Wely M, Adriaanse AU, Boss EA, *et al.* Methotrexate or expectant management in women with an ectopic pregnancy or pregnancy of unknown location and low serum hCG concentrations? A randomized comparison. *Hum Reprod* 2013;28:60–7.

52. Barnhart KT. Early Pregnancy Failure: Beware of the pitfalls of modern management. *Fertil Steril* 2012;98:1061–5.

53. Einenkel J, Handzel R, Horn L-C. Persisting Pregnancy of unknown location- Keep your eyes peeled for choriocarcinoma. *Eur J Obstet Gynecol Reprod Biol* 2010;153:224–31.

54. Cong Q, Li Guiling, Jiang W, Li B, Wang Y, Yao L, Wang S, Xu C. Ectopic choriocarcinoma Masquerading As a Persisting Pregnancy of Unknown Location: Case Report and Review of the Literature. *Journal of Clinical Oncology* 2011;29:845–8.

55. Condous G, Thomas J, Okaro E, Bourne T. Placental site trophoblastic tumour masquerading as an ovarian ectopic pregnancy. *Ultrasound Obstet Gynaecol* 2003;21:504–50.

56. Ankrum WM, Van der Veen F, Hamerlynck JV, Lammes FB. Laparoscopy: a dispensable tool in the diagnosis of ectopic pregnancy? *Hum Reprod* 1993;8:1301–6.

57. Condous G, Van Calster B, Kirk E, Haider Z, Timmerman D, Van Huffel S, Bourne T. Prediction of ectopic pregnancy in women with a pregnancy of unknown location. *Ultrasound Ostet Gynecol* 2007;29:680–7.

58. Condous G, Okaro E, Khalid A, Lu C, Van Huffel S, Timmerman D, Bourne T. A prospective evaluation of a single visit strategy to manage pregnancies of unknown location. *Hum Reprod* 2005;20(5):1398–1403.

59. The Practice Committee of the American Society for Reproductive Medicine. Medical treatment of ectopic pregnancy. *Fertil Steril* 2008;90 S206–LS212.

60. Shaunik A, Kulp J, Appleby D, Sammel MD, Barnhart KT. Utility of dilation and curettage in the diagnosis of pregnancy of unknown location. *Am J Obstet Gynecol* 2011;204:130. e1–6.

61. Chung K, Chandavarkar U, Opper N, Barnhart K. Reevaluating the role of dilation and curettage in the diagnosis of pregnancy of unknown location. *Fertil Steril* 2011;96:659–62.

62. Rubal L, Chung K. Do you need to definitively diagnose the location of a pregnancy of unknown location? The case for 'yes'. *Fertil Steril* 2012;98:1078–84.

63. Condous G, Kirk E, Lu C, Van Calster B, Van Huffel S, Timmerman D, Bourne T. There is no role for uterine curettage in the contemporary diagnostic workup of women with a pregnancy of unknown location. *Hum Reprod* 2006;21:2706–10.

64. Condous G. The term 'Pregnancy of unknown location' is staying put. *BJOG* 2011;118:1402.

65. Wilkinson H, on behalf of the Trustees and Medical Advisers. Saving Mothers' Lives. Reviewing maternal deaths to make motherhood safer: 2006–2008. *BJOG* 2011;118:1402–3.

66. Bourne T, Barnhart K, Benson CB, Brosens J, Van Calster B, Condous G. et al. NICE guidance onectopic pregnancy and miscarriage restricts access and choice and may be clinically unsafe. *BMJ* 2013;346:f197.

67. Reid S, Condous G. Is there a need to definitively diagnose the location of a pregnancy of unknown location? The case for 'n'. *Fertil Steril* 2012;98:1085–90.

Pre-implantation genetic diagnosis in oligozoospermia

Helen Bickerstaff and Srividya Seshadri

⏱ **Expert Commentary** William Ledger

Mrs and Mr Smith, aged 29 and 32 years respectively, were referred to the reproductive medicine clinic with primary sub-fertility. They had been having regular intercourse almost twice a week, without using any contraception, for over two years. For Mrs Smith, this was her first stable relationship and she was keen to conceive. She had never been pregnant before. She had a 28-day menstrual cycle, and there was no dysmenorrhoea or menorrhagia. She reported normal secondary sexual characteristic development and menarche at age 13. She had no significant past medical history and was not on any medication. There was no family history of any significant medical conditions. Her cervical smears were up-to-date and always normal, she had never had a sexually transmitted infection, and did not consume alcohol or tobacco. Her BMI was 24.

Mr Smith was in good physical health. He was non-smoker and consumed minimal alcohol. He cycled about 10 miles every day. He recalled a possible episode of mumps aged 13, although he was unsure when questioned regarding associated scrotal pain. He had never had any testicular or hernia surgery. He had not fathered any children from previous relationships.

Their relationship was stable, with no reported sexual dysfunction. They enjoyed a good and active social life. There were no financial pressures. Their inability to conceive left them anxious but they did not report any detrimental effect on their relationship or daily functioning.

✪ Learning point Epidemiology of infertility

- Infertility is defined as the failure to conceive after regular unprotected sexual intercourse for one to two years without the use of contraception in couples within the reproductive age group [1].
- The prevalence of infertility in European countries is around 14%, affecting one in seven couples [1], and rises with age (Figure 4.1). Of these, 70% will have primary infertility (neither partner has conceived previously), and 30% secondary infertility (at least one previous pregnancy together).
- The most common cause of primary infertility is male factor (35%) [2, 3].
- The most common female causes of infertility are ovarian dysfunction/anovulation (20%) and tubal factors (19.5%) [2, 3].
- Unexplained subfertility accounts for approximately 22% of cases [2, 3].
- Approximately 80% of couples will conceive within the first year (if the woman is less than 40 years of age and they have regular sexual intercourse). Of those couples who do not conceive within the first year, 50% will do so in the second year [1].
- Studies have shown that only a minority of couples with subfertility have a good understanding of ways to maximize chances of conceiving [3].

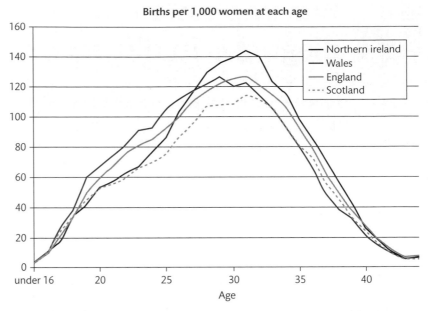

Figure 4.1 Age-specific fertility rates (ASFRs), constituent countries of the UK, 2010 [4].

Figure reproduced from Gov.UK (4) under the Open Government Licence v2.0.

❝ Expert comment

It is of paramount importance that a careful and thorough history is taken from both partners prior to infertility investigations. Particular attention should be paid to the reproductive history of the present couple and their previous relationships. Questions should be asked regarding the frequency and timing of intercourse. The timing of investigations may be directed by the age of the partners and the duration of infertility. The focus of investigations may depend on either of the partner's past history. Prior to starting the investigations, the female partner's rubella immunity status and body mass index (BMI) should be assessed, and, if necessary, she should be immunized for rubella or advised to lose weight. General advice to both partners should include eating a healthy diet, regular exercise, giving up smoking, and reducing alcohol consumption. All women who are planning a pregnancy should take 400 mcg folic acid due to its proven effect of reducing neural tube defects. 5 mg folic acid should be advised if appropriate due to comorbidities such as diabetes and renal disorders.

✚ Clinical tip Maximizing the chance of conception

As most couples presenting with subfertility continue to have a chance of conceiving naturally, advice on the timing of intercourse in order to maximize conception is important, as is maximizing the reproductive health of the couple. The following issues should be explored at the initial consultation:

Timing of intercourse

- Checking the couple's understanding of ovulation and the menstrual cycle may maximize the chance of conception. With a regular menstrual cycle, the chance of conception rises six days prior to ovulation (maximally two days prior to ovulation) and falls markedly by the day after ovulation.
- Advice to have regular intercourse two to three times a week is sufficient to cover a women's most fertile period, and may reduce anxiety or stress associated with timed intercourse for some couples.

(continued)

Weight

- Women with BMI > 30 kgm² should be provided with dietary and lifestyle advice on how to lose weight.
- Women with BMI < 20 kgm² should be advised to gain weight and reduce excessive exercise.

Pre-existing medical conditions

- Optimization of control of pre-existing medical conditions may reduce the chance of morbidity for the mother, and may reduce negative effects including prematurity on the fetus (e.g. diabetes, epilepsy, hypertension, thyroid disease, cardiac disease).
- Comorbidities should be controlled where possible using mono therapy with non-teratogenic drugs which do not interfere with fertility.

Smoking

Smoking cessation for both partners may maximize the chance of conception, and may prevent refusal of funding for artificial reproductive techniques (ART) by commissioning bodies, many of which have this as a prerequisite.

---

𝟔𝟔 Expert comment

Assessing the impact of infertility on the couple's social life, and marital and sexual relationship is important and should be addressed at this early stage of investigation. A proportion of couples when asked in the correct circumstances may admit avoidance of sexual activity, erectile or ejaculatory problems, or even non-consummated relationships. The latter may particularly be the case after female genital mutilation (FGM) type 3. Referral to psychosexual or other counselling services, teaching home self-insemination, and reversal of FGM can sometimes give enormous relief to couples having such problems.

✚ Clinical tip History and examination of the infertile woman

History

Regularity of periods

Menstrual symptoms: oligomenorrhoea or heavy menstrual bleeding, intermenstrual bleeding

Associated symptoms: dyspareunia and dysmenorrhoea

Previous history of sexually transmitted infections (STI)

History of previous gynaecology surgery, including laser loop excision treatment for abnormal cervical smears

Examination

Abdominal examination for scars and large fibroids

Speculum examination and swabs

Pelvic examination to assess the size and mobility of the uterus

---

✚ Clinical tip Clues in the history

- Ovulatory dysfunction may be suggested by a history of late menarche, amenorrhoea, oligomenorrhoea, irregular cycles, hot flushes (hypooestrogenemia due to premature ovarian failure), hirsutism, weight gain, and acne, or symptoms of thyroid dysfunction. Anovulation due to polycystic ovarian syndrome (PCOS) may be corrected by a reduction of body weight by

(continued)

5 %, although more might be advised. Anovulation due to hypothalamic hypogonadism may be corrected by reduction in excessive exercise or increase from a low BMI. A correct diagnosis and appropriate lifestyle advice or medication may restore fertility without the need for ART. Excessive regular menstrual bleeding may indicate the presence of uterine pathology such as fibroids.

- Female tubal dysfunction may be indicted by a past history of pelvic infections, previous pelvic surgery, pelvic pain, and dyspareunia.
- Delayed secondary sexual characteristic development and amennorhoea, with or without androgenism, may prompt the exclusion of karyotypic abnormalities, Kallman's syndrome, or gonadal dysgenesis.

✪ **Learning point** Infertility investigations

Baseline infertility tests

Initial tests should focus on: semen, functioning of the hypothalamic–pituitary–ovarian axis, oocyte reserve, uterine structure, and fallopian tube patency.

Female tests	Timing of the tests
FSH/LH/E2	Days 2–6 (early follicular phase)
Prolactin, testosterone	
Anti-Mullerian hormone (AMH)	Any part of the menstrual cycle
Progesterone	Mid-luteal phase, 21 days in a regular cycle or seven days before the next period
Transvaginal ultrasound	Early follicular phase
Tubal patency tests	
STI screen/HIV/Hep B/Hep C	

Male tests	Timing of the tests
Semen analysis	Sample should be collected after a minimum of two days and a maximum of seven days of sexual abstinence

---

❝ **Expert comment**

The method of testing tubal patency and the routine use of diagnostic laparoscopy for the evaluation of all cases of female infertility is debatable [5]. Where there is a history of pelvic pain, diagnostic laparoscopy and dye test allows assessment of tubal damage, and diagnosis and treatment of abnormality. Communicating hydrosalpinges are associated with a reduction in IVF success rates. Therefore, if hydrosalpinges have been diagnosed by ultrasound, a hysterosalpingogram (HSG) may be advisable prior to laparoscopy in order to establish the communication with the uterine cavity. This will enable informed consent to salpingectomy prior to laparoscopy. Where there is no pelvic pain, an hysterocontrast sonography (HyCoSy) should be performed in preference to HSG as this avoids exposure of the ovaries to ionizing radiation.

✪ **Learning point** Tests of ovarian reserve

- Early follicular phase serum follicle stimulating hormone (FSH) levels combined with oestradiol levels are a measure of ovarian reserve. A high FSH level (>10 IU/ml) is often due to reduced ovarian reserve resulting in reduced gonadal negative feedback through inhibin B from antral follicles. Normal FSH levels in the presence of high oestrogen can be falsely reassuring. High FSH/LH results in a patient with very irregular cycles must be repeated two weeks later, in case a mid-cycle peak has occurred. Very high FSH levels are associated with gonadal dysgenesis and premature ovaraian failure. Low FSH/LH levels (<2 IU/ml) are associated with hypopituitarism.

(continued)

- Anti-Mullerian Hormone (AMH) levels have the advantage of clinical reproducibility, and are not cycle-dependent. Results are stratified into normal, low, or negligible fertility [6]. AMH levels do not need repeating.
- The Antral follicle count (AFC) can be determined by transvaginal ultrasound scan, by counting the total number of follicles greater than 2 mm in both ovaries. The number of antral follicles diminishes with age. The risk of infertility with an AFC <10 is more than 20% with a 50% likelihood of inability to conceive for >one year [7].

Mrs Smith's pelvic examination was normal and a hormone profile was taken which was also normal. A transvaginal ultrasound scan was performed which was also normal with a total antral follicle count of 20. Mr Smith's semen results are shown in Table 4.1.

Table 4.1 Mr Smith's semen analysis as compared to WHO reference values for semen parameters [8]

Parameters	Normal values (lower reference limits)	Patient values 1st sample	Patient values 2nd sample
Volume in ml	1.5 (1.4–1.7)	1.8	1.8
Sperm concentration in (10^6 permL)	15 (12–16)	3.1	2.5
Motility* (a+b)%	40 (38–42)	38	35
Morphology (normal forms, %)	4 (3.0–4.0)	3	2

* Both progressive motility (a) and non-linear motility (b) in combination is taken into consideration.

Expert comment

Investigations on the male partner are important for all couples, as an abnormality in the semen analysis will be expected in over 40% of cases. A large number of couples have both female and male causes of infertility. Abnormal semen analysis should be repeated 10–12 weeks later, as there is significant temporal variation in sperm count, and it takes about 10 weeks for spermatogenesis to recover after insults such as excessive alcohol, smoking, or pyrexial illnesses. Low-volume semen analysis should raise the question of semen production following withdrawal, or loss of some of the sample.

The couple were reviewed in the clinic with the results of the investigations. Mr Smith was informed that both his semen samples were consistent with oligozoospermia. Mr Smith was examined and found to have normal secondary sexual characteristics, no varicocoeles, no hypospadia, no inguinal scars, and normal testicular sizes and consistency. On palpation, the vas deferens was present on the right side but absent on the left: congenital unilateral absence of vas deferens (CUAVD).

Clinical tip Biochemical investigation of the male with abnormal semen analysis

Gonadotrophin and testosterone levels should be taken to distinguish between causes

FSH	Testosterone	Likely mechanism
Normal	Normal	Idiopathic, sperm function, sexual dysfunction, or post-testicular causes
Raised	Normal	Testicular causes of dysfunction
Raised	Low	Testicular failure
Low	Low	Pre-testicular failure

Expert comment

There is a relationship between the degree of excessive weight and poor quality and quantity of sperm [10]. Smoking and excessive alcohol consumption are also known to affect the quality of sperm [1].

Expert comment

Micro deletions in the AZF region of the Y chromosome may be found in 10–15% of men with azoospermia or severe oligozoospermia [11]. Most NHS facilities are unable to offer molecular biochemical testing for these deletions, which are anyway not amenable to treatment.

Learning point

Intracytoplasmic sperm injection (ICSI)

ICSI is a method of fertilization which is used to improve the poor fertilization rates associated with conventional IVF and seminal fluid analysis (SFA) abnormalities, antisperm antibodies, or fertilization failure in previous IVF cycles.

Standard IVF procedures including controlled ovarian stimulation and transvaginal oocyte retrieval are performed. The cumulus cells are stripped from the oocytes to enable visual confirmation of their maturity. Mature oocytes are injected individually with single sperm under microscopic control.

Expert comment

Theoretical concerns exist regarding the potential genetic risks associated with ICSI due to the bypassing of the natural barriers to fertilization and propagation of the genetic defects. With the exception of inherited sex chromosome mutations, the relationship between ICSI and genetic defects in the offspring remain unclear. Couples should be counselled regarding this theoretical risk until there is robust data to support or refute this risk.

Learning point   Main causes of male infertility

Idiopathic (unexplained)		Constitutes the vast majority of the cases
Pre-testicular causes	Pituitary disease	• Hyperprolactinaemia • Gonadotrophin suppression (exogenous use of androgens, glucocorticoid excess) • Pituitary insufficiency (tumours, irradiation, surgery)
	Hypothalamic disease	• Gonadotrophin deficiency (Kallmans syndrome)
Testicular (defective sperm production)	Congenital	• Klinefelters syndrome (47 XXY) • Y chromosome deletions • Prader–Willi syndrome • Noonan syndrome (45 XO) • Cryptoorchidism, congenital anorchia and androgen insensitivity syndromes
	Acquired	• Vascular: varicocoele • Injury: orchitis, testicular torsion, trauma, and haematoma • Testicular tumours • Immunological: autoimmune orchitis • Iatrogenic: radiotherapy and chemotherapy, drugs (e.g. sulphasalazine)
Post testicular (defective sperm transport)	Congenital	• Congenital unilateral or bilateral absence of the vas deferens (CUAVD/CBAVD) • Cystic fibrosis • Young's syndrome
	Acquired	• Vasectomy • Viral orchitis • STI
Disorders of sperm function		• Immunological (anti-sperm antibodies) • Immotile cilia syndrome
Sexual dysfunction	Erectile Dysfunction	• Systemic illness (e.g. diabetes mellitus) • Neurological injury • Psychological
	Ejaculatory defects	• Premature ejaculation • Retrograde ejaculation • Anejaculation

Mr Smith underwent further investigations which revealed a normal hormonal profile (FSH, LH, and testosterone) and normal karyotype (46XY). The couple were advised that ART would be required to achieve a pregnancy.

In view of the finding of CUAVD in Mr Smith, and normal other investigations including karyotype and hormonal screens, genetic tests were performed to exclude a cystic fibrosis transmembrane regulator (CFTR) gene mutation. This revealed a compound heterozygote gene mutation of the gene (δ508F/5T). The couple underwent genetic counselling and CFTR screening was also offered to Mrs Smith. Mrs Smith was subsequently identified as a heterozygote carrier of the CFTR δ508F mutation. The couple received genetic counselling and were advised regarding the one in four risk of conceiving a child phenotypically affected by clinical cystic fibrosis. Pre-implantation genetic diagnosis (PGD) was discussed.

✪ Learning point Surgical sperm retrieval (SSR)

Where there is inadequate sperm in the ejaculate, ICSI must be preceded by surgical sperm retrieval.

Indications include:

1) Congenital bilateral absence of vas deferens (CBAVD)
2) Obstruction of both ejaculatory ducts
3) Azoospermia of other cause

Sperm is aspirated directly from the epididymis by percutaneous epididymal sperm aspiration (PESA) or obtained directly from the testicle either by testicular sperm aspiration (TESA) or testicular sperm extraction (TESE), also known as testicular open biopsy. These procedures are carried out under local or general anaesthesia on the day of egg collection.

The risk of birth defects after sperm retrieval with ICSI is comparable to that associated with ICSI using ejaculated sperm.

❝ Expert comment

ICSI can be used to treat couples with male factor infertility. Where inadequate numbers of motile sperm are found in the ejaculate, SSR from the testis or epididymis may be successful. In the case of CBAVD there are likely to be high numbers of sperm which can be surgically retrieved. Cases of testicular failure, particularly in association with aneuploidy or microdeletions in the AZF region 1 of the Y chromosome are far less likely to be successful. Only a handful of reported cases of successful sperm retrieval and fertilization exist in Klinefelter men.

✪ Learning point Cystic fibrosis mutations and male infertility

- Mutations in the CFTR (gene located at 7q31.2) lead to abnormalities in the structure, function, and production of a chloride channel. There are more than 100 mutations known, the most common of which is the δ508F mutation. Around 40 of the most common mutations are detected by 'extended screening' offered through most regional genetics laboratories. Homozygosity of the δ508 mutation or compound heterozygosity of two mutations may be associated with clinical cystic fibrosis. Different mutations are associated with a spectrum of phenotypic severity.
- Cystic fibrosis is the most frequent autosomal recessive genetic disorder in the Caucasian population. Incidence is 1:2500 births and CFTR gene mutations have a carrier frequency of 1:25.
- CTFR gene mutations can be associated with CUAVD or CBAVD.
- CFTR screening of the female partner should be performed for the partner of a male found to carry a CFTR mutation, to avoid phenotypically affected homozygote or compound heterozygote offspring.

✪ Learning point Pre-implantation genetic diagnosis (PGD)

PGD is considered a very early form of prenatal diagnosis and is available to couples who are at risk having a child with a specific genetic or chromosome disorder. Following IVF and ICSI, the cleavage stage embryo (at the 6–10 cell stage on day 3 post fertilization) or the blastocyst (on day 5 post fertilization) is biopsied and one or two blastomeres are removed. The representative blastomere is tested for the genetic mutation in question. Embryos predicted to be free of the specific genetic mutation are chosen for transfer. In the case of recessive disorders heterozygote carrier embryos would also be considered suitable (Figure 4.2).

❝ Expert comment

In cases where it is known that the couple carry a serious genetic condition, prenatal diagnosis (PND) after conception or pre-implantation genetic diagnosis (PGD) after ART can be offered. Cases where couples each carry a CTFR mutation may be associated with both infertility and the risk of conceiving a child phenotypically affected by cystic fibrosis. IVF and ICSI, preceded if necessary by surgical sperm retrieval, and followed by PGD or PND, may be used to treat the infertility and reduce the risk. PGD is often ethically preferable as it avoids the possible need to terminate a pregnancy if an abnormality is detected.

⊕ Clinical tip PGD testing

Currently PGD is a lengthy and complex specialized procedure for which only a small number of laboratories are licensed. The full list of conditions tested is available at <http://www.pgd.org.uk>.

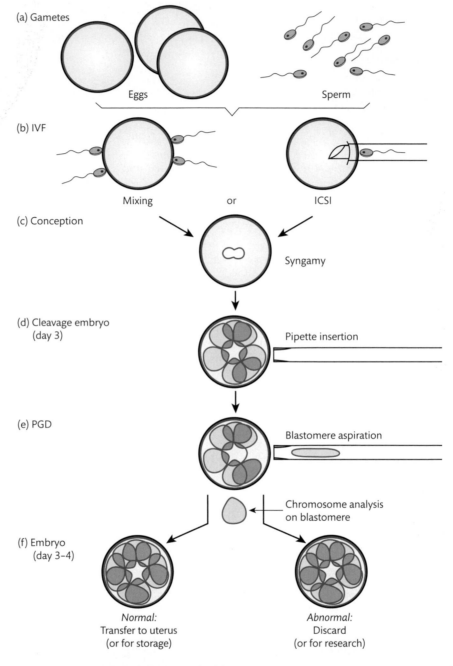

(a) Gametes

Eggs   Sperm

(b) IVF

Mixing   or   ICSI

(c) Conception

Syngamy

(d) Cleavage embryo (day 3)

Pipette insertion

(e) PGD

Blastomere aspiration

Chromosome analysis on blastomere

(f) Embryo (day 3–4)

Normal:
Transfer to uterus
(or for storage)

Abnormal:
Discard
(or for research)

Figure 4.2 The process of in-vitro fertilization (IVF) (with or without intracytoplasmic sperm injection, ICSI) and pre-implantation genetic diagnosis (PGD) at the day-3 stage. (a) Oocytes are obtained from the woman, and sperm from the man (by testicular aspiration, if necessary). (b) Oocytes and sperm are mixed in vitro; or, single sperm are injected into an oocyte (ICSI). (c) Syngamy, the fusion of male and female pronuclei, occurs. After incubation for 3 days, (d) one or two 7 blastomeres are removed from the embryo, and (e) these cells are then subject to chromosomal analysis. (f) Normal (or balanced) embryos are chosen for transfer to the uterus, or possibly for cryopreservation for a future transfer.

Reproduced from Gardner, Grant, and Shaffer, Chromosome Abnormalities and Genetic Counselling, 2011 with permission from Oxford University Press.

The couple chose ICSI and PGD. One unaffected blastocyst was implanted after PGD, a further unaffected blastocyst and one carrier blastocyst were frozen. The couple went on to conceive a singleton pregnancy without any procedural or pregnancy-related complications.

Discussion

There has been a significant increase in the numbers of couples seeking assisted reproduction techniques over the last 15 years. This increase has been driven, in part, by the availability and increased success rates of ART and a reluctance to wait for spontaneous conception after prolonged infertility. ICSI has increased the success rates of IVF for male factor infertility in couples for whom conventional IVF offered poor fertilization. A small proportion of severe male factor infertility has a genetic origin. Genetic testing for karyotype and CTFR gene mutations may identify the risk of unbalanced translocations or clinical CF in offspring, a risk which may be reduced by PGD. This clinical case highlights the need for accurate clinical assessment of a couple. The clinical diagnosis of CUAVD prompted further genetic testing of both partners, and identified the risk of a pregnancy affected by cystic fibrosis. PGD was offered to reduce this risk. This case raises the question of offering genetic testing for common recessive conditions as part of the diagnostic work up prior to IVF. There is a considerable financial and emotional cost involved in ART. According to some experts, additional genetic testing would be considered justified to avoid the rare but tragic outcomes of unexpected genetically abnormal children. However, the capability of molecular genetic diagnosis is rapidly expanding. Extended genetic testing, unless clinically directed, may result in the detection of genetic mutations of uncertain clinical importance. The least satisfactory result of this could be unnecessary PGD, with its associated risks of financial cost, emotional burden, and decreased success rates. There are ethical dilemmas raised by genetic selection. PGD has been regulated by the HFEA since its development in the late 1990s. Initially, PGD was licensed only for lethal disease, but some 15 years later the goal posts have changed and PGD is offered within the UK for late-onset conditions including Huntington Disease and BRACA 1 gene inheritance, and outside the UK for social sex selection.

> ✪ **Learning point** Counselling for ART
>
> Trying to conceive can be stressful [12]. Furthermore, some couples find the pressure of infertility, investigations, and treatment creates temporary sexual problems. Counselling is therefore an integral part of treatment and all couples embarking on ART are encouraged to see a counsellor. Counselling is often provided by HFEA-accredited counsellors who understand ART and can counsel couples regarding options and concerns. Fertility counselling is available in most assisted conception units.

A Final Word from the Expert

This case illustrates the extent to which molecular genetics have been translated into clinical practice. The correct genetic diagnosis and use of PGD reduced the risk of having a child with cystic fibrosis, a life-limiting disorder with ramifications for the whole family, and cost to the NHS. A multidisciplinary approach to such complex causes of subfertility is necessary, involving a PGD team comprising the assisted conception unit specialist doctors, nurses, embryologists, counsellors, geneticists, and scientists.

References

1. NICE Guidelines: Fertility assessment and treatment for people with fertility problems. Clinical Guideline February 2004. <http://www.nice.org.uk>

2. Maheshwari A, Hamilton M, Bhattacharya S. Effect of female age on the diagnostic categories of infertility. *Hum Reprod* 2008;23(3):538–42

3. Hull M, Glazener C, Kelly N, Conway D, Foster P, Hinton R, *et al.* Population study of causes, treatment and outcomes of infertility. *BMJ* 1985;291:1693–7.

4. Office for National Statistics (ONS), Northern Ireland Statistics and Research *Agency* (NISRA) and National Records of Scotland (NRS), Fertility Summary 2010. <http://www.ons.gov.uk/ons/dcp171780_237192.pdf>

5. Bosteels J, Herendael BV, Weyers S, D'Hooghe T. The position of diagnostic laparoscopy in current fertility practice. *Hum Reprod Update* 2007;13(5):477–85.

6. La Marca A, Sighinolfi G, Radi D, Argento C, Baraldi E, Carducci A, *et al.* Anti-Müllerian hormone (AMH) as a predictive marker in assisted reproductive technology (ART). *Hum Reprod Update* 2010;16(2):113–30.

7. Kline J, Kinney A, Kelly A, Reuss ML, Levin B. Predictors of antral follicle count during the reproductive years. *Hum Reprod* 2005;20(8):2179–89.

8. Cooper TG, Noonan E, von Eckardstein S, Auger J, Baker HW, Behre HM, Haugen TB, Kruger T, Wang C, Mbizvo MT, Vogelsong KM. World Health Organization reference values for human semen characteristics. *Hum Reprod Update* 2010; May–Jun;16(3):231–45

9. Kantartzi PD, Goulis CD, Goulis GD, Papadimas I. Male infertility and varicocele: myths and reality *Hippokratia*. 2007 Jul–Sep;11(3):99–104.

10. Kort HI, Massey JB, Elsner CW, Toledo AA, Mitchell-Leef D, Roudebush WE. Men with high body mass index values present with lower numbers of normal-motile sperm cells. Abstract no. P-355. *Fertil Steril* 2003;80, Suppl 3:S238.

11. Viswambharan N, Suganthi R, Simon AM, Manonayaki S. Male infertility: polymerase chain reaction-based deletion mapping of genes on the human chromosome. *Singapore Med J* 2007 Dec;48 (12):1140–2.

12. Griel AL. Infertility and psychological distress: a critical review of the literature. *SocSci Med* 1997;45:1679–704.

5 Recurrent miscarriage: is conservative management the best we can offer?

Ai-Wei Tang

ⓘ **Expert Commentary** Ian Greer

Case history

A 38-year-old Gravida 4 Para 1 woman was referred to the specialist recurrent miscarriage (RM) clinic by her general practitioner (GP) after 3 consecutive spontaneous miscarriages at less than 10 weeks' gestation, which followed her first successful full-term spontaneous vaginal delivery five years earlier.

Her first miscarriage had been diagnosed after she had presented to the early pregnancy unit with per vaginal spotting at nine weeks' gestation, and a transvaginal ultrasound scan confirmed a seven-week-size delayed miscarriage with absence of a fetal heart. It had been managed conservatively with spontaneous passage of products of conception after one week. She had required evacuation of products of conception under general anaesthetic for her subsequent two delayed miscarriages which all took place within the previous two years. All pregnancies had been conceived with the same regular partner. She had a normal BMI, and had no known medical problems. She was a non- smoker and drank 6–10 units of alcohol/week, from which she had abstained during her pregnancies.

> ⭐ **Learning point** Recurrent miscarriage
>
> The definition of RM by the European Human Society of Humans Reproduction and Embryology (ESHRE) is three or more consecutive early miscarriages (<12 weeks' gestation), or two late miscarriages (>12 weeks' gestation) (Table 5.1). It affects about 1% of couples trying to conceive [1]. Some clinicians consider two consecutive miscarriages as RM, and initiate investigations after the second miscarriage, on the basis that the prevalence of causes is similar in those with two, three, or more miscarriages [2]. However, with no proven intervention, investigating all women after two miscarriages at an incidence of 5% may represent a strain on the health system [3]. Furthermore, RM is associated with a range of pathologies, but few studies provide prognostic implications for future pregnancies when these conditions are identified in women with RM. There are even fewer high-quality randomized controlled trials (RCTs) that show any benefit of treatment for women with RM for subsequent pregnancy outcome.

> ⓘ **Expert comment**
>
> It is common for clinicians to request a series of investigations in women who have had RM. Where these investigations guide neither prognosis nor treatment, and may reflect association rather than causation, can these be justified?
>
> There are many factors associated with RM; few are established as causative, and there is a paucity of effective interventions. Women with this problem need specialist advice and support as often
>
> (continued)

unnecessary investigations give false hope of a definite cause and may precipitate unproven treatment with potential harm. Expert knowledge of the evidence base, good counseling and support skills are therefore necessary to provide optimal care of these women. RM clinics play a critical role in ensuring high-quality care, evidence-based practice, and optimal use of resources.

✪ **Learning point** Alcohol, smoking, and caffeine in pregnancy

Alcohol and RM

Alcohol is a teratogen that can lead to fetal alcohol syndrome in a dose-dependent relationship [4]. There is an association of alcohol consumption and spontaneous miscarriage [5]. In view of this, NICE (National Institute for Health and Clinical Excellence) recommends avoiding alcohol intake in the first three months of pregnancy, and thereafter, a limit of 1–2 UK units (1 unit = ½ pint of ordinary strength beer or 25 mls of spirit) once or twice a week [6]. At this low level, there is no clear evidence of harm to the unborn baby.

Smoking and RM

Many studies have found a dose-dependent association between miscarriage and smoking [4]. Thus, women are strongly encouraged to stop smoking prior to conceiving and should be provided smoking cessation support.

Caffeine and RM

The association is not as evident with caffeine. Although numerous studies observed a positive correlation between maternal caffeine intake and risk of miscarriage, most of these studies have methodological flaws and potential bias that do not allow a comparison of results. Hence, evidence for this causal link remains inconclusive [7].

Table 5.1 Classification of early pregnancy loss events [1]

Pregnancy loss events	Definition
Biochemical pregnancy loss	Pregnancy not located on ultrasound (US)
Empty sac loss	Gestation sac with absent structures or minimal embryonic debris without FH activity
Fetal loss	Previous identification of crown–rump length (CRL) and fetal heart (FH) activity, followed by loss of FH activity
Early pregnancy loss	USS definition of intra-uterine pregnancy with evidence of loss of FH activity, and/or failure of increase in CRL over 1 week, or persistent presence of empty gestation sac of < 12 weeks' gestation
Late pregnancy loss	> 12 weeks' gestation where CRL measurement was followed by loss of FH activity

➕ **Clinical tip** Ultrasonographic diagnosis of a first trimester miscarriage

- Should be made with a transvaginal ultrasound (TVUS) [8].
  - Mean diameter of the gestation sac is > 25 mm, with minimal embryonic structures and no fetal pole seen (Figure 5.1)
    OR
  - Crown–rump length (CRL) is > 7 mm with no fetal heart (FH) pulsations seen (Figure 5.2)
- If there is a doubt about the diagnosis, a repeat ultrasound scan at least a week apart is recommended [8,9].
- If the gestation sac is smaller than expected for gestational age, the possibility of incorrect dates should always be considered, especially in the absence of clinical features suggestive of a threatened miscarriage. In this scenario, a repeat ultrasound (US) should be performed in seven days to confirm the diagnosis [9].

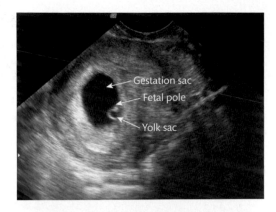

Figure 5.1 TV ultrasound scan of an early intra-uterine pregnancy.

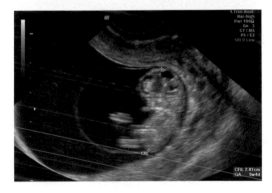

Figure 5.2 CRL measurement in early pregnancy. As this CRL is > 7 mm and no FH can be seen, a diagnosis of a miscarriage can be confidently made.

After the second miscarriage, her GP had performed a hormone profile which was normal, as was a transvaginal pelvic ultrasound scan. She was keen to discuss further investigations and management options in the specialist clinic (Table 5.2).

Further assessment in the RM clinic elicited that she had no personal or family history of venous or arterial thrombosis. Physical examination was entirely normal. Her antiphospholipid antibody screen was normal. Both parents had normal karyotypes, and she was identified as heterozygous for the Factor V Leiden (FVL) mutation. Pelvic ultrasound was performed which returned a normal result. Further imaging was therefore not indicated.

Table 5.2 Investigations in recurrent miscarriage [10]

Blood investigations	Antiphospholipid antibodies (Anticardiolipin antibodies (Ig G and Ig M) and lupus anticoagulant)
	Selective parental karyotyping (if abnormal chromosomes found in products of conceptions)
	Thrombophilia screen (if history of second trimester miscarriage)
	Blood group (to assess need for Anti-D)
	Thyroid function tests, (TFT) random plasma glucose, prolactin (if symptomatic)
Genetic testing	Cytogenetic analysis of products of conception of the third and subsequent miscarriages
Microbiological culture	High vaginal swab (HVS) if previous second trimester miscarriage
Imaging	Pelvic USS (transvaginal)
Surgical investigations	Hysteroscopy and/or laparoscopy to confirm abnormalities found on USS

⸢⸢ Expert comment

It is important to make a general assessment of the patient rather than simply performing a battery of indiscriminate investigations. Conditions such as obesity, hypothyroidism, or diabetes that are also associated with miscarriage are important especially as they can be treated with benefit to the woman's general health and not simply her reproductive problem.

⊕ **Learning point** Factor V Leiden mutation

Factor V Leiden (FVL) mutation is a hereditary thrombophilia. Activated protein C (aPC) is an anticoagulant which limits coagulation by cleaving and inactivating FVL. A single point mutation in FVL leaves it unsusceptible to proteolytic cleavage and inactivation by aPC, so leading to continued thrombin generation and increased risk of thromboembolism.

The genotypic expression of the factor V mutation is clinically important. Patients who are heterozygous for this thrombophilia have a three- to tenfold increased risk of thromboembolism, compared with an eighty- to one-hundredfold increased risk in patients with homozygous FVL mutation [11]. It is hypothesized that the thrombotic predisposition of this condition leads to placental infacts or vascular thrombosis and subsequent miscarriage risk.

Studies have shown that both heterozygous and homozygous FVL mutation are associated with miscarriage and RM [12], but treatment with antithrombotic agents in pregnancy has not been proven to significantly improve pregnancy outcomes (as highlighted later in this chapter, see 'Evidence base: Antiphopholipid antibodies and RM'). Thus, the underlying pathogenesis remains unclear.

⊘ **Evidence base** Antiphospholipid antibodies and RM

Antiphospholid syndrome (APS) is the *only* cause of RM where treatment has proven to improve subsequent pregnancy outcomes significantly. Thus, testing for antiphospholipid antibodies is the most important investigation to perform in women with recurrent miscarriage.

- A systematic review concluded that for women with RM and APS, a combination of low-dose aspirin (LDA) and unfractionated heparin (UFH) reduced the risk of subsequent pregnancy loss by 54% [13]. Unfractionated heparin combined with aspirin (two trials; $n = 40$) significantly reduced pregnancy loss compared to aspirin alone (relative risk (RR) 0.46, 95% confidence interval (CI) 0.29–0.71). Low molecular weight heparin (LMWH) combined with LDA compared to LDA alone (one trial; $n = 98$) did not significantly reduce pregnancy loss (RR 0.78, 95% CI 0.39–1.57) [14].
- A recent trial by of LMWH and aspirin in women with auto-antibodies or a coagulation abnormality, also showed similar results of comparable live birth rates in women treated with LDA and LMWH, compared with LDA alone [15].

❝ **Expert comment**

As discussed earlier, antithrombotic intervention can reduce the pregnancy loss rate in APS but increasing the dose of UFH (in combination with LDA) does not appear to decrease the risk further [13,16]. LDA alone has not been shown to reduce pregnancy loss compared with routine care or placebo [13,17–19] and interestingly, LMWH/LDA combined do not result in a reduced rate of pregnancy loss compared with LDA alone [13–15]. Although LMWH has largely replaced UFH in pregnancy because of a more favourable safety profile and once-daily dosing [20], there are only two small pilot studies comparing UFH and LMWH, and LMWH/LDA appeared equivalent to UFH/LDA for RM [21–22]. With these limited data, clinicians must weigh the better safety profile of LMWH against the greater evidence of efficacy for UFH in APS with RM. It should also be noted that heparins are heterogeneous and have a wide range of actions that could influence placentation, and thus UFH and LMW cannot be considered identical in terms of their functions [23].

⊕ **Learning point** Routine parental karyotyping is not justified

Cytogenetic analysis should be carried out, where possible, on products of conception of the third and subsequent miscarriages, as this allows for an informed prognosis for future pregnancies. An abnormal karyotype gives a better prognosis in a future pregnancy (subsequent live birth rate in

(continued)

abnormal karyotype versus normal karyotype is 68% versus 41%) and reassures the patient that this is more than likely a random event [24].

Parental karyotyping has traditionally been performed to exclude chromosomal abnormalities. The incidence of a balanced chromosomal abnormality in couples with RM is between 2–5%, commonly a Robertsonian translocation. A recent audit of routine parental karyotyping in couples with RM by Barber *et al.* in 4 UK centres (20432 couples) showed the incidence of balanced translocation to be about 1.9% (406 couples), at an estimated cost of £3–4 million to perform the karyotyping. From these, only four (0.02%) fetuses were found to have an unbalanced translocation after prenatal diagnosis [25], a result similar to that of a large case control study in six centres (278 cases, 427 controls) in the Netherlands where the risk of unbalanced translocation in offsprings to be less than 1% (4 fetuses out of 550 pregnancies) [26]. Furthermore, these couples have encouraging pregnancy outcomes with over 75% live birth rates in the subsequent pregnancy. This is similar to couples with RM without underlying chromosomal abnormality and who were offered supportive care [26,27]. Thus, routine parental karyotyping for chromosomal abnormalities is not justified and should only be offered when karyotype of the products of conception shows an unbalanced structural chromosomal abnormality [10].

✔ **Evidence base** Thrombophilia and RM

A comprehensive systematic review of the relationship between thrombophilia and adverse pregnancy outcomes showed, overall, a positive association of thrombophilia and early miscarriages [12]. The magnitude of the association is perhaps more consistent with this being a contributory rather than a causative factor. In theory, the thrombophilia may predispose the woman to placental infarcts or vascular thrombosis, but other possible mechanisms exist including thrombin impacting directly on trophoblast. The meta-analysis of 25 studies on early pregnancy loss showed a significant association for certain thrombophilias and miscarriages [12] (Table 5.3).

Table 5.3 Risk of miscarriage in women with thrombophilia

Thrombophilia	Odds ratio (95% CI)
Homozygous factor V Leiden	2.71 (1.32–5.58)
Heterozygous factor V Leiden	1.68 (1.09–2.58)
Acquired activated protein C resistance (aPCR)	4.04 (1.69–9.76)
Prothrombin gene mutation	2.49 (1.24–5.00)
Hyperhomocysteinaemia	6.25 (1.37–28.42)

✪ **Learning point** Imaging the uterine cavity

Abnormal uterine anatomy should be considered as a cause of RM, because of the high prevalence of congenital uterine anomaly in these women. A systematic review of the literature reported that women with RM had more than double the prevalence of a uterine anomaly (16.7% versus 6.7% in the general population and suggest that two-dimensional ultrasound (2D US) or hysterosalpingography (HSG) are suitable first-choice screening tools [28].

Transvaginal (TV) US provides better resolution and a clearer image, but some women consider this more invasive compared with the transabdominal approach. Careful counselling and the offer of a chaperone are key here. If uterine anomaly is suspected, hysteroscopy +/− laparoscopy, HSG, or three-dimensional (3D) US scanning can be used to confirm the findings. Three-dimensional US techniques appear promising, as they are non-invasive and offer both accurate diagnosis and classification of congenital uterine anomalies (Figure 5.3). Furthermore, 3D US techniques are highly reproducible and not operator-dependent, as volume is generated by an automatic sweep of the mechanical transducer [28]. Currently, the accuracy and role of magnetic resonance imaging (MRI) as an imaging modality for congenital uterine anomaly remains uncertain [28].

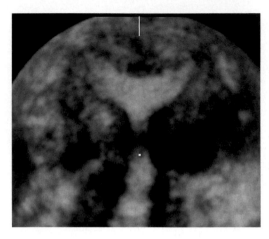

Figure 5.3 A coronal view of a septate uterus obtained from 3D US.

⊘ **Evidence base** Surgery for uterine abnormalities

Surgery to correct uterine anomalies such as arcuate or septate uterus is often offered. A systematic review of 17 observational studies (*n* = 1501) assessing hysteroscopic metroplasty or septoplasty in women with reproductive problems (RM, second trimester miscarriage, infertility, or pre-term labour) showed a pooled pregnancy rate of 60 % and live birth (LB) rate of 45 % overall, and appears safe, with a complication rate of only 1.9 % [29]. However, the women in these studies served as their own controls, and thus the benefit of surgery needs to be confirmed with randomized controlled trials. A RCT assessing this, the randomized uterine septum trans-section (TRUST) trial, is currently recruiting in Netherlands, and the results will direct future management of congenital uterine anomalies.

Three months later, she spontaneously conceived her fifth pregnancy. As advised, she attended her GP where she was prescribed low-dose aspirin and low molecular weight heparin in view of her inherited thrombophilia (heterozygous factor V Lieden). An early TVUS confirmed a viable intrauterine pregnancy of six weeks' gestation but unfortunately, she started 'spotting' eight weeks into the pregnancy. A subsequent TVUS showed a delayed miscarriage. ERPC was performed after two weeks of conservative management.

⊘ **Evidence base** Thromboprophylaxis in thrombophilia

Initial uncontrolled studies of LMWH suggested that there may be beneficial effects of improved live birth rates for women with thrombophilia and RM [30,31].

- Carp *et al.* compared the pregnancy outcomes of 37 women treated with LMWH and 48 untreated women, and there was an increased live birth rate in the treated group (70.2 % versus 43.8 %) [31].
- Brenner *et al.* found a higher live birth rate in 180 women with RM and thrombophilia after treatment with either enoxaparin 40 mg/day or 80 mg/day [30].

More recently, high-quality, randomized trials have failed to substantiate this [15,32,33].

- Laskin *et al.* randomized 88 women to LDA alone, and LDA with LMWH, and found similar live birth rates of 79.1 % and 77.8 % respectively [15].
- A subgroup analysis of women with thrombophilia in a trial by Kaandorp *et al.* (364 women) comparing treatment of LDA alone and LDA with LMWH showed similar live birth rates [33].

Thus, the evidence to support the use of LDA with or without LMWH treatment in women with thrombophilia associated RM for the sole purpose of improving pregnancy outcomes was weakened. However, anticoagulant treatment could be considered in women with second trimester miscarriages and if there is a high risk of a thromboembolic event; for example, in women homozygous for factor V Leiden mutation.

ⓕ Expert comment

The association between acquired (APS) and heritable thrombophilias and RM raised the hypothesis that unexplained RM reflected a prothrombotic phenotype with RM resulting from the effects of thrombin on trophoblast. LMWH and LDA have been used in women with unexplained RM, without evidence from randomized controlled trials. This was based on the association of RM with thrombophilia, the success of antithrombotic treatment in APS with RM, the established safety of aspirin and LMWH, and retrospective observational studies [30]. The SPIN trial [32], compared intensive pregnancy surveillance alone with LDA/LMWH in 294 women with two or more unexplained losses and found no significant reduction in the rate of pregnancy loss with the antithrombotics (OR 0.91, 95% CI 0.52–1.59) compared with surveillance alone. Kaandorp *et al.* [33] randomized women with two or more unexplained pregnancy losses, to LDA/LMWH LDA alone, or aspirin placebo. Of 364 women randomized, 299 became pregnant. Neither intervention improved live birth rates, compared to placebo in these women. (Live birth rates: LMWH/LDA 69.1% (RR 1.03, 95% CI 0.85–1.25); LDA 61.6% (RR 0.92, 95% CI 0.75–1.13); placebo 67.0%.) Although it remains possible that subgroups of women with RM of three or more losses and those with heritable thrombophilia may respond differently to antithrombotics, current evidence suggests no benefit and thus LMWH should not be recommended as a therapeutic option. As LMWH may act early in pregnancy, and in these trials it was started at six weeks' gestation, studies from assisted conception may allow the possibility of earlier intervention to be addressed [23].

✪ Learning point Management of miscarriage

Miscarriage can be managed surgically, medically, or expectantly. Surgical management is commonly a day-case procedure and is performed by using an electrical vacuum device to empty the uterus by aspiration. It can also be performed manually with a hand-held vacuum syringe [37]. Suction evacuation is a safe method and is very rarely associated with complications such as uterine perforation, cervical tears, and intra-uterine adhesions [34].

Medical management involves the initial use of mifepristone, an oral anti-progesterone used to sensitize the uterus, followed by prostaglandins such as misoprostol to induce uterine contractions. There is currently no clear evidence for the optimal dosage regime for misoprostol [38]. This method can be used on an outpatient basis, but is associated with risks of uncontrolled bleeding, which may require emergency surgical evacuation.

Expectant management involves waiting for the uterus to spontaneously expel the products of conception. Although this is the most natural method, there are risks of uncontrolled bleeding and infection. It is unclear how long follow-up can continue before the risk of infection increases.

◔ Landmark trial The miscarriage treatment (MIST) trial [39]

The largest trial of management of miscarriage was published in 2006, comparing all three methods of management of miscarriage in the first trimester. This trial included 1200 women diagnosed with missed or incomplete miscarriage, and were randomized to either:

- Expectant management for 10–14 days (399 women),
- Medical management (200 mg mifepristone orally followed by 800 mcg misoprostol vaginally one to two days later in missed miscarriage; or 800 mcg misoprostol vaginally in incomplete miscarriage) (398 women)
- Surgical management of suction curettage under general anaesthesia (403 women).

(continued)

Primary outcome—Rate of confirmed gynaecological infection within 14 days of trial entry (defined as two or more of purulent vaginal discharge, pyrexia > 38.0°C, tenderness over the uterus on abdominal examination, and a white cell count above $15 \times 109/l$).

Successful treatment—defined as no unplanned surgical evacuation within eight weeks.

Results:

- The rate of confirmed infection was similar in all three groups at 2–3%.
- Surgical management was associated with more presumed infection (defined as the prescription of antibiotics) compared with expectant management (8% versus 4%, 95% CI 1–8).
- Cessation of bleeding was sooner in the surgically managed arm, compared with medical ($p = 0.0004$) or expectant management ($p < 0.0001$), though this had no effect haemoglobin concentration at 14 days
- Expectant management had a significantly higher rate of unplanned hospital admissions compared with surgical management (49% versus 8%, 95% CI 47–36), and had higher analgesia requirements.
- 44% of women in the expectant group and 36% in the medical group ended up with an unplanned surgical evacuation. For those who underwent surgical evacuation, the rates of surgical complications were similar (1–2%).

Anxious that her reproductive potential was decreasing with her advancing age, and treatment with anticoagulation had failed, the patient began to investigate empirical treatments for RM on the internet. She presented to the consultant gynaecologist with requests for immunological investigations as well as empirical treatment with progesterone. She was counselled about the unproven nature of these interventions, and was offered the chance to participate in a trial of progesterone therapy versus placebo to prevent recurrent miscarriage. However, she was reassured that she had still about 70% chance of achieving a live birth with close monitoring and regular reassurance scans alone (Table 5.4).

Table 5.4 Predicted success rate (%) of subsequent pregnancy in relation to age and number of previous miscarriages [43]

Age (years)	Number of previous miscarriages			
	2	3	4	5
20	92	90	88	85
25	89	86	82	79
30	84	80	76	71
35	77	73	68	62
40	69	64	58	52
45	60	54	48	42

> ⊗ **Learning point** Immunotherapy and RM
>
> Pregnancy is an immunological phenomena where there is maternal adaptation of her immune system to the semi-allogenic developing embryo. In view of this, empirical immunotherapy such as intravenous immunoglobulins (IVIG) and steroids have been prescribed in an attempt to improve pregnancy outcomes in women with RM.
>
> In some cases, immunological testing for natural killer (NK) cells (peripheral NK (pNK) or uterine NK (uNK) cells) is offered to select women for immunotherapy. However, prospective studies reporting pregnancy outcomes are few, and a systematic review of the prognostic implication of pNK and uNK cells did not confirm that abnormal pNK and uNK cells density or activity is associated with subsequent miscarriage [51]. Thus, pNK and uNK cells tests should not be offered routinely to women with RM and the topic remains a subject of research [52].
>
> A recent large RCT and systematic review of IVIG therapy in RM has showed no beneficial effect in improving live births [53,54]. Similarly, there is also inadequate evidence that prednisolone reduces the risk of miscarriage. With the lack of evidence of benefit, these should not be empirically prescribed and should only be used in well-designed trials.

She contacted the RM clinic 6 months later with a positive pregnancy test. After further counselling and discussion, she opted for conservative management of regular reassurance scans with no medical intervention. She is currently 30 weeks' pregnant.

Discussion

Management of recurrent miscarriage remains challenging as there are many controversies surrounding its underlying pathophysiology. Furthermore, no cause is found in more than 50 % of cases. It is known that the risk of miscarriage increases with age and the number of previous miscarriages. However, in idiopathic recurrent miscarriage, women have an excellent prognosis, up to 75 % success of a live birth in future pregnancies, with supportive care of regular ultrasound scans for reassurance, and psychological support in a dedicated early pregnancy assessment unit (EPAU) [43]. Although the mechanism of how supportive care alone is beneficial is unknown, it is important to emphasize this fact when counselling women seen in RM clinics, avoid prescribing empirical treatment [10].

In view of the benefit of antithrombotic in RM associated with APS, such therapy has been assessed in RM in general. There have been two large RCTs of thromboprophylaxis versus no treatment in women with RM (2 losses). These randomized trials have shown similar live-birth rates in women treated with LDA or LMWH/LDA versus supportive treatment with no pharmacological intervention [32,33,55]. Two other RCTs compared different anti-thrombotic intervention, i.e. there was no untreated control arm and the outcomes were similar for both groups [15,56]. Another randomized trial of low-dose aspirin versus placebo [19] that included 54 women with three or more pregnancy losses did not find a significant difference in miscarriages (RR 1.00; 95 % CI, 0.78–1.29). Thus while screening for APS is warranted in women with RM, heritable thrombophilia screening is not, in view of limited data on association and lack of an effective intervention. There remains a case to assess the association between heritable thrombophilia and three or more losses or a second trimester loss and the benefits of intervention in these specific groups [55]. In line with this, RCOG has recommended that thromboprophylaxis should not be prescribed in the absence of APS [10,57]. It should however be considered if these women give a personal history of thromboembolism.

Although women with idiopathic recurrent miscarriage have a very good prognosis, with about a 50 % chance of a successful pregnancy even at the age of 40 with five previous miscarriages [43], they should be informed of the potential obstetric complications later in pregnancy. Women with RM have an increased risk of preterm delivery (< 34 weeks' gestation), preterm pre-labour ruptured of membranes (PPROM), placenta praevia, and low birthweight (< tenth centile) [59], and therefore should be considered for consultant-led antenatal care

Clinicians may be persuaded by women to prescribe empirical treatments in an attempt to improve subsequent pregnancy outcomes when there are no reasons found for the recurring miscarriages. An alternative would be to encourage these women to participate in methodologically sound studies and trials to provide more evidence for the management of couples with RM. It is also important to highlight again the good prognosis in subsequent pregnancy, and beneficial effect of regular reassurance scans and support of a dedicated EPAU.

A Final Word from the Expert

Women with RM present many challenges, not least because of our inability to identify a clear cause in the majority and the lack of effective interventions. All too often we raise these women's hopes of a successful pregnancy by providing unproven treatment, which is later found to be ineffective. Optimal management requires specialist care and specific clinics for these women to support them through their patient journey. To enhance the evidence base and so improve our understanding of the condition and identify effective interventions, it is important that such specialist clinics also focus on research. An effective network of such clinics would offer us the opportunity to provide sufficient power in studies and trials to ensure that new evidence is produced in a timely manner, and so address the challenge of RM for the future.

References

1. Farquharson RG, Jauniaux E, Exalto N. Updated and revised nomenclature for description of early pregnancy events. *Hum Reprod* Nov 2005; 20(11):3008–11.
2. Habayeb OM, Konje JC. The one-stop recurrent miscarriage clinic: an evaluation of its effectiveness and outcome. *Hum Reprod* Dec 2004; 19(12): 2952–8.
3. Rai R, Regan L. Recurrent miscarriage. *Lancet* Aug 12 2006; 368(9535): 601–11.
4. Gardella JR, Hill JA, 3rd. Environmental toxins associated with recurrent pregnancy loss. *Semin Reprod Med* 2000; 18(4): 407–24.
5. Kline J, Shrout P, Stein Z, Susser M, Warburton D. Drinking during pregnancy and spontaneous abortion. *Lancet* Jul 26 1980; 2(8187): 176–80.
6. Antenatal care: routine care for the healthy pregnant woman. In: (NICE) NIfHaCE (ed.) 2008.
7. Signorello LB, McLaughlin JK. Maternal caffeine consumption and spontaneous abortion: a review of the epidemiologic evidence. *Epidemiology* Mar 2004; 15(2): 229–39.
8. The Management of Early Pregnancy Loss. RCOG Green-top Guidelines. 2006.
9. Hately W, Case J, Campbell S. Establishing the death of an embryo by ultrasound: report of a public inquiry with recommendations. *Ultrasound Obstet Gynecol* May 1995; 5(5): 353–7.
10. The Investigation and Treatment of Couples with Recurrent First-trimester and Second-trimester Miscarriage. RCOG Green-top Guidelines. 2011.

6 Lethal congenital abnormalities: the importance of a multidisciplinary approach

Lisa Story

✆ **Expert Commentary** Pippa Kyle

Case history

A 24-year-old woman, Gravida 3, Para 2 booked her pregnancy at 12 weeks'. She had previously undergone two emergency caesarean sections at term. The second pregnancy was complicated by a uterine scar rupture after an attempted vaginal delivery. The current pregnancy was conceived with the same partner who was a second cousin. She reported a regular menstrual cycle and the calculated estimated date of delivery was equal to that given by a dating ultrasound scan at 13 + 6 weeks' gestation. Screening tests gave a low risk for trisomy 18, 21, and 13. Nuchal translucency was 1.13 mm (Figure 6.1) and PAPP-A was 1.05.

⭐ **Learning point** Screening tests for aneuploidy

Both the nuchal translucency scan and maternal serum blood tests contribute to a formal screening test for chromosomal abnormalities, particularly Down syndrome (trisomy 21). A nuchal scan is performed between 11 and 13 + 6 weeks and measures the amount of fluid at the back of the neck of the fetus the nuchal translucency. High readings may be seen in chromosomal abnormality or congenital heart disease. Low levels of plasma-associated plasma protein A (PAPP-A), and high levels ßHCG (analytes measured from maternal serum) in the first trimester have been shown to correlate with Down syndrome. Risk of trisomy 21 is calculated by multiplying the background maternal age and gestation-related risk by a likelihood ratio derived from the nuchal translucency (NT) measurement and the two blood tests.

An anatomy scan was performed at 20 + 3 weeks' at which point a number of abnormalities were detected including micrognathia (Figure 6.2), polyhydramnios, and fibula, tibia, humerus, ulna, and femur measurements all plotting below the third centile. The femur was bowed in shape (Figure 6.3).

She was referred to the fetal medicine unit where the scan findings were confirmed. There was bowing/fractures of the long bones and an abnormal skull shape. She was informed that these findings most likely represented a skeletal dysplasia. She was counselled regarding the risk of intrauterine/neonatal death or disability and was offered invasive karyotype testing and termination of pregnancy. These were both declined. She also was referred to a geneticist for further counselling.

She was followed up in the fetal medicine unit on a two to four weekly basis. At 32 + 1 weeks', growth of the long bones remained below the third centile. The AFI had increased to 34 and she was offered formal amniodrainage if she became

⊕ **Clinical tip** Ensuring an accurate nuchal transluscency measurement

- A scan assessing nuchal translucency should be performed between 11 and 13 + 6 weeks' gestation
- The fetus should be visualized in the sagittal section
- The head should be in neutral position
- The fetus should be enlarged to fill approximately 75% of the screen
- The maximum thickness is measured from leading edge to leading edge
- The nuchal lucency should be distinguished from the amniotic membrane

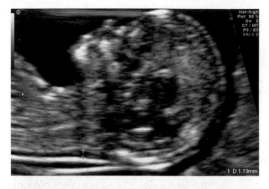

Figure 6.1 An ultrasound image demonstrating measurement of nuchal transluscency.

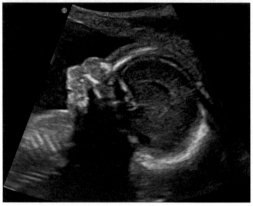

Figure 6.2 Profile view of the fetal head demonstrating micrognathia.

> ✪ **Learning point** Assessment of the fetus with a suspected skeletal dysplasia
>
> As with any condition, a full history is necessary to elucidate risk factors, including a family history, drug history, and any relevant maternal disease.
>
> • Increased nuchal translucency/nuchal fold and skin thickening is associated with many skeletal dysplasias [4].
> • Long bones: a short femur may be identified at the anomaly scan. This should prompt assessment of other long bones and measurements should be checked against appropriate charts. The pattern of abnormality i.e. whether there is generalized shortening affecting the proximal bones more prominently may aid diagnosis. Abnormalities in the shape of the bones may indicate fracturing and specific position of the limbs should be noted. Bowing of the femur is illustrated in Figure 6.2. The texture of bones may also appear abnormal, short, and thick, and with an abnormal texture is often found in osteogenesis imperfecta.
> • Hands: polydactyly and the presence of short fingers/trident hands should be noted.
> • Skull: the shape should be noted and extent of mineralization. Abnormalities of skull shape can be noted in some craniosyntosis syndromes. Frontal bossing, depressed nasal bridge, cleft palate, and micrognathia may also be present in some skeletal dysplasias. A hypolucent skull may suggest osteogenesis imperfecta.
> • Spine: the degree of mineralization should be noted, ectopic calcification, and malformation of vertebrae.
> • Thorax: the shape and circumference of the thorax should be noted and plotted on relevant charts. The thorax may be small as a result of a short spine associated with spondylodysplasias. Ribs should be examined and beading which may result from fractures may indicate osteogenesis imperfecta.
> • A full anatomy scan should be formed to check for other markers suggestive of a syndrome.
> • If a condition with a known gene mutation is suspected, genetic testing may be offered; e.g. FGFR-3 mutations for achondroplasia and thanatophoric dysplasia.

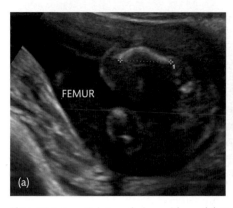

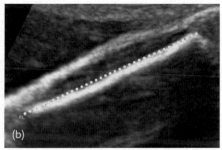

Figure 6.3 A sagittal view of a bowed femur (A). Note curvature compared to a normal femur (B).

> ⭐ **Learning point** Types of skeletal dysplasia
>
> There are many different forms of skeletal dysplasia. The most common lethal and non lethal forms are listed briefly as follows:
>
> *Thanatophoric dysplasia* this is the most common lethal dysplasia complicating 1:20 000 pregnancies. Two subgroups exist, I and II, and they are characterized by short long bones +/- bowing (particularly of the femur), short ribs and fingers, macrocephaly with frontal bossing, and a cloverleaf skull may be seen.
>
> *Achondrogenesis* this is a group of lethal skeletal dysplasias complicating 2:10 000 pregnancies and is associated with limb and shortening with conservation of head growth. Two subtypes exist. Type I is associated with micrognathia, short limbs, fractures, and lack of spinal and cranial ossification. Type II is not associated with rib fractures and skull development appears normal. Both subtypes may be associated with increased nuchal translucency and preserved abdominal and head growth in comparison to small limbs and chest. Polyhydramnios is a common feature.
>
> *Osteogeneisis imperfect* this is a connective tissue disorder of type I collagen and comprises a number of subtypes with an incidence of 1.6-3.5:100 000 livebirths. Most severe cases are new dominant mutations but some cases are autosomal recessive. Type I may present with one or two fractures with slightly shortened bones. Callus formation may be present with bone angulation or bowing. This subtype is often diagnosed postnatally. Type II is the most severe and lethal. It is associated with hypomineralization, beaded ribs, small chest, and short long bones and hypomineralization of the skull. Type III is severe but compatible with life characterised by progressive deformation beginning in utero: limb shortening and bowing evident by 20 weeks, chest and ribs often appear normal with no beading, head shape is normal. Type IV is a diverse group and prenatal detection is often difficult.
>
> *Achondroplasia* is the most common non lethal skeletal dysplasia, affecting up to 15:100 000 births, due to mutations in the fibroblast growth factor receptor 3 gene. Limb length is often normal until 22 weeks and diagnosis is normally in the third trimester. Other sonographic findings may include frontal bossing of the skull, short fingers, macrocephaly, small thorax, and mild ventriculomegaly. Polyhydramnios is a common feature. In the homozygous form achondroplasia is lethal.

symptomatic. She declined this. The progression of the polyhydramnios can be seen in Figure 6.4 which charts the amniotic fluid index. It spontaneously stabilized.

At 34 + 3 weeks, these findings persisted and considerable concern was raised in the fetal medicine unit again regarding prognosis. An appointment was also made with the neonatologists in order to counsel her with regards to the expected neonatal course and prognosis and potential options for management in light of the expected poor outcome of the baby following delivery.

> 🔎 **Expert comment** Skeletal dysplasias
>
> Skeletal dysplasias are a heterogeneous group of disorders. Although certain types are lethal, others do not prevent individuals from leading productive lives requiring minimal intervention. They complicate 2.4/10 000 births; perinatal death occurring in 55% of cases [1]. A number of different classifications have been proposed for skeletal dysplasias. These may be based on clinical/radiological grounds or by the genetic/molecular basis of the disease (as described in the related learning point) [2,3].

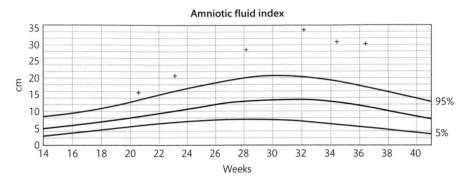

Figure 6.4 Progression of the amniotic fluid index in the pregnancy.

> **⊗ Learning point** Polyhydramnios
>
> Polyhydramnios is a common ultrasound finding, complicating 1% of pregnancies. Polyhydramnios is defined as an increase in the amniotic fluid and is gestation dependent. Normal ranges of amniotic fluid can be also be seen in Figure 6.4. The aetiology is varied and prognosis is often linked to both the cause and extent. Causes may be subdivided into maternal and fetal:
>
> - Idiopathic
> - Maternal causes
>   - Maternal diabetes may be associated with fetal macrosomia.
>   - Maternal obesity may be associated with fetal macrosomia.
> - Fetal Causes
>   - Increased urine output such as in fetal macrosomia associated with diabetes, Fetal cardiac overload such as seen in twin-to-twin transfusion (TTTS).
>   - Abnormal swallowing/absorption:
>   - Obstruction of the gastrointestinal tract may be found in conjunction with signs of obstruction of the gastrointestinal tract, i.e. dilated bowel loops, an abdominal or thoracic mass.
>   - Impediment to fetal swallowing may be associated with cleft lip/palate or muscular abnormalities such as myotonic dystrophy.
>   - Karyotype abnormalities should be considered although these are more common when the polyhydramnios is associated with other abnormalities or fetal growth restriction. This is often detected earlier in gestation.
>
> A number of complications can result as a consequence of polyhydramnios. These include:
>
> - Maternal:
>   - Maternal respiratory compromise and discomfort.
>   - Post-partum haemorrhage.
> - Fetal
>   - Pre-term labour.
>   - Malpresentation.
>   - Abruption associated with sudden decompression.
>   - Cord prolapse at the time of rupture of membranes.
>
> Management is dependent on the aetiology, gestation, and extent of the polyhydramnios. Diabetes should be excluded and assessment of the likelihood of chromosomal abnormalities. Mild polyhydramnios may require no further intervention other than serial ultrasounds to monitor the AFI and to assess for associated malformations. Severe cases of polyhydramnios may warrant amnioreduction. Non-steroidal anti-inflammatory drugs (NSAIDS) have also been used in the research setting for the treatment of polyhydramnios, however these are not widely used in clinical practice due to side effects for both mother and fetus[5].

⊘ **Evidence base** Amniodrainage

Amnio-reduction (AR) and NSAIDS have not been assessed in randomized controlled trials. The aim of AR to remove 2-3 litres over a short period of time before the mother feels discomfort from contractions. Usually there is considerable relief of symptoms for the mother following the procedure. Complications are rare but have been reported, including placental abruption and expansion of the placenta as the fluid is removed, resulting in hypotension in the fetus which may have sequelae on the nervous system and heart. Indomethacin and sulindac have been assessed in a few small case studies. Their mechanism of action is on the renal vasculature resulting in a reduction in fetal urine output; however, side effects include premature closure of the ductus arteriosus and decreased renal perfusion. These significant fetal side effects and the lack of large randomized controlled studies means that their therapeutic applications are limited [6].

The couple were very keen for active management and a plan was made for a thorough assessment of the baby's condition at the time of delivery allowing further discussion with parents at that time.

Due to the maternal history of two previous caesarean sections (the second complicated by scar dehiscence in labour), a third caesarean section was performed electively at 38 weeks' gestation. The couple had undergone full counselling with regards to the poor prognosis of the condition from the fetal medicine unit, geneticists, and the neonatal team.

An uncomplicated caesarean section was performed with the neonatal team in attendance. The baby was born in poor condition showing significant respiratory compromise. The parents were keen for active management and so intubation was attempted but not possible due to severe micrognathia associated with the skeletal dysplasia. The baby was transferred to the neonatal unit and was supported with continuous positive airway pressure (CPAP). Neonatal examination and chest X-ray confirmed the severe skeletal dysplasia. The baby persistently remained hypoxic and sadly died at 48 hours.

The parents declined a full postmortem examination but consented to a full skeletal radiological survey and also accepted blood to be taken for DNA investigations. These confirmed thanatophroric dysplasia.

⊕ **Clinical tip** Counselling for future pregnancies

A correct diagnosis may have significant implications for future pregnancies. Post-mortem examination should be offered including a radiological skeletal survey, and even if the full postmortem is not wanted, the radiological skeletal survey may be accepted and this may be key to making an accurate diagnosis. The increasing identification of genes associated with skeletal dysplasias is facilitating enhanced prenatal diagnosis and more accurate prognostic information. Tissue storage of DNA is recommended and this will facilitate more prompt diagnosis in future pregnancies. Review by a clinical geneticist is then imperative to guide recurrence risks for future pregnancies.

Discussion

Fetal medicine is a challenging area within obstetrics. It raises numerous ethical dilemmas with regard to prenatal diagnosis, uncertainty of prognosis, and interventions which may risk shortening of the pregnancy.

A good clinical history, particularly with regards to previous medical, obstetric, family, and drug history and any consanguinity is vital. Information regarding screening tests accepted in early pregnancy and risks of chromosomal abnormalities are important in conjunction with any abnormalities detected on a detailed anatomy scan of the fetus.

Where an abnormality is detected, the importance of counselling from the multi-disciplinary team is paramount to provide patients and their families with the most up-to-date information from which they can make informed decisions about their care.

The patient should be supported in the decisions she makes, particularly if she chooses to continue with a pregnancy that has a very poor prognosis.

A Final Word from the Expert

Five per cent of pregnancies are complicated by congenital abnormalities and of these 15 % prove lethal [7]. Although termination of pregnancy is legal at any gestation if there is deemed to be a significant risk of physical or mental disability to the fetus, not all parents wish to proceed with ending the pregnancy. It has been suggested that providing a choice for the family lessens the emotional and physiological effects which can be associated with termination, and indeed certain religious and cultural beliefs may mean that terminating the pregnancy may not be acceptable for some women. If parents chose to continue with a pregnancy associated with poor prognosis palliative planning is often required.

Palliative care is defined as the active, total approach to care which embraces physical, emotional, social, and spiritual elements, providing an enhanced quality of life for the child, support for the family, management of symptoms, and the provision of respite and care through death and bereavement[8]. Palliative planning may be used in a number of situations: neonates that are born pre-term on the limits of viability, or in cases such as this one where there is a known lethal congenital abnormality. Holistic palliative care requires a clear definition of the pathology of the condition, agreement of a multidisciplinary team regarding the diagnosis, and its certainty, as well as the prognosis. Involvement of the family is a crucial part of this process and family centred care is key. Psychological, spiritual, and social support is required throughout. Formal written plans should be made with regards to the mode of delivery and fetal monitoring. In many cases, spontaneous labour may be awaited, partly due to the implications for future pregnancies; however, caesarean section may be indicated for maternal reasons or if the family wish the child to be born alive. Clear postnatal plans should also be made with regard to resuscitation, analgesia, and sedation. Communication with both the family and members of the multidisciplinary team and community healthcare providers is essential. Perinatal bereavement involvement should also be provided.

References

1. Papadatos CJ (ed.) *Birth Prevalence of Skeletal Dysplasias in the Italian Multicentric Monitoring System for Birth Defects*. New York: Alan R Liss, 1982, 441–9.
2. Hall, CM. International nosology andclassification of constitutional disorders of bone(2001). *Am J Med Genet* 2002;113(1):65–77.
3. Spranger J. International classification of osteochondrodysplasias. The International Working Group on Constitutional Diseases of Bone. *Eur J Pediatr* 1992;151(6):407–15.

4. Makrydimas G et al. Osteogenesis imperfecta and other skeletal dysplasias presenting with increased nuchal translucency in the first trimester. *Am J Med Genet* 2001;98(2):117–20.

5. Peek MJ, et al. Medical amnioreduction with sulindac to reduce cord complications in monoamniotic twins. *Am J Obstet Gynecol* 1997;176(2):334–6.

6. Harman CR. Amniotic fluid abnormalities. *Semin Perinatol* 2008;32(4):288–94.

7. Kilby MD, Pretlove SJ, Bedford Russell AR. Multidisciplinary palliative care in unborn and newborn babies. *BMJ* 2011;342:d1808.

8. Leuthner SR. Fetal palliative care. *Clin Perinatol* 2004;31(3):649–65.

Monochorionic diamniotic twin pregnancy complicated by twin–twin transfusion syndrome

7

Muna Noori

Expert Commentary Sailesh Kumar

Case history

A 25-year-old woman with a naturally conceived monochorionic twin pregnancy was referred to the fetal medicine unit at 17+2 weeks gestation with twin-to-twin trans-fusion syndrome (TTTS). Her pregnancy had been uncomplicated up to that point. She had had a low risk for Down syndrome on first trimester combined screening with no discordancy in crown–rump lengths or nuchal translucency measurements. This was her third ongoing pregnancy, the first two resulting in spontaneous vaginal deliveries at 40 weeks' gestation without complications.

Ultrasound assessment confirmed a monochorionic diamniotic twin (MCDA) pregnancy (Figure 7.1). The recipient (Twin A) was active with normal biometry. This twin's bladder was enlarged with associated polyhydramnios (deepest pool of liquor measuring 8.3 cm). All fetal Dopplers were normal.

The biometry of Twin B (the donor) was on the third centile. This twin's blad-der was not visualized and there was marked oligohydramnios, with a deepest pool of liquor of only 1.9 cm. There was intermittently absent end-diastolic flow in the umbilical artery but the ductus venosus waveform was normal. The scan findings were therefore suggestive of stage 2 TTTS with concomitant fetal growth restriction.

> ✪ **Learning point** Monozygotic and dizygotic twin pregnancies
>
> - The incidence of monozygotic twin births is 3.5 per 1000 pregnancies, 30% of which are dichorionic and 70% of which are monochorionic.
> - Monozygotic pregnancies occur at similar frequencies in all ethnic groups and are unaffected by parity or maternal age. Conversely, dizygotic twinning occurs more commonly in African and Asian ethnic groups, is more frequent in older or multiparous women, and is more common following ovulation induction and other assisted reproduction techniques.
> - Perinatal outcomes are largely determined by chorionicity, with monochorionic pregnancies carrying a much higher risk.
> - Accurate assignment of chorionicity is critical to managing the pregnancy and this is most accurately determined in the first trimester. Detection of the 'T-sign', which represents two thin layers of amnion, suggests the presence of a monochorionic placenta whereas a 'lambda sign', which comprises four membranes (two chorions and two amnions), indicates a dichorionic pregnancy (Figure 7.1).

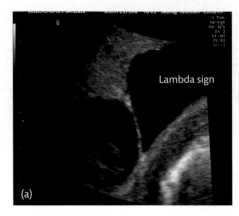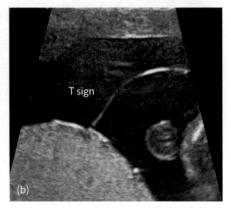

Figure 7.1 (A) Dichorionic twin pregnancy demonstrated by a 'lambda' or 'twin peak' sign.
(B) Monochorionic twin pregnancy characterized by a 'T sign'. The inter-twin septum in a monochorionic pregnancy is thinner than that in a dichorionic pregnancy. The presence of discordant gender also usually confirms a dizygotic pregnancy.

Courtesy of Dr Gowrishankar Paramasivam.

✪ Learning point First trimester screening and risk assessment in multiple pregnancy

The current recommended method of screening for Down syndrome in multiple pregnancies is by measurement of nuchal translucency in combination with maternal plasma PAPP-A (pregnancy-associated placental protein-A) and βhCG (beta human chorionic gonadotrophin) biochemistry (combined test) between 11 +0 and 13 +6 weeks gestation, as in singleton and dichorionic diamniotic pregnancies [1].

The detection rate for trisomy 21 (Down syndrome) in the first trimester has been shown to be lower in twin pregnancies, particularly monochorionic pregnancies, compared to singletons, as PAPP-A and βhCG in maternal plasma are derived from both twins and are usually twice as high [2] Furthermore, NT measurements can be discrepant in 20–25% of monochorionic twins [3], particularly as an elevated NT may hint towards early TTTS and may therefore not be as useful a screening tool compared to singleton pregnancies. The use of a mean NT has previously been suggested to be a more effective screening measure for trisomy 21 [4] Nevertheless, combined screening should be offered to all women with monochorionic twins, and NT discrepancies should prompt additional surveillance for TTTS.

---

❻ Expert comment

Venous Doppler is critical in the assessment of the cardiovascular impact of TTTS. Absence of forward flow in the ductus venosus 'a' wave implies progression of TTTS from volume imbalance to overt cardiovascular compromise.

✪ Learning point The pathophysiology of twin-to-twin transfusion syndrome (TTTS)

TTTS is a complication unique to monochorionic twin pregnancies. It occurs in 6–17% of MCDA pregnancies, and if managed conservatively, is associated with a mortality rate of 80–100% [5]. It is usually diagnosed between 16 and 25 weeks gestation although the diagnosis can also be suspected in the first and third trimesters.

The mechanism of TTTS is most often explained on an angioarchitectural basis. A monochorionic twin placenta contains a number of placental anastomoses which can be arterio-arterial (AA), arterio-venous (AV) or veno-venous (VV). AA and VV anastomoses are typically superficial and bidirectional, with the direction of flow depending on the relative interfetal vascular pressure gradients. AV anastomoses by contrast, are typically deeper and occur on a capillary level within a shared cotyledon. In most monochorionic pregnancies, interfetal transfusion across placental AA and AV anastomoses is a constant but balanced phenomenon with no net gain or loss in either fetus. However, in a proportion of cases a chronic net flow imbalance develops and TTTS results [6]. The donor twin

(continued)

develops oligohydramnios, hypovolaemia, and becomes oliguric whereas the recipient becomes hypervolaemic, polyuric, and has polyhydramnios, which eventually culminates in circulatory overload and hydrops. TTTS is also more common when the cord insertion is peripheral or velamentous.

The renin–angiotensin system is also activated with various neurohormonal mechanisms coming into play because of the circulatory imbalances between the two fetuses. This together with the cardiac overload seen in the recipient may explain some of the longer-term cardiovascular phenotypes seen in these children.

The couple were counselled regarding scan findings and advised that close monitoring was required with a high probability that the TTTS would progress necessitating intervention.

✚ Clinical tip Diagnosing TTTS

The diagnosis of TTTS is based on ultrasound findings of:

Recipient	Donor
Polyhydramnios A distended (polyuric) bladder	Oligohydramnios Small bladder*
Evidence of circulatory overload (cardiac hypertrophy, cardiomegaly, systolic dysfunction, atrioventricular regurgitation, or frank hydrops)	The donor not infrequently has umbilical artery waveform abnormalities (absent or reversed end-diastolic flow).

*When there is anhydramnios in the donor sac, the inter-twin membrane is usually wrapped around this fetus giving it a 'stuck' appearance (Figure 7.2). In more severe cases, fetal Dopplers can become abnormal with the recipient having ductus venosus abnormalities or a pulsatile umbilical vein. A five-stage classification system of disease severity was proposed by Quintero in 1999 [7] (Table 7.1).

Table 7.1 Quintero staging system

Quintero stage	Ultrasound features
1	Polyhydramnios in the recipient's sac (DVP > 8 cm prior to 20 weeks and > 10 cm after 20 weeks) and oligohydramnios in the donor's sac (DVP < 2 cm). The bladder of the donor twin is still visible.
2	The bladder of the donor twin remains empty and the inter-twin membrane is wrapped around it (stuck twin).
3	Abnormal fetal Dopplers in either twin, including absent or reversed end-diastolic flow in the umbilical artery of the donor fetus or abnormal venous Doppler waveforms in the recipient, such as reverse flow in the ductus venosus or pulsatile umbilical venous flow.
4	Fetal hydrops in either twin (usually recipient).
5	Fetal death of one or both twins.

Repeat scan a week later showed clear progression to stage 3 TTTS. The recipient now had a markedly distended bladder, increasing polyhydramnios (deepest pool 11 cm), and worsening fetal Dopplers (absent and occasionally reversed 'a' wave in the ductus venosus). The donor's bladder was not visible, anhydramnios was now present, and the umbilical artery Dopplers showed persistent absent end-diastolic flow.

> **⊕ Clinical tip** Differentiating TTTS from discordant growth
>
> Monochorionic twins may be discordant in size, with the smaller twin producing smaller amounts of urine resulting in discordance in amniotic fluid volume. In severe cases, the smaller twin may develop oligohydramnios with the deepest vertical pool of liquor measuring < 2 cm. In isolated discordant growth, the bladder in the smaller twin may be smaller but is usually still visible. It is unusual to see a 'stuck' twin in pure isolated discordant growth. Not infrequently, both TTTS and discordant growth can coexist, and in this situation the donor will have an increased risk of demise following any fetoscopic laser procedure because of its reduced placental territory after ablation of any anastomoses.
>
> The distinction between isolated discordant growth and TTTS is made by the absence of polyhydramnios in the larger, appropriately grown twin. Fetal size discrepancy is not a prerequisite for TTTS, although it is important to consider that 20 % of twin pairs with discordant growth progress to TTTS. For this reason, the diagnosis can sometimes only be made at the end of the pregnancy, either at birth or in the event of fetal demise. Careful fetal surveillance is therefore necessary.

> **✪ Learning point** Monitoring for progression of TTTS
>
> TTTS can develop acutely so regular ultrasound assessment (usually every two weeks) is essential to monitor the pregnancy. More frequent monitoring may be required if there are any earlier concerns, particularly if discordance in liquor volume or bladder sizes is present as this may represent a pre-clinical manifestation of the disease. Both NICE and the RCOG have guidelines that pertain to monitoring of monochorionic pregnancies [1, 8].
>
> Ultrasound monitoring of the pregnancy should include the following:
>
> **Biometry for growth**—although not a prerequisite for making a diagnosis of TTTS, a proportion of twin pairs with discordant growth progress to develop TTTS. Measurement of biparietal diameter (BPD), head circumference (HC), abdominal circumference (AC), and femur length (FL) should be performed on a fortnightly basis to monitor fetal growth.
>
> **Liquor volume**—assessment of the overall amniotic fluid index should be performed at each visit. A deepest vertical pool (DVP) in each sac should also be measured.
>
> **Appearance of fetal bladders**—fetal bladders should be examined at each visit to determine discordancy in their sizes (a polyuric bladder in the recipient twin and an oliguric bladder in the donor twin will be evident in TTTS).
>
> **Appearance of the inter-twin membrane**—in non-TTTS cases, the inter-twin membrane is readily visible and appears to float freely due to evenly distributed liquor volumes in each sac. When TTTS develops, the inter-twin membrane can appear folded or subsequently 'wrapped' around the donor twin due to the significant oligo/anhydramnios (Figure 7.2).
>
> **Fetal Dopplers**—abnormalities in the umbilical artery, ductus venosus, or umbilical vein may be present. The donor frequently has absent or reversed end-diastolic flow in the umbilical artery (Figure 7.3) whereas the recipient tends to have abnormal ductus venosus (Figure 7.4) or umbilical vein waveforms.
>
> **Fetal echocardiography**—abnormal cardiac phenotype may be present in the recipient fetus. The main features include an increased cardiothoracic ratio (CTR), atrioventricular valve regurgitation, ventricular hypokinesia, hydrops, and right ventricular outflow tract obstruction. Scoring systems (CHOP—Children's Hospital of Philadelphia) have been developed to determine their prognostic value in TTTS [6]. The efficacy of such scoring systems is uncertain.

The couple were counselled about the scan findings and various management options were discussed. Fetoscopic laser ablation of placental anastomoses (FLAP) was offered and accepted by the couple. It was performed under local anaesthetic with antibiotic prophylaxis (750 mg Cefuroxime intravenously) and tocolysis (Indomethacin 100 mg rectally).

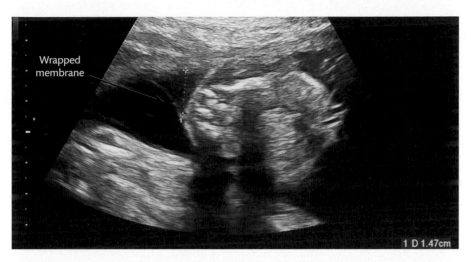

Figure 7.2 Inter-twin membrane 'wrapped' around the donor twin.

Courtesy of Dr Gowrishankar Paramasivam.

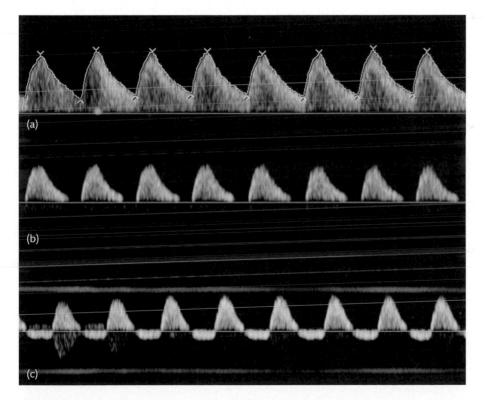

Figure 7.3 Umbilical artery Doppler waveforms. (a) Positive end-diastolic flow; (b) Absent end-diastolic flow; and (c) Reversed end-diastolic flow.

Courtesy of Dr Gowrishankar Paramasivam.

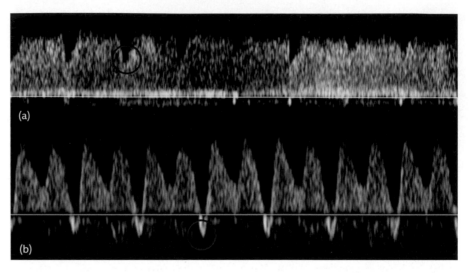

Figure 7.4 Doppler waveforms in the ductus venosus. (a) Positive 'a' wave; (b) Reversed 'a' wave.
Courtesy of Dr Gowrishankar Paramasivam.

The procedure was uncomplicated with seven arterio-venous (AV) anastomoses identified and ablated. The placenta was posterior in location which facilitated mapping of the chorionic plate vessels. At the end of the procedure an amniodrainage of 1500 mL was performed leaving a deepest pool of 6 cm in the recipient's sac. Following this the patient was admitted overnight for observation.

✪ **Learning point** Management options for TTTS

Without treatment, more advanced disease results in the death of one or both fetuses with a risk of brain injury in the survivor.

1. Serial amnioreduction

Serial amnioreduction was initially the mainstay treatment of TTTS with survival rates of 50–70%. However, this treatment only addresses the symptoms related to uterine overdistension from polyhydramnios but fails to treat the underlying pathological process (i.e. unbalanced interfetal transfusion). Furthermore, survivors of amnioreduction have been found to have a higher incidence of major neurodevelopmental handicap [10]. Amnioreduction may still be useful in a setting of TTTS not meeting the criteria for laser surgery (stage 1 or stage 2 disease), where laser surgery is not technically possible, or as a treatment option for those situations in which the expertise for laser coagulation is not available.

2. Septostomy

This technique involves the deliberate creation of a puncture in the inter-twin membrane in order to allow amniotic fluid from the polyhydramniotic sac to flow freely into the oligohydramniotic sac, thereby relieving the pressure in the recipient's sac [11]. However, like serial amnioreduction, this technique does not treat the underlying cause of the disease. Septostomy can give rise to serious complications that relate to pseudo-monoamnionicity such as cord entanglement, and it has no place in the treatment of TTTS.

3. Fetoscopic laser ablation of vascular anastomoses – non-selective and selective procedures

Fetoscopic laser ablation aims to interrupt the placental anastomoses which are the cause of the disease and thereby resolves the haemodynamic imbalance that defines the syndrome. It was originally
(continued)

performed by laparotomy under general anaesthetic but technological advances have enabled a minimally invasive approach under local anesthaesia to be used. A purpose-designed fetoscope is introduced transcutaneously into the uterine cavity to visualize the chorionic plate vessels, and coagulation of the inter-twin anastomoses is achieved with a laser fibre (Nd:YAG or diode) (Figure 7.5). The procedure is generally performed under antibiotic cover and tocolytic therapy (in our unit, we administer rectal indomethacin an hour before and for four to five days following the procedure). Cervical length assessment should be performed prior to fetoscopic laser surgery as a cervical length of < 15 mm is generally believed to increase the risk of preterm labour in twins. Some advocate cervical cerclage in these circumstances [12], although there is no good evidence base for such additional procedures prior to FLAP.

Some authorities recommend a selective approach, in that only anastomoses are ablated. Using this technique, placental surface vessel mapping is undertaken to identify vascular communications between the donor and recipient. Vessels are followed systematically from the point they cross the inter-twin membrane until it can be verified whether they are normal or if they culminate in an anastomosis with the co-twin [13]. Although the selective technique is more time-consuming, it has been shown to be associated with a higher survival rate. In the non-selective technique, all vessels crossing the inter-twin membrane are coagulated [14].This approach is associated with a higher fetal loss rate than a selective technique, particularly if there is a significant discordance in placental territory which is often the case in advanced disease [15]. Concomitant amnioreduction at the end of the laser procedure is sometimes necessary. A follow-up scan should be performed 24 hours following the procedure and weekly thereafter, to monitor fetal growth, liquor volume, and Doppler waveforms in the umbilical artery, ductus venosus, and middle cerebral artery. Survival rates of at least one twin following laser therapy range from 76–88% have been reported [1,16].

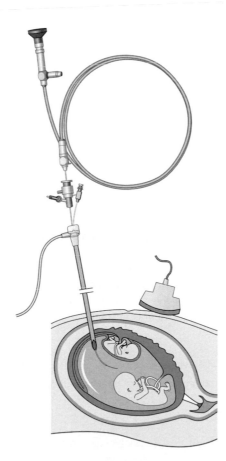

Figure 7.5 The technique of fetoscopic ablation of placental anastomoses. A purpose-designed fetoscope is inserted into the uterine cavity under local anaesthetic to visualise the chorionic plate. Inter-twin anastomoses are identified and photocoagulated using a laser fibre (taken from http://www.eurofoetus.org/eurotwin2twin/public/ttts.php).

© KARL STORZ–Endoskope, Germany.

> **❻ Expert comment**
>
> Although the Quintero staging system provides clinicians with a useful framework against which disease can be monitored and treatment tailored to severity, it is important to remember that TTTS may not always progress from one stage to the next in a sequential fashion. TTTS may present with advanced ultrasonographic features, or with mild features that do not progress. Furthermore, stages 1 and 2 may overlap or occur transiently in normal monochorionic twin pregnancies [17]. Although regression is possible, even with more advanced disease, this is only more likely to occur with stage 1 TTTS and therefore a conservative approach with stage > 2 disease must be taken with caution [18]. When progression to higher stages does occur, the outcome is often poor with perinatal survival ranging from 46–58%.
>
> The Eurofetus study [16], along with clinical case series [19,20] and a more recent meta-analysis [21], have shown comparable perinatal survival but improved neurological outcomes with laser therapy compared to conservative management. As the decision to intervene surgically in stage 1 TTTS remains controversial, an international RCT has been established to clarify whether fetoscopic laser therapy is superior to conservative management in stage 1 TTTS.

The next day, 20 hours following the laser procedure, repeat scan confirmed both fetuses were alive, with normal umbilical artery and ductus venosus Dopplers. The ex-donor now had a deepest pool of liquor of 2 cm in its sac with a normal-size bladder.

The patient was discharged home and a follow-up scan was arranged for the following week. She was warned that in the event of bleeding, leakage of fluid, or sudden distension of her abdomen, she should seek medical attention prior to her next scheduled appointment.

> **➕ Clinical tip** Complications associated with fetoscopic laser surgery
>
> - Preterm rupture of membranes (10%) [16].
> - Treatment failure (2–14%) [22]. This is more common with anterior placentae when visualization of the chorionic plate vessels is more difficult.
> - Recurrence of TTTS following initial resolution after FLAP (14%) [23].
> - Demise of one or both fetuses (13–30%) [13, 16].
> - Brain injury in one or both fetuses (13–17%) [24, 25].
> - Twin anaemia polycythaemia sequence (TAPS) (2–13%) [5, 26].
> - Reversal of TTTS, where the donor becomes the recipient and vice versa (5%) [27].

A week later, the TTTS had completely resolved and the patient was referred back to her local unit for subsequent follow-up, including a fetal brain MRI scan at 24 weeks' gestation.

Serial scans in her local unit confirmed that both babies continued to grow normally albeit the ex-donor remained on the third centile for weight. The fetal MRI was reported as normal.

> **✔ Evidence base** Management options for twin-to-twin transfusion syndrome
>
> **Septostomy versus amnioreduction**
>
> This trial, which included 71 women with TTTS at < 24 weeks' gestation, found no significant differences between septostomy and amnioreduction with regard to fetal or neonatal death, although
>
> (continued)

there was a significantly higher need for a combination of therapies such as laser coagulation, cord occlusion or serial amnioreductions in the septostomy arm of the trial (40% versus 8%) [28].

Amnioreduction versus fetoscopic laser ablation procedures

Fetoscopic laser ablation of anastomotic vessels is the first-line treatment of TTTS diagnosed before 26 weeks. The first randomized trial comparing amnioreduction with fetoscopic laser surgery included 142 women with TTTS between 15 and 26 weeks' gestation. The results showed that fetoscopic laser ablation resulted in higher survival rates and lower rates of neurological complications at six months of age than did serial amnioreduction in severe TTTS presenting before 26 weeks' gestation. The trial concluded early as soon as a clear benefit was demonstrated in the laser group [16].

A recent meta-analysis including 442 cases of TTTS from 5 case series treated with laser showed an overall survival rate of 57–77% following laser surgery and of 38–81% following serial amnioreduction. They also observed a non-significant trend towards better survival in stages 1 and 2 compared with stages 3 and 4 [21].

An NIH sponsored trial, which included 40 women with TTTS stages 2–4 who all underwent amnioreduction prior to randomization, and were subsequently randomized and treated before 24 weeks' gestation, showed neonatal outcomes (survival at 30 days and survival of one or both twins) to be equivalent in both arms, although the incidence of fetal recipient mortality was significantly higher in the laser arm of the trial, particularly for stages 3 and 4 TTTS [29]. However, the trial concluded early due to poor recruitment and results must be interpreted with caution.

⭐ **Learning point** Selective fetocide

For some patients the risks associated with FLAP may be unacceptable and they may prefer selective fetal reduction instead. Although the standard technique of selective fetocide in dichorionic twins is intra-cardiac potassium chloride (KCl) injection, this cannot be used in monochorionic twins due to the risk of the cardiotoxic agent affecting the co-twin because of the shared placental anastomoses. Techniques that occlude the vessels in the umbilical cord are required instead.

Bipolar diathermy cord occlusion is an effective method for selective fetocide in monochorionic twins, and is associated with a high rate of single survival (> 80%) in most series, with normal neurological outcome in approximately 90% of cases. The procedure carries a number of risks including preterm pre-labour rupture of membranes (PPROM) and placental abruption. A prospective observational study of 59 patients reported a 93% co-twin single survival rate following bipolar cord occlusion [30]. The 7% fetal loss rate in this study was due to abruption and intra-amniotic haemorrhage, which occurred within 24 hours of the procedure. The rate of PPROM was reported as 20% within three weeks of the procedure. This procedure is only available at selected fetal medicine centres and is generally an option up to 28 weeks' gestation.

When cord occlusion is being considered as a management option in TTTS, the choice of which fetus to terminate remains controversial. Although the donor is most often growth-restricted and has abnormal Doppler flow, the recipient is more likely to be hydropic. It has been suggested that either fetus can be equally appropriate choices for fetocide with similar perinatal outcomes [30].

More recently, **radiofrequency ablation** (RFA) has been used to perform selective fetal reduction in monochorionic twin pregnancies with good perinatal outcomes [31] (Figure 7.6).

At 36 weeks the patient was admitted in preterm labour and underwent an emergency Caesarean section because the leading twin was breech. Both babies were delivered in good condition. The ex-recipient weighed 2.3 kg and the ex-donor weighed 1.4 kg respectively. Cranial ultrasound scans following delivery were normal. Both twins were discharged well, after a few weeks in hospital.

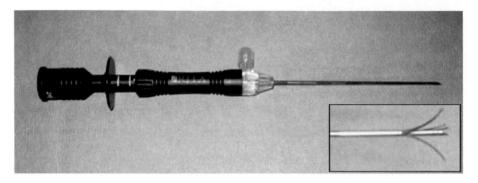

Figure 7.6 A radiofrequency ablation needle. The needle is inserted with the tines withdrawn. Once it has been inserted in the correct location (the fetal abdominal cord insertion) the tines are deployed to enable even, concentric coagulation of fetal tissue when an alternating current is applied (inset).

Courtesy of Dr Gowrishankar Paramasivam.

⚐ Expert comment Unexpected fetal death in monochorionic twin pregnancies

It has been suggested that fetal death in monochorionic twin pregnancies is highest prior to 24 weeks' gestation, and is often a consequence of TTTS or IUGR [32]. However, despite intensive fetal surveillance, unexpected late fetal death has been observed in up to 4.6% of seemingly uncomplicated monochorionic twin pregnancies beyond this gestation [33]. In this study, postmortem assessments were carried out following fetal demise and subacute TTTS was noted in two out of seven pregnancies, the remaining five being unexplained. A more recent population study of 387 monochorionic pregnancies delivered after 24 weeks' gestation showed a 6.2% prospective risk of fetal death after 33 weeks [34]. More intensive antenatal monitoring has been suggested, as has earlier delivery, in an attempt to avoid late unexpected fetal loss. However, larger studies are needed to justify a change in current practice.

⚐ Expert comment Timing of delivery

The optimal timing and mode of delivery of monochorionic twins remains controversial. Delivery of monochorionic twins is generally planned between 36 and 37 weeks' gestation unless there are other factors that indicate earlier delivery [1,8]. Although there is a risk of an acute interfetal transfusion occurring during labour the exact level of this risk remains unknown. Both NICE and the RCOG suggest that vaginal delivery is not contraindicated and Caesarean section should be performed for standard obstetric indications. If vaginal birth is the chosen mode of delivery, continuous electronic fetal monitoring should be undertaken [8].

✪ Learning point Neurological injury in monochorionic twins

The risk of neurodevelopmental abnormality is known to be high in monochorionic pregnancies complicated by TTTS or following death of a co-twin. A recent systematic review has shown that following the death of one twin after the first trimester, the odds of death of the co-twin and neurological abnormality among survivors is four to sixfold higher in monochorionic compared with dichorionic pregnancies [35]. Fetal growth restriction is also known to increase the risk of cerebral palsy and impaired neurological development as does prematurity and low birthweight.

It has been suggested that monochorionicity itself is a risk factor for cerebral damage. The presence of placental anastomoses confers a greater risk of perinatal morbidity and mortality to monochorionic compared with dichorionic twins.

The mechanism of brain injury is believed to be secondary to severe fetal hypotension when one fetus partially exsanguinates into its dying co-twin through the shared placental anastomoses. If this fetus survives the hypotension and recovers, severe brain injury is possible [36]. Such lesions are characteristically cystic changes in watershed areas of the fetal brain and can result in considerable long-term neurological handicap. Other potential mechanisms for *in utero* cerebral damage in monochorionic twins include passage of thrombotic material from the dead to the healthy twin secondary to coagulopathy due to the death of one twin [37]. Patterns of brain injury seen in monochorionic fetuses include cystic periventricular leukomalacia (PVL) (diagnosed either *in utero* or postnatally), intraventricular haemorrhage (IVH), or cerebrovascular lesions secondary to emboli. These can result in blindness, deafness, and significant neurological impairment including cerebral palsy.

> ⊘ **Evidence base** Neurodevelopment outcomes following intrauterine treatment for TTTS
>
> - Studies assessing neurological outcomes after conservative management of TTTS or serial amniodrainage suggest major neurodevelopmental impairment occurs in a similar proportion of surviving neonates (14.3–26 %) [10, 24, 38, 39].
> - Adverse neurodevelopmental outcome in monochorionic twins with TTTS successfully managed with fetoscopic laser ablation has been reported in 1.9–16 % of neonates [10, 40, 41]. In the longer term, the incidence of severe neurodevelopmental impairment at 2 and 5 years of age is reported as 13–17 %, including a cerebral palsy rate of 6–7 % [25, 28, 42].

> ❝ **Expert comment**
>
> The mechanism of brain injury following FLAP is poorly understood with both hypotensive and embolic mechanisms postulated. While long-term neurodevelopmental follow-up data continues to be collected, uncertainty about long-term neurological outcome following *in utero* treatment remains a major concern for physicians and parents.

Discussion

Monochorionic twin pregnancies can be associated with considerable morbidity and mortality, particularly if complicated by TTTS. Therapeutic strategies that have been developed to ameliorate or treat TTTS are also not without risk. There is now international consensus that fetoscopic laser surgery is the only *in utero* treatment that optimizes fetal survival whilst minimizing morbidity in severe TTTS and should be the treatment of choice for more advanced disease [43].

A prospective observational study of 100 consecutive MC pregnancies with stage 2–4 TTTS treated with fetoscopic laser reported perinatal survival rates of 75.5 % with 85 % survival of at least one twin. The mortality rate for donors and recipients was not significantly different but the fetal death rate was higher among donor twins. Severe neurological abnormalities were evident in 2.8 % of surviving twins [10]. In another report of more than 1300 fetoscopic laser ablation procedures, the mean survival rate at birth following a laser ablation procedure was 66 % with cerebral lesions occurring at one to six months postnatally in 2–7 % of cases [45]. Long-term neurological outcomes in surviving monochorionic twin pregnancies remain an area of concern for physicians and parents alike. Follow-up data continue to be collected which will facilitate counselling of parents when discussing management options.

MCDA multiple pregnancies are at risk of a number of other complications:

Isolated discordant growth occurs in 12–25 % of all monochorionic pregnancies and a 25 % cut-off in weight discrepancy is widely accepted to make the diagnosis of isolated discordant growth. Fetal growth restriction occurs more frequently in donors (85 %), but may be evident in both twins in 14 % of cases, and in 7 % of recipients. There seem to be two patterns of isolated discordant growth in monochorionic twins, early onset (before 20 weeks) and late onset (after 26 weeks and often undiagnosed until birth). Early-onset discordant growth carries a higher mortality (15 %) and there is often abnormal umbilical artery blood flow in the smaller twin. Late-onset discordant growth has a lower mortality rate (4 %) and umbilical artery Dopplers are usually normal [46]. The distribution of the placental territories plays a major role in the onset of discordant growth. If these territories are unevenly distributed, the risk increases tenfold [47]. Furthermore, it is not the number of anastomoses that plays a role in the onset of discordant growth or for that matter TTTS, but the nature of anastomoses, with deep AV anastomoses being the usual culprit.

Twin reversed arterial perfusion (TRAP) sequence or 'acardiac twinning' complicates 1 % of MC pregnancies [48]. Circulatory failure occurs in one of the twins between eight and 12 weeks, and usually results in an abnormal twin mass (the acardiac or perfused twin). The TRAP sequence is characterized by the flow of blood from the umbilical artery of the 'pump' (normal) twin in a reverse direction into the umbilical artery of the acardiac fetus via an AA anastomosis. This blood is poorly oxygenated and results in underdevelopment of the head, heart, and upper limbs of the acardiac fetus, although the lower half of the body is often better developed. Two criteria must be fulfilled for the TRAP sequence to develop. Firstly, an AA anastomosis must exist, and secondly, there must be discordant development or *in utero* fetal death of one twin that allows flow reversal to take place. The acardiac twin is a true parasite and would not exist without the presence of the 'pump' twin. The pump fetus is at risk because the demands on its heart may be considerable as it has to perfuse not only itself but also the acardiac fetus. Hydrops of the pump twin may ensue which carries a very poor prognosis.

Twin anaemia-polycythaemia sequence (TAPS) may occur in up to 13 % of cases following laser therapy. In such cases, the former recipient becomes progressively anaemic following FLAP and the donor becomes polycythaemic. Almost 50 % of cases of TAPS are seen when anastomoses remain following FLAP, and are typically located near the placental margin. Such complications are less likely to occur if placental anastomoses are coagulated in a selective manner. TAPS may present at birth with a small plethoric twin and a larger, anaemic twin. The presence of polycythaemia in the ex-donor and chronic anaemia with a reticulocytosis in the ex-recipient, in the absence of hypovolaemic shock, aids in differentiating this condition from a more acute inter-fetal transfusion. TAPS may also occur spontaneously, in the absence of treatment TTTS. [45]

Discordant structural and karyotypic anomalies—Structural malformations are reported to be two to three times more frequent in monochorionic twins compared to dizygotic twins and five times more common than in singletons. The likely cause for this is the potentially teratogenic effect of embryo cleavage or the consequence of a shared placental circulation. Anomalies include midline malformations (as seen in conjoined twins or acardiac twinning), neural tube defects, facial clefting, cloacal and abdominal wall anomalies, and limb reduction defects. Structural cardiac abnormalities are particularly prevalent in monochorionic twins [49]. It is important to note that although extremely rare, monochorionic twins can be discordant for chromosomal abnormalities and discordancy for all common aneuploidies have been reported. Most of these cases involve one twin with Turner (45,XO) syndrome and the other with either a female or male phenotype but usually a mosaic karyotype. This phenomenon is known as 'heterokaryotypic monozygotism' and reflects either a postzygotic mitotic event or a prezygotic meiotic error. The incidence of karyotypic abnormalities is also significantly higher in acardiac twins with some studies suggesting a 30 % incidence of aneuploidy.

A Final Word from the Expert

This case highlights some of the clinical challenges encountered whilst managing monochorionic twin pregnancies, specifically when complicated by TTTS. Once diagnosed, careful ultrasound surveillance is vital in order to plan the timing of an appropriate therapeutic intervention.

Although pregnancy outcome in this particular monochorionic pregnancy was favourable, this is not always the case. Fetoscopic laser ablation is a highly specialised technique. It can be associated with immediate procedure-related complications, including premature rupture of membranes and inadequate ablation, resulting in fetal demise, as well as neurological injury which may not become apparent until childhood. Fetal outcome following fetoscopic laser therapy has been shown to improve with centre and operator experience [45] and on this basis, should only be offered in specialist centres by experienced operators.

References

1. Multiple pregnancy: the management of twin and triplet pregnancies in the antenatal period. National Collaborating Centre for Women's and Children's Health. Commissioned by the National Institute for Health and Clinical Excellence. 2011; June:83–93.

2. Nicolaides K. Screening for fetal aneuploidies at 11 to 13 weeks. *Prenat Diag* 2011;31:7–15.

3. Monni G, Zoppi MA, Ibba RM, Putzolu M, Floris M. Nuchal translucency in multiple pregnancies. *Croat Med J* 2000;41:266–9.

4. Vandecruys H, Faiola S, Auer M, Sebire N, Nicolaides KH. Screening for trisomy 21 in monochorionic twins by measurement of fetal nuchal translucency thickness. *Ultrasound Obstet Gynecol* 2005;25:551–3.

5. Habli M, Lim FY, Crombleholme T. Twin-to-twin transfusion syndrome: a comprehensive update. *Clin Perinatol* 2009;36:391416 x.

6. Galea P, Jain V, Fisk NM. Insights into the pathophysiology of twin-twin transfusion syndrome. *Prenat Diagn* 2005;25:777–85.

7. Quintero RA, Morales WJ, Allen MH, Bornick PW, Johnson PK, Kruger M. Staging of twin-twin transfusion syndrome. *J Perinatol* 1999;19:550–5.

8. Management of monochorionic twin pregnancy. *RCOG Green-top Guideline No. 51. Dec* 2008.

9. Stirnemann JJ, Nasr B, Proulx F, Essaoui M, Ville Y. Evaluation of the CHOP cardiovascular score as a prognostic predictor of outcome in twin-twin transfusion syndrome after laser coagulation of placental vessels in a prospective cohort. *Ultrasound Obstet Gynecol* 2010;36:52–7.

10. Cincotta RB, Gray PH, Gardener G, Soong B, Chan FY. Selective fetoscopic laser ablation in 100 consecutive pregnancies with severe twin-twin transfusion syndrome. *ANZJOG* 2009;49:22–7.

11. Saade GR, Belfort MA, Berry DL, Bui TH, Montgomery LD, Johnson A, *et al.* Amniotic septostomy for the treatment of twin oligohydramnios-polyhydramnios sequence. *Fetal Diagn Ther* 1998;13:86–93.

12. Salomon LJ, Nasr B, Nizard J, Bernard JP, Essaoui M, Bussieres L, *et al.* Emergency cerclage in cases of twin-to-twin transfusion syndrome with a short cervix at the time of surgery and relationship to perinatal outcome. *Prenat Diagn* 2008;28:1256–61.

13. Quintero RA, Comas C, Bornick PW, Allen MH, Kruger M. Selective versus non-selective laser photocoagulation of placental vessels in twin-to-twin transfusion syndrome. *Ultrasound Obstet Gynecol* 2000;16:230–6.

14. Ville Y, Hyett J, Hecher K, Nicholaides K. Preliminary experience with endoscopic laser surgery for severe twin-twin transfusion syndrome. *N Engl J Med* 1995;332:224–7.

15. Ville Y, Hecher K, Gagnon A, Sebire N, Hyett J, Nicolaides K. Endoscopic laser coagulation in the management of severe twin-to-twin transfusion syndrome. *Br J Obstet Gynecol* 1998;105:446–53.

16. Senat MV, Deprest J, Boulvain M, Paupe A, Winer N, Ville Y. Endoscopic laser surgery versus serial amnioreduction for severe twin-to-twin transfusion syndrome. *New Engl J Med* 2004;351:136–44.

17. Bebbington MW, Tiblad E, Huesler-Charles M, Wilson RD, Mann SE, Johnson MP. Outcomes in a cohort of patients with Stage 1 twin-to-twin transfusion syndrome. *Ultrasound Obstet Gynecol* 30 (Abstract OP10.04).

18. O'Donoghue K, Cartwright E, Galea P, Fisk NM. Stage 1 twin-twin transfusion syndrome: rates of progression and regression in relation to outcome. *Ultrasound Obstet Gynecol* 2007;30:958–64

19. Huber A, Diehl W, Bregenzer T, Hackelöer BJ, Hecher K. Stage-related outcome in twin-twin transfusion syndrome treated by fetoscopic laser coagulation. *Obstet Gynecol* 2006;108:333–7.

20. Wagner MM, LoprioreE, KlumperFJ, OepkesD, VandenbusscheFP, MiddeldorpJM. Short- and long-term outcome in stage 1 twin-to-twin transfusion syndrome treated with laser surgery compared with conservative management. *AJOG* 2009;201:286.e 1–6.

21. Rossi AC, D'Addario V. The efficacy of Qunitero staging system to assess severity of twin-twin transfusion syndrome treated with laser therapy: a systematic review with meta-analysis. *Am J Perinatol* 2009;26:537–44.

22. Baschat A, Chmait RH, Deprest J, Gratacós E, Hecher K, Kontopoulos E, *et al.* WAPM consensus group on twin-to-twin transfusion syndrome. *J Perinatal Med* 2011;39:107–12.

23. Robyr R, Lewi L, Salomon LJ, Yamamoto M, Bernard JP, Deprest J, *et al.* Prevalence and management of late fetal complications following successful selective laser coagulation of chorionic plate anastomoses in twin-to-twin transfusion syndrome. *Am J Obstet Gynecol* 2006;194:796–803.

24. Lopriore E, Nagel HTC, Vandenbussche FPHA, Walther FJ. Long-term neurodevelopmental outcome in twin-to-twin transfusion syndrome. *Am J Obstet Gynecol* 2003;189:1314–19.

25. Graeff C, Ellenrieder B, Hescher K, Hackeloer BJ, Huber A, Bartmann P. Long-term neurodevelopmental outcome of 167 children after intrauterine laser treatment for severe twin-twin transfusion syndrome. *Am J Obstet Gynecol* 2006;194:303–8.

26. Slaghekke F, Kist WJ, Oepkes D, Pasman SA, Middeldorp JM, Klumper FJ, *et al.* Twin Anaemia-Polycythemia Sequence: diagnostic criteria, classification, perinatal management and outcome. *Fetal Diagn Ther* 2010;27:181–90.

27. Wee LY, Taylor MJ, Vanderheyden T, Wimalasundera R, Gardiner HM, Fisk NM. Reversal of twin-twin transfusion syndrome: frequency, vascular anatomy, associated anomalies and outcome. *Prenat Diagn* 2004 Feb; 24(2):104–10.

28. MoiseJr KJ, Dorman K, Lamvu G, Saade GR, Fisk NM, Dickinson JE, *et al.* A randomized trial of amnioreduction versus septostomy in the treatment of twin-twin transfusion syndrome. *Am J Obstet Gynaecol* 2005;193:701–7.

29. Crombleholme TM, Shera D, Lee H, Johnson M, D'Alton M, Porter F, *et al.* A prospective, randomized multicentre trial of amnioreduction vs selective fetoscopic laser photocoagulation for the treatment of severe twin-twin transfusion syndrome. *Am J Obstet Gynecol* 2007;197:396.e 1–396. e 9.

30. Taylor MJ, Govender L, Jolly M, Wee L, Fisk NM. Validations of the Quintero staging system for twin-twin transfusion syndrome. *Obstet Gynecol* 2002;100:1257–65.

31. Paramasivam G, Wimalasundera R, Wiechec M, Zhang E, Saeed F, Kumar S. Radiofrequency ablation for selective reduction in complex monochorionic pregnancies. *BJOG* 2010;117:1294–8.

32. Sebire NJ, Snijers RJ, Hughes K, Sepulveda W, Nicolaides KH. The hidden mortality of monochorionic twin pregnancies. *Br J Obstet Gynecol* 1997;104:1203–7.

33. Barigye O, Pasquini L, Galea P, Chambers H, Chappell L, Fisk NM. High risk of unexpected late fetal death in monochorionic twins despite intensive ultrasound surveillance: a cohort study. *PLoS Med* 2005;2(6):eP 172.

34. Tul N, Verdenik I, Novak Z, *et al.* Prospective risk of stillbirth in monochorionic-diamniotic twin gestations: a population based study. *J Perinat Med* 2011 Jan;39(1):51–4.

35. Ong SSC, Zamora J, Khan KS, Kilby MD. Prognosis for the co-twin following single-twin death: a systematic review. *BJOG* 2006;113:992–98.

36. Bajoria R, Kingdom J. The case for routine determination of chorionicityand zygosity in multiple pregnancy. *Prenat Diagn* 1997;17:1207-25.

37. Benirschke K. Intrauterine death of a twin: mechanisms, implications for surviving twin, and placental pathology. *Semin Diagn Pathol* 1993;10:222–31.

38. Dickinson JE, Duncombe GJ, Evans SF, French NP, Hagan R. The long term neurologic outcome of children from pregnancies complicated by twin-to-twin transfusion syndrome. *Br J Obstet Gynecol* 2005;112:63–8.

39. Frusca T, Soregaroli M, Fichera A, Taddei F, Villani P, Accorsi P, Martelli P. Pregnancies complicated by twin-twin transfusion syndrome: outcomeand long term neurological follow-up. *Eur J Obstet Gynecol Reprod Biol* 2003;107:145-50.

40. Dickinson JE, Evans SF. Obstetric and perinatal outcomes from the Australian and New Zealand Twin-Twin Transfusion Registry. *Am J Obstet Gynecol.* 2000;182;706–712.

41. Lenclen R, Paupe R, Ciarlo G, Couderc S, Castela F, Ortqvist L, Ville Y. Neonatal outcome in preterm monochorionic twins with twin-twin transfusion syndrome after intrauterine treatment with amnioreduction or fetoscopic laser surgery: comparison with dichorionic twins. *Am J Obstet Gynecol* 2007;196:450.e 1–450. e 7.

42. Lopriore E, Van Wezel-Meijler G, Middeldorp JM, Sueters M, Vandenbussche FP, Walther FJ. Incidence, originand character of cerebral injury in twin-to-twin transfusion syndrome treated with fetoscopic laser surgery. *Am J Obstet Gynecol* 2006;194:1215-20.

43. Roberts D, Gates S, Kilby M, Neilson JP. Interventions for twin-twin transfusion syndrome: a Cochrane review. *Ultrasound Obstet Gynecol* 2008;31:701–11.

44. Yamamoto M, Ville Y. Laser treatment in twin-to-twin transfusion syndrome. *Semin Fetal Neonatal Med* 2007;12:450–7.

45. Morris R, Selman T, Harbidge A, Martin WI, Kilby MD. Fetoscopic laser coagulation for severe twin-to-twin transfusion syndrome: factors influencing perinatal outcome, learning curve of the procedure and lessons for new centres. *BJOG* 2010;117:1350–7.

46. Lewi L, Gucciardo L, Van Mieghem T, de Koninck P, Beck V, Medek H, *et al.* Monochorionic diamniotic pregnancies: natural history and risk stratification. *Fetal Diagn Ther* 2010;27:121–33.

47. Quintero RA, Martinez JM, Lopez J, Bermúdez C, Becerra C, Morales W, *et al.* Individual placental territories after selective laser photocoagulation of communicating vessels in twin-twin transfusion syndrome. *Am J Obstet Gyneol* 2005;192:1112–18.

48. Chalouhi GE, Stirneman JJ, Salomon LJ, Essaoui M, Quibel T, Ville Y. Specific complications of monochorionic twin pregnancies: twin-twin transfusion syndrome and twin reversed arterial perfusion sequence. *Semin Fetal and Neonatal Med* 2010;15:349–56.

49. Rustico MA, Baietti MG, Coviello D, Orlandi E, Nicolini U. Managing twins discordant for fetal anomaly. *Prenat Diagn* 2005;25:766–71.

8 'Rescue' cerclage after bulging membranes at 22 weeks: delaying the inevitable?

Natasha Hezelgrave

ⓒ Expert Commentary Andrew Shennan
ⓒ Guest Expert Geraint Lee

Case history

A 30-year-old Gravida 2 Para 0 woman was referred to the preterm surveillance ante-natal clinic by her midwife at 18 weeks' gestation. At the age of 24, she underwent a large loop excision of the transformation zone (LLETZ) under local anaesthetic for cervical intraepithelial neoplasia grade 2 (CIN 2) extending into the endocervical glands with clean margins and with normal smear tests thereafter. One year earlier she experienced a mid-trimester miscarriage, having presented with abdominal pain and bleeding at 22 weeks followed by spontaneous passage of fetus and placenta. The fetus was structurally and chromosomally normal at postmortem and no cause for miscarriage was identified. There was no clinical or histological evidence of chorioamnionitis. She had no other significant past medical history and was not taking any regular medication.

Her current pregnancy was spontaneously conceived with a long-term partner, and had been uneventful. She had a normal dating ultrasound at 12 weeks' gestation and all her booking investigations had been normal thus far.

In clinic she appeared well, with no abdominal pain or per vaginal loss. The patient's obstetric history and background of LLETZ prompted close monitoring with cervical length assessments. A trans-cervical ultrasound was normal (Figure 8.1), revealing a cervical length measurement of 28–30 mm. She was reassured and given an appointment to be seen at 22 weeks for a repeat cervical length and fetal fibronectin test.

> **ⓒ Expert comment**
>
> The role of preterm clinics is undefined. A few centres have developed them, driven by the large number of women with a previous mid-trimester or preterm birth (occurring in 7% of pregnancies). Other risk factors are also prevalent, such as previous destructive procedures on the cervix estimated to involve up to 1 in 10 women in some populations, and higher order multiple pregnancies. Unlike many other specialist clinics (e.g. diabetes), management protocols and interventions in high-risk asymptomatic women are not established. However, powerful predictive tools for early birth now exist, both for symptomatic and asymptomatic women, such as transvaginal ultrasound of the cervix and cervicovaginal fetal fibronectin. Their use is increasingly prevalent in Europe and North America, but less so in the UK. The challenge is to link their use with improved outcome.

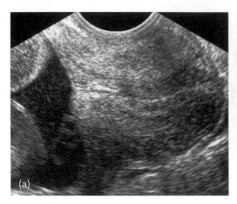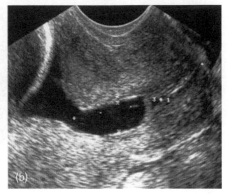

Figure 8.1 Transvaginal ultrasound of (a) a normal cervix, and (b) a short cervix with funnelling.

Reprinted from *Best Practice & Research Clinical Obstetrics & Gynaecology*, Rachel Simcox and Andrew Shennan, Cervical cerclage in the prevention of preterm birth, 2007, with permission from Elsevier.

⭐ **Learning point** Cervical incompetence after cervical surgery

Cervical surgery, including cold-knife and laser conization and loop electrosurgical excision procedure (LEEP), performed for treatment of cervical intraepithelial neoplasia has been shown to increase the likelihood of cervical weakness, thereby increasing risk of mid-trimester miscarriage, premature rupture of membranes, and preterm delivery.

In a prospective study ($n=132$), women with a history of LEEP, cold-knife conization, and cryotherapy all independently had shorter cervical lengths than low-risk controls and similar lengths to women with previous spontaneous preterm birth. LEEP and cold-knife conization, but not cryotherapy, were associated with spontaneous preterm birth less than 37 weeks (odds ratio 3.45, 95% confidence interval 1.28–10.00, $p=0.02$; and odds ratio 2.63, 95% confidence interval 1.28–5.56, $p=0.009$, respectively) [1]. It is likely that an increased number and greater depth of biopsy confers greater risk, although results of studies are conflicting.

A diagnosis of precancerous change in the cervix is also thought to be independently associated with an increased risk of preterm birth; both treated and untreated women are thought to be at increased risk, with treated women more likely than untreated women to deliver prematurely [2].

💬 **Expert comment**

The exact mechanism of increased risk associated with cervical surgery is unclear. The simplistic view that weakness results in incompetence is not borne out by the clinical observations that very short cervices often are associated with term pregnancies, and that mid-trimester losses are rarely recurrent; both of these occur even without intervention. Ascending 'infection', once the barrier between vagina and uterus is breeched, will frequently cause labour or rupture of membranes. There is increasing evidence that the role of the cervix and endocervix is more complex, including biochemical and immunological elements. Whether supporting the cervix with a suture will reduce risk in women with prior cervical surgery is simply not known, but it is a logical intervention. However, the use of cerclage, including different techniques such as occlusion sutures (which close the endocervix), or abdominal sutures (higher placed), are in desperate need of more evidence and these un-established procedures should probably only be performed as part of clinical trials except in extraordinary circumstances. Their role in primiparous women with risk factors such as cervical surgery is particularly lacking; there is some evidence that '"low-risk' women with an incidental finding of a short cervix do not benefit from cerclage.

➕ **Clinical tip** Cervical length (CL) assessment by ultrasound

- CL assessment is the only screening test that allows early identification of internal cervical os opening; the first physical change of cervical ripening that precedes labour.
- Measurements should be taken from the internal to external os along the entire cervical canal. Most studies have used a cut-off length of ≤25 mm to predict risk of preterm labour or indicate the need for the insertion of a cervical cerclage in high-risk women.
- Pressure effect, funneling of the cervix, and the presence of 'sludge' are documented during the procedure, but evidence is sparse regarding their sensitivity and specificity for predicting preterm birth.

✅ **Evidence base** Prior history predicts spontaneous preterm birth (sPTB)

The current simplest predictor of sPTB is a previous pregnancy history of preterm delivery, preterm premature membrane rupture, or spontaneous second trimester miscarriage. The risk of a preterm delivery < 35 weeks' in a subsequent pregnancy with a history of the aforementioned is 8.6 % [3].

✅ **Evidence base** Cervical length predicts sPTB

Measurement of cervical length has been demonstrated to be a sensitive predictor of preterm delivery in both low-risk and high-risk pregnancies.

Risk of preterm birth is inversely related to cervical length; the shorter it is, the higher the risk of preterm birth. Several studies have demonstrated that the risk of preterm delivery is substantially higher in high-risk women with cervical length less than 25 mm, at 14–24 weeks of gestation, than in those with a longer cervix.

- Observational studies have shown, in high-risk pregnancies between 15–24 weeks' gestation, the incidence of preterm birth <34 weeks is between 19.8–75 % in those women with a CL <25 mm, compared to 7–23 % of women with cervical length >25 mm [4–8].
- The risk of preterm delivery increases exponentially with decreasing cervical length, from less than 1 % at 30 mm to almost 80 % at 5 mm [9].

More than half of all spontaneous preterm births occur in low-risk women. Several studies have demonstrated that the risk of preterm delivery is substantially higher in women with cervical-length shortening than in those with a longer cervix.

- Hassan *et al.* ($n=6877$) demonstrated that even in low-risk women, a cervix of <15 mm between 14–24 weeks' gestation results in a nearly 50 % chance of delivering prior to 32 weeks' gestation [10].

At 22 + 1 weeks she returned to the clinic for review, having remained well in the preceding four weeks. On speculum examination, prior to performing a fetal fibronectin test, her cervix was 2 cm dilated with visible bulging fetal membranes. She was asymptomatic, apyrexial, and clinically well.

✴️ **Learning point** Bulging fetal membranes

The onset of labour and delivery is typically characterized by the progressive effacement and dilation of the cervix. Threatened second trimester miscarriage (delivery between 13–24 weeks' gestation) and preterm delivery (delivery between 24 and 37 completed weeks' gestation) have multi-factorial maternal and fetal aetiologies that, as yet, have been poorly defined. Nevertheless, they are characterized by premature cervical effacement and dilation, ultimately resulting in delivery of the fetus.

As the cervix progressively shortens, the membranes around the fetus may prolapse through the internal and external cervical os so that on presentation fetal membranes may well be seen herniating through the cervical canal on ultrasound or speculum examination (Figure 8.2). Women may present asymptomatically, as part of routine cervical-length screening, or present symptomatically with pain, a feeling of pressure in the vagina, or watery vaginal loss, thought to be related to a transudate across the exposed membrane.

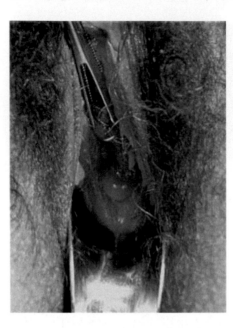

Figure 8.2 Dilated cervical os and visible membranes.

Manju Chandiramani and Andrew H Shennan, Premature cervical change and the use of cervical cerclage, 2007, *Fetal and Maternal Medicine Review*, Cambridge University Press.

> ✔ **Evidence base** Fetal fibronectin (fFN) predicts sPTB
>
> - fFN is an extracellular matrix glycoprotein thought to be produced by extra villous chorionic trophoblasts which allows the amniotic sac to adhere to the uterine decidua. It is normally detectable in the cervico-vaginal secretions of pregnant women up until 22 weeks. After this period, the fetal membranes are strongly adherent and isolated from the cervix by the thick secretions of the cervical canal, and fFN should be undetectable.
> - The presence of fFN indicates that there is choriodecidual disruption, possibly associated with the fetal membranes separating from the decidua, suggesting that events that pre-empt labour are occurring. Fetal fibronectin is commonly present after about 35 weeks' gestation and this presence is probably physiological rather than pathological. Therefore the presence of fFN in cervico-vaginal secretions between 22–35 weeks' gestation is indicative of a higher risk of preterm labour.
> - The excellent negative predictive value of fibronectin is hugely valuable.
>   - In women who are symptomatic of preterm birth between 22–34 weeks' gestation, a negative fibronectin test confers a 99.5% negative prediction value that delivery would not occur within seven days, 99.2% within 14 days, and 84.5% before 37 weeks [11].
>   - In women who are asymptomatic but are high-risk for preterm birth, a negative fetal fibronectin test at 24 weeks confers a <1% probability of delivery before 30 and 34 weeks and <2% before 37 weeks [12].
> - The positive predictive value of fibronectin is less accurate.
>   - A positive fFN confers a relative risk of preterm labour of 3.2 in symptomatic women though the positive prediction value remains under 50% for most gestational end-points, even in high-risk populations [11].
>   - A positive fibronectin in asymptomatic high risk women at 24 weeks' gestation confers probabilities of 46–58% chance of delivery at 30–37 weeks' gestation [12].
> - A Cochrane meta-analysis suggests that knowledge of fFN results in lower sPTB rates by identifying a much higher-risk group, which suggests that targeting interventions at women more likely to benefit could be beneficial [13].

❝ Expert comment

Fetal fibronectin has traditionally been used to predict delivery in symptomatic women in threatened preterm labour. The use of fetal fibronectin in asymptomatic women (after 22 weeks) is currently not recommended. However, its prediction is comparable to that of cervical length, and some studies suggest even better. Combining ultrasound and fetal fibronectin gives the best prediction. For example a short cervix with a negative fetal fibronectin will generally have a good outcome. Research needs to establish the interventions that ensue following this information, but it is likely that targeting the highest risk women is an effective strategy, and this has been recommended in an HTA review in 2010.

✛ Clinical tip Fetal fibronectin testing

- Usually a rapid qualitative test which gives a positive/negative results
- Quantitative bedside tests exist and are currently under evaluation in research environments
- Speculum is inserted and swab is rotated in posterior fornix until tip is saturated with secretions (approx. 10 seconds)
- False positive results more likely if:
  - Intercourse within the last 24 hours
  - Presence of vaginal bleeding
  - Performed after a digital vaginal examination

Diagnosis, management options, and likely outcome were discussed with the patient at length. The following options were offered:

1) Expectant management with bed-rest as an outpatient or inpatient.
2) Admission with same-day insertion of a rescue cerclage, followed by bed-rest.

The patient chose the latter. A 'rescue cerclage' was inserted by modified Macdonald technique (Figure 8.3) under spinal anaesthesia on the same day. One dose of intravenous (IV) co-amoxiclav 1.2 gram was administered intra-operatively. The procedure was uneventful and she was admitted to the ward for bed-rest, with a plan to administer steroids at 24 weeks once fetal viability was reached.

✪ Learning point Indications for transvaginal cervical cerclage

- History indicated cerclage
  - Prophylactic measure in asymptomatic women, inserted as a result of risk factors in a woman's obstetric history.
  - Usually performed between 12–14 weeks' gestation, following assessment of viability and risk of aneuploidy.
  - Of benefit to women with 3 or more preterm births (See Evidence Base).
- Ultrasound indicated cerclage
  - Inserted following transvaginal ultrasound scan between 16–24 weeks which demonstrates a 'short' cervix (< 25 mm) in the presence of a history of spontaneous preterm delivery or second trimester loss [16, 17]; has not been proved to be beneficial for an incidental finding of a short cervix, in the absence of a prior history.
  - The differential benefit of ultrasound indicated cerclage-benefit observed in high- and low-risk women is difficult to explain and requires more research.
  - The role of cerclage in women with other risk factors such as previous cervical surgery, with or without a short cervix, is not clear.

(continued)

◆ Landmark trial The Preterm Prediction study [3]

Prospective observational cohort study of 2929 women (22–24 weeks' gestation) between 1992–1994, to determine risk factors for spontaneous preterm birth. The most clinically reliable, readily measurable, and thus strongest predictors of preterm birth were fFN, cervical length, and past history. If the fFN test was positive, cervical length was less than 25 mm and there was a history of spontaneous preterm birth (sPTB), there was > a 50% risk of delivery before 32 weeks.

❝ Expert comment

If an asymptomatic high-risk women has a negative fibronectin test and a cervix > 25 mm at 24 weeks' gestation, I would discharge her from preterm surveillance clinic with a < 1% chance of delivery < 34 weeks'.

✛ Clinical tip Quantitative fFN

Quantitative fibronectin (qfFN), which utilizes thresholds other than the traditional 50 ng/ml 'positive cut-off', enhances the positive predictive power of the test in women symptomatic of PTB, whilst maintaining excellent negative prediction [14]. The qfFN test is gradually replacing the qualitative (positive/negative) test used in clinical practice to assess risk in symptomatic women.

❝ Expert comment

There is no good evidence to support the use of tocolysis, non-steroidal anti-inflammatory drugs, or antibiotics in the peri-operative period. Their routine use is not currently recommended. The RCOG recommend that the decision to administer intra-operative antibiotics should be at the clinician's discretion [15].

⊘ **Evidence base** History
indicated cerclage

An international multi-centre
trial [18] (n=1292) of high-risk
women demonstrated that
women with a history of three or
more pregnancies ending before
37 weeks (n=104) benefitted
from cerclage, which halved the
incidence of preterm delivery prior
to 33 weeks (15% versus 32%,
p<0.05.) No other outcomes,
including perinatal death, favoured
cerclage, and some outcomes,
including infection, were worse in
the cerclage group.

- Rescue Cerclage
  - Insertion of a McDonald or a purse string suture into the cervix of women who present with a dilated cervix and bulging membranes.
  - Usually done with as little delay as possible once the diagnosis of bulging membranes has been made.

⊘ **Evidence base** Rescue cerclage

Poor evidence exists regarding the benefit of rescue cerclage; only one RCT evaluating rescue cerclage and bed-rest plus peri-operative indomethacin versus bed-rest alone (n=23, mean gestation 22–23 weeks) [19]. Preterm delivery before 34 weeks' gestation was significantly reduced in the cerclage group versus bed rest alone (7/13 versus 10/10; p=0.02). There was a trend towards improvement in neonatal survival (56% versus 28%) and a significant reduction in compound neonatal morbidity (71% versus 100%, RR 1.6, 95%, CI 1.1–2.3). However, the authors did not provide any data on the incidence of chorioamnionitis or neonatal morbidity.

While it appears that rescue cerclage may delay delivery, there are limited data to support improvement in neonatal mortality or morbidity. Chorioamnionitis is reported to complicate 5–80% of pregnancies treated with emergency cerclage [20]. Thus, there is concern regarding prolonging a pregnancy with sub-clinical chorioamnionitis with the associated risk of fetal inflammatory brain injury, as well as prolonging a pregnancy from pre-viability to severe prematurity. There are no long-term follow-up studies to show the effect of 'rescue' cerclage on the development and behaviour of these children. There is also the maternal risk of infection both in the short-term and the long-term effect on fertility.

⟨⟩ **Expert comment**

Gestational age is highly related to outcome, both in terms of mortality and morbidity. Prolonging gestation is a desirable goal. However, this may not always be the case and it is clear when there are clinical signs of chorioamnionitis, delivery should be expedited to avoid serious morbidity or mortality in both mother and baby. As inflammation *in utero* is known to cause neurological damage and cerebral palsy, delivery under these circumstances is likely to improve outcome even at early gestations, as continued *in utero* exposure will increase risk. This may even occur in asymptomatic women. Maternal signs of chorioamnionitis are relatively late (e.g. pyrexia or abdominal tenderness). Interventions that prolong gestation at these critical gestations, such as cerclage or possibly progesterone, may inadvertently increase risk. In addition, late miscarriages maybe converted into severe preterm birth with serious morbidity. Studies need to include evaluation of baby outcome, preferably at older ages, and include neuro-developmental outcomes. We cannot assume that prolonging gestation is always desirable. Performing these long-term studies is difficult.

⟨⟩ **Expert comment**

Cervical cerclage is a relatively common surgical intervention performed by many obstetricians despite the lack of a well-defined population for whom there is clear evidence of benefit. In addition, there is little consensus on the optimal procedure, or technique (low/high vaginal, abdominal, tape/nylon, single/multiple, endocervical/purse string), or timing of insertion (elective, ultrasound indicated, pre-conceptual). In addition, the mechanism of action is not clearly understood; cerclage may provide structural support, but is also likely to assist in maintaining a biochemical barrier, protecting membranes against exposure to ascending pathogens. The role of cerclage may differ depending on underlying pathophysiology, e.g. prior cervical surgery, cervical shortening, or multiple pregnancy.

Whilst there may be some evidence that a history-indicated cerclage is beneficial to women with 3 or more previous preterm births, the desire for the clinician to help, coupled with the desperate need of the woman to receive a beneficial intervention, understandably leads to non-evidence-based practice.

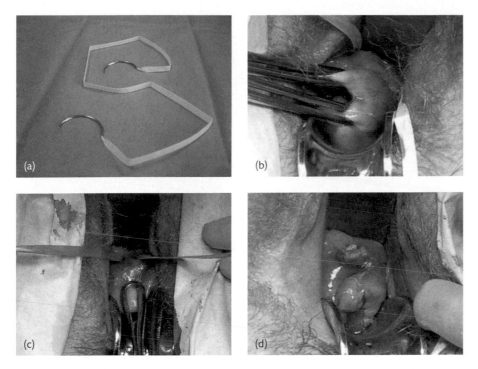

Figure 8.3 Insertion of a purse-string (McDonald) cervical suture (a) using Mersilene tape. (b) The cervix is grasped with sponge forceps and the suture is inserted from the 12 o'clock to the 3 o'clock position. (c) An anterior knot is tied, and (d) a double knot facilitates removal.

Reprinted from *Obstetrics, gynaecology and reproductive medicine*, Manju Chandiramani, Rachel M Tribe, and Andrew H Shennan, Preterm labour and prematurity, 232–7, 2007 with permission from Elsevier.

She remained well, and a repeat trans-cervical ultrasound performed 1 week after the procedure revealed a shortened closed cervix measuring 14 mm, with a funnel measuring 5×7 mm at the level of the internal os, and 8 mm of cervix above the suture.

> ⊕ **Clinical tip** Cerclage technique
> - Macdonald suture (transvaginal cerclage) (Figure 8.3)
>   - Purse-string suture placed at the cervico-vaginal junction, without bladder mobilization.
>   - Usually removed easily without need for regional anaesthesia.
> - Shirodkar suture (high transvaginal cerclage)
>   - Transvaginal purse-string suture placed following bladder mobilization, to allow insertion above the level of the cardinal ligaments.
>   - Frequently requires regional anaesthesia for removal.
> - Rescue cerclage
>   - McDonald suture inserted (as previously referred to).
>   - Deep Trendelenberg position required for insertion.
>   - Foley catheter may be inserted into the cervix and balloon filled with water until membranes retract back into uterine cavity.
> - Abdominal suture
>   - Purse-string cerclage inserted at laparotomy (Pfannenstiel incision) either pre-conceptually or in early pregnancy.
>   - Laparoscopic insertion possible pre-conceptually.

> ✓ **Evidence base** Choice of cerclage
>
> In the absence of evidence to recommend either Shirodkar or McDonald cervical suture as superior over the other, the choice of technique is at the discretion and experience of the operating surgeon.
>
> There are no randomized controlled trials comparing the effectiveness of abdominal cerclage with transvaginal cerclage. Whilst a systematic review [21] of 13 case series and one controlled non-randomized trial showed a lower risk of delivery at less than 24 weeks in women with an abdominal cerclage in situ ($n=117$) compared with transvaginal cerclage ($n=40$), there was also a higher incidence (3.4% versus none) of serious operative complications.
>
> Consequently, with a lack of compelling evidence to convince clinicians of its superiority, and the small, albeit significant risk of morbidity associated, transabdominal cerclage should be reserved for judicious use in the appropriate patient. Further research in this area is needed.

> ✪ **Learning point** Post-cerclage follow-up
>
> Following insertion of an emergency cerclage, there is usually some degree of re-modelling of cervical tissue; transvaginal cervical assessment confirms this by a closed length above and below the suture. Post-operative upper cervical length (length above the stitch) is an independent predictor of outcome [22].
>
> Women can be managed with regular transvaginal ultrasound assessment post-cerclage insertion to ascertain the upper cervical length allowing clinicians to counsel women appropriately of impending preterm birth while instigating therapy with antenatal corticosteroids if indicated to decrease neonatal morbidity associated with respiratory distress syndrome.

At 24+0 weeks she received 2 doses of betamethasone 12 mg intramuscularly 24 hours apart, and was counselled by the neonatologist regarding gestation and specific risks of death and disability to the baby if it was to be premature. She enquired about the use of vaginal progesterone to prolong pregnancy.

> ✪ **Learning point** Antenatal corticosteroids
>
> - Respiratory distress syndrome is a complication of preterm birth (PTB) and is a leading cause of neonatal morbidity and mortality.
> - It is well established that antenatal corticosteroids to accelerate fetal lung maturation should be administered to women between 24 and 34 weeks' gestation with any symptoms of threatened preterm labour, as well as antepartum haemorrhage, preterm rupture of membranes, and any condition requiring elective preterm delivery.
> - A Cochrane systematic review demonstrated that the effect of steroid treatment is optimal if the baby is delivered more than 24 hours and less than seven days after the start of treatment [23].
> - Robust data on the benefit of steroid administration over 28 days before preterm delivery is lacking.
> - Although frequent practice amongst many clinicians, there is increasing evidence that the administration of repeated doses of steroids may be beneficial in terms of fetal lung function but may have adverse effects on brain function and fetal growth.

> ❝ **Expert comment**
>
> The use of antenatal corticosteroids to reduce respiratory morbidity is one of the few interventions to improve fetal mortality in obstetrics. The timing maybe critical, as if given too soon (<24 hours before delivery) or too late (>14 days) may not be as effective. There are concerns that repeat courses may be harmful, and these do reduce fetal growth marginally. Predictive tests for delivery therefore maybe useful in targeting steroids, particularly as the combination of a long cervix and a negative fetal fibronectin has a very high negative prediction. Less than 1% of preterm women will deliver in two weeks with a negative fetal fibronectin and cervix >25 mm, even if contracting. Steroids could be withheld in most of these women.

✪ Learning point Vaginal progesterone to prevent preterm birth

Physiologically, progesterone is responsible for maintaining myometrial quiescence during pregnancy. As a result, it has been advocated in the prevention of preterm birth in singleton pregnancies. The evidence supporting the optimum dose, agent, timing, and effects on short- and long-term maternal and neonatal outcomes (including adverse effects) is, however, limited.

- A Cochrane systematic review revealed that progesterone (intramuscular and vaginal administration) was associated with a significant reduction in preterm birth < 34 weeks (one study; 142 women; risk ratio (RR) 0.15; 95% confidence interval (CI) 0.04–0.64) and preterm birth at less than 37 weeks (four studies; 1255 women; RR 0.80; 95% CI 0.70–0.92) [24].
- A systematic review and meta-analysis of individual patient data (n=775) in 2012 revealed that vaginal progesterone administration to women with a sonographically short cervix < 25 mm was associated with a significant reduction in the risk of preterm birth < 33 weeks (12.4% versus 22.0%; RR 0.58; CI 0.42–0.80) [25].
- Further UK trials are ongoing.

❝ Expert comment

Prolonging gestation does not necessarily result in improved fetal outcome. Use of vaginal progesterone can be considered in women with a short cervix, but studies confirming longer-term benefit to the neonate to justify such practice are awaited.

She was discharged from hospital at 28 weeks, however she was readmitted at 28+6 with lower abdominal pain and PV discharge. On arrival, she had mild but palpable contractions, approximately once every 10 minutes. She was afebrile and otherwise well. On speculum, the os was closed, stitch was visible, and clear liqour was seen pooling in the vagina. Fetal lie was longitudinal and cephalic, cardiotocograph (CTG) was normal, as were maternal inflammatory markers and white cell count. Contractions steadily increased in frequency over the next hour and the decision was taken to remove the cervical stitch.

➕ Clinical tip Removal of cervical stitch

- A transvaginal cervical cerclage should be removed at 37 weeks in the absence of labour.
- A Macdonald (low cervical) suture is usually removed without anaesthetic, via speculum examination and cutting of the suture knot with sterile scissors. Grasping the knot with sponge holding forceps may make this easier.
- The incidence of difficulty in removing a cervical suture is 1% [26].
- A high vaginal (Shirodkar) suture needs removal under spinal anaesthetic.
- If a woman is symptomatic for preterm labour it must be removed before labour becomes established to prevent cervical trauma.
- Whilst PPROM is not an indication for stitch removal in itself, a clinical diagnosis of chorioamnionitis is a clinical indication for stitch removal.

Five hours after the stitch was removed, a live male infant weighing 1005g was delivered vaginally without complication. The infant was born in good condition and was transferred to NICU on nasal continuous positive airways pressure (nCPAP). He remained on nCPAP for two weeks and did not require intubation. He received parenteral nutrition whilst slowly establishing enteral breastmilk feeds. He had one episode of central-line sepsis, for which he received 5 days' intravenous antibiotics and the line was removed. He was discharged, in air and fully breastfeeding at 35 weeks' corrected gestational age. Serial cranial ultrasounds performed at the bedside demonstrated a small unilateral germinal matrix haemorrhage in the first days of life. This resolved on subsequent scans and his ultrasound at term was normal. Neurological examination at term was gestation appropriate.

❝ Guest expert comment (neonatology)

This describes a typical course for a baby born at 28–29 weeks gestation. Despite the use of exogenous surfactant being shown to increase survival and to reduce the incidence of chronic lung disease, many centres attempt to avoid intubation and mechanical ventilation in moderately preterm infants as this can also reduce respiratory morbidity.

> **❝ Guest expert comment (neonatology)**
>
> Breastmilk is a vital component of neonatal nutrition. Children who are preterm are at increased risk of necrotizing enterocolitis (NEC) and sepsis. Formula milk increases the risk of NEC significantly. All mothers should be encouraged to express as soon as they are able after birth. Following discharge, these infants will be seen in follow-up clinics until at least two years corrected age. They have increased healthcare utilization during childhood. Some of the more subtle developmental and behavioural difficulties may not present until later in childhood and into secondary education.

Histology report of the placenta demonstrated the presence of acute infective changes (infiltration of polymorphonuclear leucocytes) though no organism was cultured.

> **❝ Guest expert comment (neonatology)**
>
> Chorioamnionitis and sepsis are associated with adverse outcomes for preterm infants. At 27–28 weeks, survival is 78–88% [27, 28]. Maternal chorioamnionitis may lead to increased fetal mortality [29]. Additionally, those infants exposed to chorioamnionitis are more likely to have cerebral palsy compared to their peers [30]. In particular, they may have periventricular white matter changes, which are often not evident at birth and may only evolve with time. Despite improvement in neonatal survival at all gestations, there is still a significant burden of long-term neurodisability, which has remained relatively constant. It is possible to have an adverse neurological outcome with a normal-term cranial ultrasound.

Discussion

Although the insertion of a rescue suture has become common practice among some clinicians, considerable controversy exists as to the benefit of such an intervention, and significant variation in practice exists both within and between tertiary centres, with some clinicians advocating the routine use of rescue cerclage, and others favouring expectant management of such women.

Such variation in practice has been maintained by the lack of robust evidence to support or refute the placement of a rescue cerclage in these women. There are concerns that, as compared with an ultrasound indicated elective cerclage, the degree of dilatation and exposure of fetal membranes to vaginal micro-organisms, which subsequently stimulates the inflammatory process resulting in miscarriage or severe preterm delivery, may be independent of pathology causing dilatation initially. Thus, there is concern that any further intervention, such as the placement of a cerclage, may result in further inflammation and delivery at a lower gestation than would have happened with expectant management.

With advanced degrees of dilatation, insertion of a cervical suture must be done after lengthy consideration that reaching viability with an intervention may inadvertently result in an increase in overall morbidity. With the insertion of a cerclage, there is also the possibility of intra-operative complications including rupture of membranes, infection, and bleeding. Thus it is speculated that insertion of a rescue suture may result in earlier miscarriage or, at later gestations, the survival of a more damaged baby, either by virtue of lower gestational age, or by the increased risk of chorioamnionitis and neonatal sepsis.

A Final Word from the Expert

The high-risk nature of exposed fetal membranes at pre-viable gestations will often justify action with little evidence of benefit. This is probably warranted given the anecdotal evidence of extremely poor outcome without action. Observational data showing some good outcome with action, suggest the need for larger controlled trials, which should include longer-term outcomes. For such a common condition, with such potential for substantive long-term and costly morbidity, it is surprising that there is such little evidence in this area. New tests to diagnose *in utero* inflammation, such as cytokines (IL6), will soon be commercially available, and may aid in targeting such interventions. As always, more research is needed, however, all clinicians need to engage with this process and be brave enough to enroll their patients if we are really going to improve outcomes in the future.

References

1. Crane JM, Delaney T, Hutchens D. Transvaginal ultrasonography in the prediction of preterm birth after treatment for cervical intraepithelial neoplasia. *Obstet Gynecol* 2006;107(1):37–44

2. Castanon A, Brocklehurst P, Evans H, Peebles D, Singh N, Walker P, *et al.* PaCT Study Group. Risk of preterm birth after treatment for cervical intraepithelial neoplasia among women attending colposcopy in England: retrospective-prospective cohort study. *BMJ* 2012;345:e5174.

3. Goldenberg RL, Iams JD, Mercer BM, Meis PJ, Moawad AH, Copper RL, *et al.* The preterm prediction study: the value of new vs standard risk factors in predicting early and all spontaneous preterm births. NICHD MFMU Network. *Am J Public Health* 1998; 88(2): 233–8.

4. Guzman ER, Walters C, Ananth CV, O'Reilly-Green C, Benito CW, Palermo A, *et al.* A comparison of sonographic cervical parameters in predicting spontaneous preterm birth in high-risk singleton gestations. *Ultrasound Obstet Gynecol* 2001;18:204–10.

5. Owen J, Yost N, Berghella V, Thom E, Swain M, Dildy GA 3rd, *et al.* National Institute of Child Health and Human Development, Maternal-Fetal Medicine Units Network. Mid-trimester endovaginal sonography in women at high risk for spontaneous preterm birth. *JAMA* 2001;286:1340–8.

6. Watson WJ, Stevens D, Welter S, Day D. Observations on the sonographic measurement of cervical length and the risk of premature birth. *J Matern Fetal Med* 1999;8:17–19.

7. Berghella V, Tolosa JE, Kuhlman K, Weiner S, Bolognese RJ, Wapner RJ. Cervical ultrasonography compared with manual examination as a predictor of preterm delivery. *Am J Obstet Gynecol* 1997;177:723–30.

8. Andrews WW, Copper R, Hauth JC, Goldenberg RL, Neely C, Dubard M. Second-trimester cervical ultrasound: associations with increased risk for recurrent early spontaneous delivery. *Obstet Gynecol* 2000;95:222–6.

9. Heath VC, Southall TR, Souka AP, Elisseou A, Nicolaides KH. Cervical length at 23 weeks of gestation: prediction of spontaneous preterm delivery. *Ultrasound Obstet Gynecol* 1998; 12(5): 312–17.

10. Hassan, SS, Romero, R, Berry, SM, Dang, K, Blackwell, SC, Treadwell, MC, *et al.* MDa Patients with an ultrasonographic cervical length ≤15 mm have nearly a 50 % risk of early spontaneous preterm delivery *Am J Obstet Gynecol* 2000; 182(96): 1458–67

11. Peaceman AM, Andrews WW, Thorp JM, Cliver SP, Lukes A, Iams JD, *et al.* Fetal fibronectin as a predictor of preterm birth in patients with symptoms: a multicenter trial. *Am J Obstet Gynecol* 1997; 177(1): 13–18.

12. Shennan A, Jones G, Hawken J, Crawshaw S, Judah J, Senior V, *et al*. Fetal fibronectin test predicts delivery before 30 weeks of gestation in high-risk women, but increases anxiety. *BJOG* 2005; 112(3): 293–8.

13. Berghella V, Hayes E, Visintine J, Baxter JK. Fetal fibronectin testing for reducing the risk of preterm birth. *Cochrane Database Syst Rev* 2008, Oct 8;(4): CD006843.

14. Abbott DS, Radford SK, Seed PT, Tribe RM, Shennan AH. Evaluation of a quantitative fetal fibronectin test for spontaneous preterm birth in symptomatic women. *Am J Obstet Gynecol* 2013 Feb; 208(2): 122.e1–6.

15. Royal College of Obstetricians and Gynaecologists. Cervical Cerclage: Green-top Guideline. 2011.

16. Berghella V, Odibo AO, To MS, Rust OA, Althuisius SM. Cerclage for short cervix on ultrasonography: meta-analysis of trials using individual patient-level data. *Obstet Gynecol* 2005;106:181–9.

17. Owen J, Hankins G, Iams JD, Berghella V, Sheffield JS, Perez-Delboy A, *et al*. Multicenter randomized trial of cerclage for preterm birth prevention in high-risk women with shortened midtrimester cervical length. *Am J Obstet Gynecol* 2009;201:375 e1–8.

18. MRC/RCOG Working Party on Cervical Cerclage. Final report of the Medical Research Council/Royal College of Obstetricians and Gynaecologists multicentre randomised trial of cervical cerclage. *Br J Obstet Gynaecol* 1993; 100(6): 516–23.

19. Althuisius SM, Dekker GA, Hummel P, van Geijn HP. Cervical incompetence prevention randomized cerclage trial: emergency cerclage with bed rest versus bed rest alone. *Am J Obstet Gynecol* 2003 Oct; 189(4): 907–10.

20. Cockwell HA, Smith GN. Cervical incompetence and the role of emergency cerclage. *J Obstet Gynaecol Can* 2005; 27(2): 123–9.

21. Zaveri V, Aghajafari F, Amankwah K, Hannah M. Abdominal versus vaginal cerclage after a failed transvaginal cerclage: a systematic review. *Am J Obstet Gynecol* 2002;187:868–72.

22. Groom KM, Shennan AH, Bennett PR. Ultrasound-indicated cervical cerclage: Outcome depends on preoperative cervical length and presence of visible membranes at time of cerclage. *Am J Obstet Gynecol* 2002: 187(2); 445–9.

23. Roberts D, Dalziel S. Antenatal corticosteroids for accelerating fetal lung maturation for women at risk of preterm birth. *Cochrane Database of Syst Rev* 2006, Issue 3. Art. No. CD004454.

24. Dodd JM, Flenady V, Cincotta R, Crowther CA. Prenatal administration of progesterone for preventing preterm birth in women considered to be at risk of preterm birth. *Cochrane Database Syst Rev* 2006 Jan 25;(1): CD004947.

25. Romero R, Nicolaides K, Conde-Agudelo A, Tabor A, O'Brien JM, *et al*. Vaginal progesterone in women with an asymptomatic sonographic short cervix in the midtrimester decreases preterm delivery and neonatal morbidity: a systematic review and meta-analysis of individual patient data. *Am J Obstet Gynecol* 2012 Feb; 206(2): 124.e1–19.

26. MRC/RCOG Working Party on Cervical Cerclage. Final report of the Medical Research Council/Royal College of Obstetricians and Gynaecologists multicentre randomised trial of cervical cerclage. *Br J Obstet Gynaecol* 1993;100:516–23.

27. Larroque B, Bréart G, Kaminski M, Dehan M, André M, Burguet A, *et al.*, on behalf of the Epipage study group. Survival of very preterm infants: Epipage, a population based cohort study. *Arch Dis Child Fetal Neonatal Ed* 2004;89:F139–F144.

28. Acolet D, Elbourne D, McIntosh N, Weindling M, Korkodilos M, Haviland J, *et al*. Project 27/28: Inquiry Into Quality of Neonatal Care and Its Effect on the Survival of Infants Who Were Born at 27 and 28 Weeks in England, Wales, and Northern Ireland. *Pediatrics* 2005; 116; 1457.

29. Lau J, Magee F, Qiu, Z, Houbé J, Von Dadelszen P, Lee SK. Chorioamnionitis with a fetal inflammatory response is associated with higher neonatal mortality, morbidity, and

resource use than chorioamnionitis displaying a maternal inflammatory response only. *Am J Obstet Gynecol* 2005;193:708–13.

30. Soraisham AS, Trevenen C, Wood S, Singhal N, Sauve R. Histological chorioamnionitis and neurodevelopmental outcome in preterm infants. *Journal of Perinatology* 2013;33:70–5.

Early-onset fetal growth restriction

Lisa Story and Sze Jean Wang

ⓘ Expert Commentary Ed Johnstone
ⓘ Guest Expert Commentary Neil Marlow

Case history

A 25-year-old Caucasian woman booked into antenatal care at 10 weeks' gestation. Her only previous obstetric history was a miscarriage at eight weeks' gestation, one year prior to the current pregnancy. She had no previous medical history of note and was not on any regular medication. She was a regular smoker, but declined referral to the NHS smoking cessation service at booking. Body mass index was 22.4, blood pressure was 105/56, and no abnormalities were detected in the routine pregnancy blood tests, or urine analysis. Prenatal screening for aneuploidy was declined and a dating scan confirmed the menstrual date-calculated gestation.

At 19 + 1 weeks' gestation, a routine anomaly scan was performed, demonstrating a fetus that was globally small with all measurements (biparietal diameter [BPD], head circumference [HC], abdominal circumference [AC], and femur length [FL]) below the 5th centile. No anatomical abnormalities were detected. Further assessment was performed at the regional tertiary fetal medicine centre confirming previous findings. In addition to a grossly abnormal placenta (that was enlarged, irregular, and occupying 50 % of the uterine cavity), bilateral notched uterine artery Doppler's and absent umbilical artery end-diastolic flow were found (Figure 9.1). An amniocentesis was performed revealing a normal male karyotype 46XY. The differential diagnosis was severe early-onset fetal growth restriction (FGR) or genetic abnormality. A poor prognosis was given and termination of pregnancy offered, but the patient elected to continue the pregnancy.

✪ Learning point Aetiology of FGR

FGR may be divided into maternal, fetal, and placental causes.

Fetal causes of FGR

- Genetic abnormalities are associated with 5–20 % of cases of FGR.
  - Trisomies 18 and 13, can result in growth restriction through a reduction in the number of small muscular arteries in the tertiary stem villi of the placenta [1].
  - Single-gene disorders, partial chromosomal deletions, specific placental mosaics, and uniparental disomy have all also been associated with abnormal fetal growth [1].
  - A reduction in growth velocity is also a common finding in fetal infections, accounting for 10 % of cases of FGR. Examples include cytomegalovirus, rubella, syphilis, toxoplasmosis, and malaria [2].

(continued)

Maternal causes of FGR

- Smoking
- Prenatal smoking is strongly correlated with low birthweight and FGR [3]. This effect is also noted with other maternal conditions that cause a reduction in oxygen-carrying capacity including lung disease, anaemia, cyanotic heart disease, and life at high altitude [1].
- Pre-eclampsia (as described)
- Pre-existing maternal disease, e.g. autoimmune, vascular.

Placental causes of FGR

- Compromised supply of nutrients and oxygen through the placenta.

A compromised supply of nutrients and oxygen through the placenta to the fetus is the commonest cause of FGR; this has been reported to account for up to 90% of cases [4]. Placental dysfunction results in a reduction in fetal cell size and is associated with another pregnancy specific condition, pre-eclampsia. This is a multi-system disease and can result in increased systemic vascular resistance, increased platelet aggregation, endothelial dysfunction, and activation of the coagulation system [5]. Early-onset pre-eclampsia is often association with fetal growth restriction as the two conditions share common pathophysiology [5].

❝ Expert comment

The association between FGR and thrombophilia is unclear. Specific genetic mutations leading to a maternal thrombophilic state resulting in an increased risk of placental thrombosis [6]. However, a meta-analysis found there was a statistically significant association only between factor V Leiden and FGR, and this was in case control studies only [6]. Further research needs to be undertaken to assess true associations between thrombophilia and FGR to eliminate the effects of publication bias.

❝ Expert comment

Always check agreement with previous dating scan measurements and menstrual dates when presented with globally small fetuses in the mid-trimester. Chromosomal or genetically abnormal pregnancies are often small by the first trimester, but this is often not appreciated and the menstrual dates are wrongly changed. This can cause great confusion later, particularly if fetuses are symmetrically small. Abnormal uterine and umbilical artery Doppler waveforms have a poor positive predictive value for FGR at 18–20 weeks' gestation; however, the converse of this is that normal uterine and umbilical artery Doppler waveforms have a good negative predictive value for severe early-onset FGR due to placental failure. This means that these additional tests can be helpful before the third trimester. Examination of the placenta can also be useful and a depth >4 cm and diameter <10 cm may be associated with FGR [9].

✚ Clinical tip Establishing cause

When early-onset FGR is identified, an amniocentesis should be offered to establish the fetal karyotype as well as screening maternal blood for intrauterine infection. If the history is suggestive, screening for maternal thrombophilias may be considered. Smoking cessation advice should be offered as there are significant improvements in outcome for women who stop smoking in early pregnancy, and likely dose response effects on pregnancy outcome at all gestations [7]. In addition to FGR, abnormal placentation is also associated with pre-eclampsia and placental abruption [8].

The patient continued to undergo close surveillance, although it was explained that the baby was not expected to attain a viable weight. She underwent weekly ultrasound scans of viability, and growth measurements were taken fortnightly. During this period, the fetus continued growing under the fifth centile, with normal amniotic fluid volume (AFI) and intermittent absent end-diastolic flow (EDF) in the umbilical artery.

At 29 weeks, the fetus was estimated to weigh 509 g and fetal circulatory assessment via Doppler ultrasound was instituted on a weekly basis. The results initially

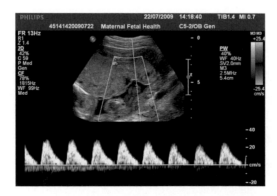

Figure 9.1 Grossly thickened and irregular placenta occupying more than 50% of the uterine cavity in association with absent umbilical end-diastolic flow at 19 weeks' gestation.

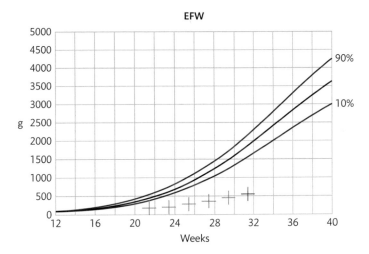

Figure 9.2 Estimated fetal weight (EFW) chart of the monitored fetus described. Severe early-onset FGR is associated with declining growth velocity and increasing deviation from the mean, as demonstrated here.

showed normal middle cerebral artery and ductus venosus (DV) wave patterns, but this deteriorated; at 31 + 4 weeks the ductus venosus 'a' wave became absent. Estimated fetal weight at this gestation was 530 g (Figure 9.2). Betamethasone was administered over 24 hours and a live male infant weighing 520 g was delivered by planned lower segment caesarean section, as the baby was unlikely to tolerate labour. The baby was transferred to the neonatal unit and the woman made an uneventful recovery from the operation.

✪ Learning point Ultrasound findings in FGR

Where abnormal placentation has occurred, abnormal vascularisation with maladaptation of the uterine spiral arteries and failure of trophoblast development results in deficient blood supply and inadequate nutrient and oxygen transfer to the fetus. These physiological maladaptations correlate with a number of ultrasound findings.

● Uterine artery notching and raised resistance index (RI)

Failure of spiral artery remodelling correlates with uterine artery notching, and abnormal trophoblast development correlates with raised resistance progressing to absent or reversed end-diastolic flow in the umbilical arteries, thus both of these changes are frequently seen with FGR pregnancies [10].

● Arterial and venous Dopplers

Abnormal placentation may lead to decreased fetal oxygen availability and hypoxia. As these changes are generally chronic, the fetus has some ability to compensate which can be detected by changes in blood flow in the arterial and venous umbilical artery Dopplers.

● Middle cerebral artery pulsatility index

The primary compensation in response to fetal hypoxia is to redistribute oxygenated blood towards the cerebral circulation. This is achieved by cerebral vasodilatation and is reflected in the decreased middle cerebral artery (MCA) pulsatility index (PI) [8].

● Fetal abdominal circumference

In response to hypoxia, the fetus increases the proportion of oxygen-rich blood going from the umbilical vein to the right atrium, by altering the diameter of the ductus venosus [11]. This occurs at

(continued)

the cost of blood reaching the portal circulation. Clinically this is expressed in the form of reduced fetal liver (and consequently abdominal circumference) growth velocity.

● Reversal of the ductus venosus 'a' wave

As the disease progresses, and the fetus becomes increasingly hypoxic, due to the build-up of lactic acid decreasing myocardial activity, a reversal of the DV 'a' wave becomes apparent. Evidence suggests that analysis of the DV waveform effectively identifies those preterm FGR fetuses that are at high risk for adverse outcome (particularly stillbirth) and this is a more accurate predictor of perinatal outcome compared to umbilical or middle cerebral artery measurements alone [12].

⊘ **Landmark trial** Growth restriction intervention trial (GRIT)[13]

The timing of delivery is controversial in FGR. The risks of continuation of the pregnancy and heightened risk of intra-uterine death have to be weighed against preterm delivery and risks of neonatal complications. The GRIT study aimed to evaluate this by assessing the effect of early delivery to pre-empt terminal hypoxia versus delaying delivery to prolong gestation. Fetuses ranged from 24–36 weeks, and the median length of delay was 4.9 days in the delay group, and 0.9 days in the immediate group. However, results showed a lack of difference in overall mortality between the immediate and the delay group (10% versus 9% mortality) [13].

❝ **Guest expert comment (neonatology)**

GRIT demonstrated that there was no benefit in delaying versus immediate delivery in situations where the obstetrician had doubt about management. Not only was there no difference in mortality but also there was also no difference in two-year [29] or school-age outcomes for survivors [30]. More recent publications from a small study have suggested that short-term outcomes for fetal growth restriction delivered < 30 weeks may not be as bad as originally thought [14], although there is a high rate of neonatal chronic lung disease [14], and long-term outcomes remain impaired [15]. More recent data still suggest that for pregnancies presenting 26–32 weeks with FGR, mortality is low (7%) and severe neonatal morbidity may be as low as 25% [31]. Given the improving situation for such pregnancies it is important that babies are delivered in as good condition as possible.

❝ **Expert comment**

There is no clear consensus on how frequently patients with below-viability estimated weights in the third trimester should be seen, but although there is often a sense of hopelessness around the outcomes of such pregnancies, it is extremely difficult to predict outcome. As a result clinicians should remain open-minded in such circumstances, and provide as much support and scan time as is practicable. Even though most such pregnancies will have poor outcomes, developing a good relationship with the patient at this stage can make reaching management decisions in the future much easier for all parties.

Three months following delivery, the patient returned to the obstetric clinic for review. Her thrombophilia profile was normal. Future pregnancies were discussed and she was counselled that the risk of FGR in future pregnancies was around 25%. It was recommended that she take pre-conceptional folic acid 400 mcg and aspirin 75 mg, starting in the first trimester of her next pregnancy.

❝ **Expert comment**

It is worth noting that the studies included in the meta-analysis demonstrating reduction in FGR associated with aspirin use were performed in women at risk of pre-eclampsia. It is unclear what benefit aspirin has in preventing IUGR in the absence of coexisting risk factors.

★ **Learning point** FGR recurrence

● The recurrence rates for severe early-onset FGR are high and should not be underestimated, estimated at 22–28% [23–25].
● Prophylactic aspirin started early in the pregnancy is recommended: the largest and most recent meta-analysis suggesting clear benefit (Reduction in FGR RR 0.44, 95% CI 0.30–0.65, incidence 7% treated versus 16.3% control [16].
● Periconceptional folic acid reduces the incidence of neural tube defect (NTD) formation, but recent evidence suggests that it may also ameliorate some of the harmful effects on fetal growth of smoking [17]. It should therefore be strongly recommended to high-risk, smoking women, and continued past the first trimester (when its use for NTD prevention ceases).

Unfortunately, following a long period of care on the NICU and various complications of prematurity and growth restriction, the baby boy died aged 5 months and 6 days, following an episode of sepsis.

> ✪ **Learning point** Outcome of FGR fetuses
>
> - FGR is associated with significant morbidity and mortality, the severity of which correlates to the degree of *in utero* compromise [18].
> - Many pregnancies with FGR are delivered preterm, which independently confers significant morbidity and mortality. There is some debate as to the extra morbidity from FGR.
> - A meta-analysis has shown that FGR fetuses are at a fifteenfold increase risk of intra-uterine death [19].
> - The severity of FGR is directly related to an increase risk of fetal demise; fetuses with absent or reversed end-diastolic flow on antenatal Doppler velocimetry having higher mortality rates [20]. This is independent of gestational age [21].
> - If survival beyond the antenatal period occurs there is also a significantly increased risk of neonatal death [19].
> - Growth restricted fetuses are susceptible to intrapartum asphyxia, particularly if vaginal delivery occurs due to transient interruptions to blood supply during labour which is poorly tolerated by the FGR fetus with poor reserves [18].
> - Preterm (less than 37 weeks' gestation) FGR fetuses tend to have lower Apgar scores at birth, and depending upon severity of FGR, there is increased risk of complications such as intracranial haemorrhage, sepsis, necrotising enterocolitis, and bronchopulmonary dysplasia compared with appropriately grown preterm babies ($p<0.01$) [19].
> - FGR neonates are at increased risk of hypoglycaemia and polycythaemia [18].
> - The risk of complications decreases with advancing gestation; however, FGR fetuses are still at risk of perinatal complications even at later gestations.

> ❝ **Guest expert comment (neonatology)**
>
> FGR is associated with an increased risk of nosocomial infection, and is associated with low neonatal granulocyte levels. However, attempts to reduce the risk with granulocyte macrophage colony stimulating factor (GM-CSF) have not been successful [22]. FGR confers an increased risk of gut ischemia and necrotizing enterocolitis, but again this is difficult to quantify and inconsistent in a range of studies. Newer strategies such as the use of early colostrum feeding, slow advancement of breastmilk feed volumes, and the use of probiotics, may be effective in reducing this risk.

The patient subsequently booked with her third pregnancy at 8 + 4 weeks' gestation, less than a year after her previous caesarean section. She was still smoking and her BMI had increased to 27. Her booking bloods were normal and blood pressure was 116/56. She was taking folic acid 400 mcg and was started on oral aspirin, 75 mg daily. An early dating scan at 9 + 4 weeks' showed crown–rump length (CRL) in agreement with menstrual dates.

At 14 + 4 weeks', an ultrasound scan performed revealed that the AC and femur length (FL) of the fetus were below the fifth centile, while the BPD and HC were between the fifth and tenth centile. EDF of the umbilical artery was negative and there was notching in both the right and left uterine artery.

Serum screening for Down syndrome was performed at 15 + 6 weeks' which revealed a raised alpha fetoprotein (αFP) level. Ultrasound biometry showed that both the BPD and HC had now dropped below the fifth centile, and there was once again evidence of a global severe FGR. The placenta was also noticed to be bulky. Although the raised αFP level was most likely due to severe FGR there was still a possibility of a chromosomal disorder (calculated risk 1:35 from mid-trimester serum screening). As a result she was offered an amniocentesis. Termination of pregnancy was also offered in view of previous history and poor outcome, but this was declined. Amniocentesis was performed which revealed a normal 46XX karyotype.

She had close surveillance between 19 weeks and 31 weeks, and once again growth remained below the fifth centile with abnormal uterine and umbilical artery Dopplers. At 32 weeks' gestation the DV waveform once again became abnormal, betamethasone was administered and a live female infant weighing 688 g was delivered.

Despite developing similar complications to her brother, she was discharged from NICU after a three-month stay. Initial development was within normal limits for an infant born at this weight and gestation, but between 12–24 months of age, weight gain fell behind expected centiles, and although the child remains to have a definitive diagnosis, initial assessment by clinical geneticists suggests a form of primordial dwarfism is present.

Discussion

FGR is an obstetric condition associated with significant morbidity and mortality. Although placental causes account for the largest proportion, karyotype and genetic abnormalities and congenital infections should also be considered, and testing offered where appropriate, particularly when onset is early.

Monitoring should be undertaken using fetal biometry, with intervals of at least two weeks to assess growth, and interim Doppler and liquor assessment where indicated. The timing of delivery and intensity of surveillance is governed by the individual clinical scenario as well as the gestation of the pregnancy. When delivery is thought to be imminent, prior to 34 weeks, steroids should be administered to facilitate fetal lung maturity. Due to the fact there is a high association of FGR with pre-eclampsia, close surveillance of women should be undertaken to monitor not only fetal growth but maternal blood pressure and urinalysis, especially in cases where uterine artery Dopplers have also been abnormal.

Patients should be counselled that there is an increased risk of recurrence of FGR in future pregnancies. Lifestyle modifications such as smoking cessation should be encouraged, and folic acid should be started pre-conceptually and aspirin in early pregnancy. Subsequent pregnancies should be considered high risk and consequently, care should be consultant-led with increased surveillance of both the mother and fetus.

A Final Word from the Expert

At the current time it is difficult to provide accurate counselling information to patients presenting with severe early-onset FGR. After excluding aneuploidy, gross fetal abnormality, and infection it is sensible to observe growth over a two-week period as typically placental failure will usually demonstrate a significant decline in growth velocity during this time. In the absence of such decline, it is very difficult to predict long-term outcome, and parents and health professionals are left with the very difficult and highly individual choice as to whether to continue pregnancy or not. Improvements in prenatal diagnostic testing will most likely aid this situation in the next decade, but fundamentally better longer-term follow-up studies of this rare, but significant problem are required.

The baby with FGR faces a range of neonatal challenges, the risk of which really depends on the condition of the baby at the time of birth; where there is acute fetal deterioration with abnormal CTG variability and poor ductus venosus Doppler flows, the baby is likely to be in poorer condition and develop significant respiratory disease, and is at high risk of developing necrotising enterocolitis. Where the baby is delivered more electively, the risk of these conditions seems to be less and modern neonatal care provides a good chance of neonatal survival without major morbidity.

Although the short-term outcomes are of immediate interest, it is important to understand the longer-term issues for babies born after FGR [26, 27]. The literature is confusing for babies born SGA and very restricted for babies born after well-documented FGR. In essence, there is increased risk of cerebral palsy at low weights for gestation and of cognitive impairment from a range of studies. Among longitudinal studies of babies born very preterm identified using fetal assessment with FGR, the studies are small but there is evidence of a significant reduction in mean cognitive scores [26], and thus an increased risk of learning difficulties, although the numbers studied are too small to be quantified. The issues with impaired childhood lung function [28] relate to the sequelae of neonatal bronchopulmonary dysplasia. There is a general risk increase for cardiovascular disease in adult life but this remains unquantified for babies born after abnormal fetal growth.

References

1. Hendrix N, Berghella V. Non-placental causes of intrauterine growth restriction. *Semin Perinatol* 2008;32(3):161–5.
2. Luesley DM, Baker PN (eds.) *Obstetrics and Gynaecology An Evidence-Based Text for MRCOG*. RCOG: London, 2004.
3. Wang X, Zuckerman B, Pearson C, Kaufman G, Chen C, Wang G, *et al.* Maternal cigarette smoking, metabolic gene polymorphism, and infant birth weight. *JAMA* 2002;287(2):195–202.
4. Bauer R, Walter B, Brust P, Füchtner F, Zwiener U. Impact of asymmetric intrauterine growth restriction on organ function in newborn piglets. *Eur J Obstet Gynecol Reprod Biol* 2003;110 Suppl 1:S40–9.
5. Sibai B, Dekker G, Kupferminc M. Pre-eclampsia. *Lancet* 2005;365(9461):785–99.
6. Facco F, You W, Grobman W. Genetic thrombophilias and intrauterine growth restriction: a meta-analysis. *Obstet Gynecol* 2009;113(6):1206–16.
7. Bickerstaff M, Beckmann M, Gibbons K, Flenady V. Recent cessation of smoking and its effect on pregnancy outcomes. *Aust N Z J Obstet Gynaecol* 2012;52(1):54–8.

8. Dikshit S. Fresh look at the Doppler changes in pregnancies with placental-based complications. *J Postgrad Med* 2011;57(2):138–40.

9. Toal M, Keating S, Machin G, Dodd J, Lee Adamson S, *et al.* Determinants of adverse perinatal outcome in high-risk women with abnormal uterine artery Doppler images. *Am J Obstet Gynecol* 2008;198(3):330 e1–7.

10. Espinoza J, Romero R, Mee Kim Y, Kusanovic JP, Hassan S, Erez O, *et al.* Normal and abnormal transformation of the spiral arteries during pregnancy. *J Perinat Med* 2006;34(6):447–58.

11. Kiserud T, Jauniaux E, West D, Ozturk O, Hanson MA. Circulatory responses to maternal hyperoxaemia and hypoxaemia assessed non-invasively in fetal sheep at 0.3-0.5 gestation in acute experiments. *BJOG* 2001;108(4):359–64.

12. Baschat AA, Gembruch U, Harman CR. The sequence of changes in Doppler and biophysical parameters as severe fetal growth restriction worsens. *Ultrasound Obstet Gynecol* 2001;18(6):571–7.

13. When do obstetricians recommend delivery for a high-risk preterm growth-retarded fetus? The GRIT Study Group. Growth Restriction Intervention Trial. *Eur J Obstet Gynecol Reprod Biol* 1996;67(2):121–6.

14. Brodszki J, Morsing E, Malcus P, Thuring A, Ley D, Marsál K. Early intervention in management of very preterm growth-restricted fetuses: 2-year outcome of infants delivered on fetal indication before 30 gestational weeks. *Ultrasound Obstet Gynecol* 2009;34(3):288–96.

15. Morsing E, Gustafsson P, Brodszki J. Lung function in children born after foetal growth restriction and very preterm birth. *Acta paediatrica* 2012;101(1):48–54.

16. Bujold E, *et al.* Prevention of preeclampsia and intrauterine growth restriction with aspirin started in early pregnancy: a meta-analysis. *Obstet Gynecol* 2010;116(2 Pt 1):402–14.

17. Bakker R, Timmermans S, Steegers EA, Hofman A, Jaddoe VW. Folic acid supplements modify the adverse effects of maternal smoking on fetal growth and neonatal complications. *J Nutr* 2011;141(12):2172–9.

18. Pallotto EK, Kilbride HW. Perinatal outcome and later implications of intrauterine growth restriction. *Clin Obstet Gynecol* 2006;49(2):257–69.

19. Damodaram M, Story L, Kulinskaya E, Rutherford M, Kumar S. Early adverse perinatal complications in preterm growth-restricted fetuses. *Aust N Z J Obstet Gynaecol* 2011;51(3):204–9.

20. Kramer MS, Olivier M, McLean FH, Willis DM, Usher RH. Impact of intrauterine growth retardation and body proportionality on fetal and neonatal outcome. *Pediatrics* 1990;86(5):707–13.

21. Divon MY, Haglund B, Nisell H, Otterblad PO, Westgren M. Fetal and neonatal mortality in the postterm pregnancy: the impact of gestational age and fetal growth restriction. *Am J Obstet Gynecol* 1998;178(4):726–31.

22. Marlow N, Morris T, Brocklehurst P, Carr R, Cowan FM, Patel N, *et al.* A randomised trial of granulocyte-macrophage colony-stimulating factor for neonatal sepsis: outcomes at 2 years. *Arch Dis Child Fetal Neonatal Ed* 2013;98(1):F46–53.

23. Morris RK, Cnossen JS, Langejans M, Robson SC, Kleijnen J, ter Riet G, *et al.* Serum screening with Down's syndrome markers to predict pre-eclampsia and small for gestational age: systematic review and meta-analysis. *BMC Pregnancy Childbirth* 2008;8:33.

24. Beta J, Bredaki FE, Rodriguez Calvo J, Akolekar R, Nicolaides KH. Maternal serum alpha-fetoprotein at 11-13 weeks' gestation in spontaneous early preterm delivery. *Fetal Diagn Ther* 2011;30(2):88–93.

25. Gagnon A, Wilson RD, Audibert F, Allen VM, Blight C, Brock JA, *et al.* Obstetrical complications associated with abnormal maternal serum markers analytes. *J Obstet Gynaecol Can* 2008;30(10):918–49.

26. Morsing E, Asard M, Ley D, Stjernqvist K, Marsál K. Cognitive function after intrauterine growth restriction and very preterm birth. *Pediatrics* 2011;127(4):e874–82.

27. Walker DM, Marlow N. Neurocognitive outcome following fetal growth restriction. *Arch Dis Child Fetal Neonatal Ed* 2008;93(4):F322–5.

28. Morsing E, Gustafsson P, Brodszki J. Lung function in children born after foetal growth restriction and very preterm birth. *Acta Paediatr* 2012;101(1):48–54.

29. Thornton JG, Hornbuckle J, Vail A, Spiegelhalter DJ, Levene M. Infant wellbeing at 2 years of age in the Growth Restriction Intervention Trial (GRIT): multicentred randomised controlled trial. *Lancet* 2004;364(9433):513–20.

30. Walker DM, Marlow N, Upstone L, Gross H, Hornbuckle J, Vail A, *et al.* The Growth Restriction Intervention Trial: long-term outcomes in a randomized trial of timing of delivery in fetal growth restriction. *Am J Obstet Gynecol* 2011;204(1):34 e1–9.

31. Lees C, Marlow N, Arabin B, Bilardo CM, Brezinka C, Derks JB, *et al.* Perinatal morbidity and mortality in early-onset fetal growth restriction: cohort outcomes of the trial of randomized umbilical and fetal flow in Europe (TRUFFLE). *Ultrasound Obst Gyn* 2013;42(4):400–8.

10 Dilemmas of preterm birth

Danielle Abbott

ⓘ **Expert Commentary** Andrew Shennan
ⓘ **Guest Expert** Neil Marlow

Case history

A 32-year-old primiparous British Asian woman, presented to the assessment unit at 27 + 1 week gestation, with a history of clear fluid draining vaginally and intermittent lower back pain. At the time of booking at 11 weeks' gestation, she had a BMI of 22, was a non-smoker and considered low-risk. Her booking bloods, combined screening test, and anomaly scan were all normal.

On examination she was afebrile with a blood pressure of 105/77, and her pulse was 73 beats per minute. Her abdomen was soft and non-tender and the fetus was palpated as lying longitudinally and cephalic. A speculum examination revealed clear liquor draining from the cervix. A cardiotocograph (CTG) was performed and was assessed as normal.

She was admitted to hospital with a diagnosis of preterm prelabour rupture of membranes (PPROM). Dexamethasone 12 mg imtramuscularly and erythromycin 250 mg bd orally was prescribed. Blood tests on admission revealed a C-reactive protein (CRP) of 8 and white cell count (WCC) of 9.1. A high vaginal swab (HVS) grew no demonstrable pathogens. Inpatient monitoring to detect presence of clinical chorioamnionitis was commenced which included four-hourly observations and twice-weekly blood tests for markers of inflammation. Fetal ultrasound confirmed oligohydramnios (Figures 10.1 and 10.2) and an estimated fetal weight (EFW) of 1.1 kg.

⊗ **Learning point** Preterm prelabour rupture of fetal membranes

- Preterm prelabour rupture of the fetal membranes (PPROM) is defined as the rupture of the amniotic membranes with release of the amniotic fluid more than 1 hour prior to the onset of labour prior to 37 weeks' gestation.
- PPROM occurs in 2% of pregnancies and is associated with 30–40% of preterm deliveries [1–3].
- The causes of PPROM are likely to be multifactorial with recognized associations between ascending infection from the the genital tract and subclinical chorioamnionitis. The three main causes of neonatal death associated with PPROM are prematurity, sepsis, and pulmonary hypoplasia (associated with oligohydramnios).
- Theoretical concerns about abruption are rarely reported [4].
- Around one-third of women with PPROM have positive amniotic fluid culture, although the prevalence of infection is likely to be underestimated [5].
- Women with intra-uterine infection associated with PPROM deliver earlier than those without infection [6].

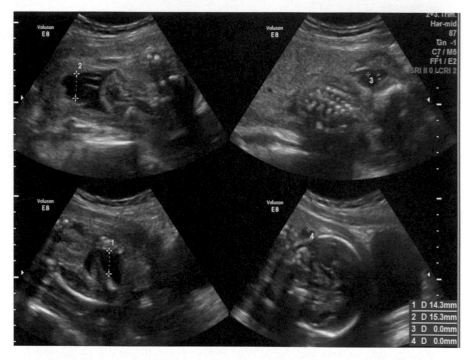

Figure 10.1 Severe oligohydramnios in 2nd trimester consistent with PPROM.

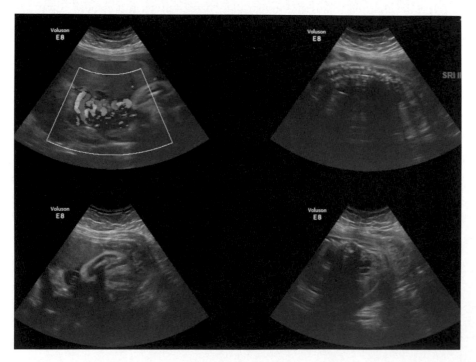

Figure 10.2 Severe oligohydramnios in 3rd trimester consistent with PPROM.
Note, the measurements for amniotic fluid index (AFI) includes the vertical pockets of amniotic fluid which does not contain umbilical cord or fetal parts. With thanks to Dr Surabhi Nanda at St Thomas' Hospital for supplying the images

⭐ **Learning point** Diagnosis of PPROM

The diagnosis of PPROM is made by a combination of clinical suspicion, patient history, and some simple tests. The presence of a pool of fluid in the vagina during a sterile speculum examination is highly suggestive of amniotic fluid and rupture of membranes. A range of historic tests have been used to confirm rupture of membranes including Nitrizine (which detects a change in pH) and ferning tests (characteristic ferning of the crystalline pattern of dried amniotic fluid) with a sensitivity of 90% for detection of amniotic fluid [13].

Commercial tests include Amnisure™, a rapid immunoassay which detects the presence of placental α-microglobulin-1(PAMG-1), which is accurate in the diagnosis of ruptured membranes with a sensitivity and specificity of 98.9% and 100% respectively [14], and Actim PROM™, which detects insulin-like growth factor binding protein-1 [15]. Comparative studies of the two in clinical settings are limited with small numbers, but it appears PAGM-1 may be more accurate [16]. Use of these tests in the NHS setting is limited by cost, and interest has turned to a pantyliner (which uses Nitrizine to turn amniotic fluid blue) which has a sensitivity of 98% and costs around £1.50 [17]. Ultrasound findings of oligohydramnios with an amniotic fluid index (AFI)≤10 cm may confirm a diagnosis with sensitivity and specificity values of 89.2% and 88.5% respectively [18].

➕ **Clinical tip** Monitoring after PPROM

Monitoring after PPROM is focused on the detection of clinical chorioamnionitis, due to its maternal and fetal implications. Symptoms include abdominal pain, fever, and offensive vaginal discharge. Signs include maternal and fetal tachycardia, pyrexia, uterine tenderness, leucocytosis, and rising inflammatory markers.

Maternal temperature, pulse, and fetal heart rate should be monitored every four to eight hours. Since positive genital tract cultures predict around half of positive amniotic fluid cultures with a false positive rate of 25%, weekly culture of high vaginal swabs from the vagina should not be routinely performed [10]. Given the poor sensitivities (< 50%) and false-positive rates (8%) for leucocytosis in the detection of clinical chorioamnionitis, blood tests should be taken and interpreted judiciously [7, 8, 9].

Regular fetal auscultation/cardiotocography is recommended, since a fetal tachycardia predicts around 20–40% of cases of intra-uterine infection, although this is often a late sign [11, 12].

❝ **Expert comment**

In the case of a good clinical history and positive speculum finding, such tests to detect rupture of membranes are probably unnecessary. Whether they may help in the context of an equivocal case is less clear [18]. We currently do not have a test which can reliably tell us if the baby is infected. Risk–benefit is related to infection versus prematurity. Some commercial companies are developing point-of-care markers such as inflammatory cytokines which may help us in the future. These should pre-date clinical symptoms and potentially make the management far safer.

➕ **Clinical tip** Digital vaginal examination

When PPROM is suspected, digital vaginal examination should be avoided to help prevent transfer of vaginal micro-organisms to the cervix and sterile uterine cavity, prostaglandin release, and potential preterm labour. A study of 271 women demonstrated that the latency interval between rupture of membranes and delivery was significantly shorter after vaginal examination than if speculum examination alone was performed [20].

🔘 **Landmark trial**

Broad-spectrum antibiotics for preterm pre-labour rupture of fetal membranes: the ORACLE I randomized trial [21]

- A large multi-centre randomized controlled trial (RCT) of 4826 women (with no clinical evidence of infection) admitted with PPROM <37 weeks' to co-amoxiclav + erythromycin, co-amoxiclav + placebo, erythromycin + placebo, or placebo only.
- The primary outcome measure was a composite of neonatal death, chronic lung disease, or major cerebral abnormality on ultrasonography before discharge from hospital.

(continued)

⊕ **Clinical tip** Erythromycin in PPROM

The Royal College of Obstetricians and Gynaecologists (RCOG) UK Green-top Guidelines recommend that erythromycin be given for 10 days following diagnosis of PPROM [22].

Results

○ Fewer infants whose mothers were randomized to erythromycin had the composite primary outcome than those allocated to placebo (12.7% versus 15.2%, p = 0.08).

○ Co-amoxiclav only and co-amoxiclav + erythromycin had no benefit over placebo with regard to this outcome.

○ Women randomized to erythromycin had reduced chance of delivery within seven days from randomization.

○ Although co-amoxiclav only and co-amoxiclav + erythromycin were associated with prolongation of pregnancy, they were also associated with a significantly higher rate of neonatal necrotizing enterocolitis (NEC).

⊘ Landmark trial

Broad spectrum antibiotics for spontaneous preterm labour ORACLE II [23]

● Multi-centre RCT randomizing 6295 women with suspected spontaneous preterm labour with intact membranes and no evidence of clinical infection to co-amoxiclav + erthryomycin, co-amoxiclav + placebo, erythromycin + placebo, or placebo only.

● The primary outcome measure was a composite of neonatal death, chronic lung disease, or major cerebral abnormality on ultrasonography before discharge from hospital.

Results

○ None of the trial antibiotics were associated with a lower rate of the composite primary outcome compared with placebo.

○ A non-significant increase in the rate of NEC in women prescribed co-amoxiclav was noted.

○ Seven-year follow-up of the infants in this trial revealed that the prescription of erythromycin (with or without co-amoxiclav) was associated with an increase in the proportion of children with any level of functional impairment and cerebral palsy [24].

❝ Guest expert comment (neonatologist)

The later outcomes for ORACLE give valuable insight into the effects of perinatal interventions at an age when most people are not really concerned about the relationship with perinatal care. It is critical that we continue to monitor long-term outcomes for the babies of women enrolled in trials designed to prolong pregnancy for just the reasons demonstrated by the study discussed. It is also important to remember that because ORACLE was such a large study, it was able to detect these differences although on a secondary analysis. These important effects may be small and missed in smaller studies.

❝ Expert comment

Very preterm birth (<32 weeks') is commonly associated with infection and micro-organisms usually gain access to the sterile uterine cavity by ascending from the vagina. It would seem logical to use antibiotics to treat this insult and thereby reduce preterm birth and improve outcome.

However, certain antimicrobials have been linked to adverse events. ORACLE I showed that co-amoxiclav was associated with an increased risk of neonatal necrotizing enterocolitis, and thus erythromycin became the preferred choice for women with preterm ruptured membranes [21]. However, the increased use of erythromycin has been linked to a substantial increase in antibiotic resistance. Follow-up of participants in the ORACLE II found an increased risk of cerebral palsy at seven years in the children of women with intact membranes who received antibiotics for spontaneous preterm labour [24]. The theory is that treating women who may have subclinical infection could increase risk by masking this infection, so that the fetus has

(continued)

increased exposure to a hostile in utero environment. In addition, if infection goes undetected the need for an early delivery will be missed. Metronidazole has been associated with an increased risk of preterm delivery when given prophylactically to high-risk women [25], thus vaginally administered clindamycin may be a better choice for bacterial vaginosis. Finally, the effects of antibiotics on neonatal gut flora have been linked to immune intolerance and increases in allergy, although breastfeeding may help limit antibiotic induced abnormal colonization of the neonatal intestine [26].

🍴 Guest expert comment (neonatologist)

Once delivered, the conundrum posed by infection and preterm birth continues. We know that we can isolate ureaplasma urealyticum from the respiratory tract of many babies [27]. The relationship with ongoing lung disease and with ongoing inflammatory activation is not well understood, and treatment with conventional antibiotics such as erythromycin in conventional doses is ineffective in eradicating the organism or in the reduction of clinical symptoms. Better understanding of this relationship and its treatment offers the prospect for antenatal treatment and prevention of chronic lung disease and other sequelae.

✪ Learning point Pathophysiology of PPROM

Several major aetiologic factors have been linked to PPROM. These include:

- Maternal infection of the reproductive tract (bacterial vaginosis, trichomoniasis, gonorrhoea, chlamydia, and sub-clinical chorioamnionitis).
- Behavioural factors (smoking, substance abuse).
- Obstetric complications (multiple gestation, polyhydramnios, cervical weakness).
- Genetic (Ehlers-Danos syndrome, Marfans).

Weakening of the amniochorion extracellular matrix by collagen degradation is one of the key events leading to rupture of membranes. Contributing factors include the effects of bacterial metabolism and maternal or fetal host inflammatory response. Infection-induced activation of membrane matrix-specific enzymes (matrix metalloproteinases) is associated with membrane weakening and rupture.

Intra-uterine infection, as defined by positive amniotic fluid cultures, is demonstrated in around a third of women with PPROM, although this is likely to be an underestimate since not all pathogens are detected by conventional method of culture [28].

Positive amniotic fluid cultures are associated with preterm delivery, and increased neonatal morbidity including neonatal sepsis, respiratory distress syndrome, chronic lung disease, periventricular malacia, intraventricular haemorrhage, and cerebral palsy. This is thought to be a result of the 'fetal inflammatory syndrome', which occurs in the fetus in response to intra-amniotic infection; a syndrome which is associated with high levels if IL-6 (an inflammatory cytokine) within the fetus and severe neonatal morbidity [28].

🍴 Expert commentary

Screening for or treating women with abnormal vaginal flora such as bacterial vaginosis has no benefit [29]. Treatment seems to eradicate bacterial vaginosis but has no effect on preterm birth and its consequences, although the results of different studies vary; different trials have reported that treatment both extended and reduced gestational age at delivery. More research is needed to establish the factors related to benefit, including the populations to be screened, antimicrobials to be used, and the gestational age to target. Currently, the National Institute for Health and Clinical Excellence (NICE) does not recommend screening for bacterial vaginosis in pregnancy, even in women at high risk [30].

> ✪ **Learning point** Timing of delivery
>
> The decision to deliver or manage cases of PPROM expectantly is dependent upon an assessment of the risks of potential uterine infection versus the risks associated with prematurity.
>
> There have been a number of studies which evaluated maternal and neonatal outcome following expectant and immediate delivery [31–33]. Most have demonstrated benefits of expectant management for gestations less than 34 weeks, in the absence of infection or other obstetric or medical complications, a view that is supported by NICE guidance and RCOG Green-top Guidelines.
>
> Management of pregnancies complicated by PPROM between 34 and 37 weeks remains controversial; in light of a lack of significant neonatal benefit with prolongation of pregnancy until 37 weeks, early delivery may avoid the subsequent risk of chorioamnionitis. NICE and RCOG state that delivery should be considered at 34 weeks [34].
>
> The publication of a recent randomized controlled trial comparing induction of labour versus expectant management between 34 and 37 weeks included 536 women. The primary endpoint was neonatal sepsis. Neonatal sepsis occurred in 2.6% and 4.1% (non-significant) of the neonates born in the induction and the expectant management groups respectively. The authors concluded that this study, in addition to a recent meta-analysis, confirmed that induction of labour did not substantially improve pregnancy outcome when compared with expectant management [35, 36]. However, many methodological weaknesses exist within the available studies with insufficient power to detect meaningful measures of infant and maternal morbidity.
>
> **Management at home**
>
> There is currently insufficient published literature to make recommendations for monitoring and management at home. In one randomized study of home versus hospital management, latency period and gestational age of delivery were similar in both groups, with no significant difference in the number of chorioamnionitis or neonatal sepsis. However, in this study only 18% of women were eligible for randomization, and those randomized had an amniocentesis for gram stain and culture which differs from usual UK practice [35].

Two days later, Ms PS started to experience lower abdominal pain, and developed a foul-smelling vaginal discharge. She also developed a temperature of 38°C and felt unwell. A diagnosis of clinical chorioamnionitis was made, and a decision was made to deliver her by emergency caesarean section.

> ✪ **Learning point** Chorioamnionitis
>
> The definition of chorioamnionitis varies according to the diagnostic criteria. (1) Clinical, with the presence of typical clinical findings including maternal fever, abdominal tenderness, offensive liquor, or (2) histological, with microscopic evidence of infection (microabscesses, neutrophils, and macrophages) or inflammation on examination of the placenta, villi (villitis), and umbilical cord (funisitis).
>
> Clinical chorioamnionitis is the most common maternal complication associated with PPROM. The earlier the gestation of PPROM, the more likely it is that infection is the causative factor. Histological studies suggest that infection and inflammation of the intra-amniotic cavity and fetal membranes frequently precede PPROM. Furthermore, histological evidence of inflammatory changes is often noted adjacent to the site of membrane rupture. Chorioamnionitis is significantly associated with development of cerebral palsy [37]. Most scientists now believe that bacterial infection may initiate events, but ultimately it is the host inflammatory response which is responsible for PPROM and preterm labour.
>
> Despite the impact of histological chorioamnionitis and intra-amniotic infection on pregnancy outcome, the RCOG doesn't currently recommend performing routine amniocentesis to establish diagnosis prior to the onset of clinical chorioamnionitis, or fetal sepsis which may inevitably occur later, although this practice is more common in the USA [21].

> ✪ **Learning point** Delivery of the preterm infant
>
> The optimal mode of delivery of the preterm infant has remained a controversial point. Large robust randomized controlled trials in this area are lacking, making it more difficult to dictate clinical management accurately. In particular, evidence informing delivery of the breech infant cannot be extrapolated directly from the results of the Term Breech Trial, which as the title clearly states, involved term infants.
>
> The largest available study published in 2012 looked at 2885 small for gestational age (SGA), singleton, live-born, vertex neonates delivered between 25 and 34 weeks of gestation (known congenital anomalies and birth weight less than 500 g were excluded). Of these, 42.1% were delivered vaginally, and 57.9% were delivered by caesarean (non-randomized). There was no significant difference in intraventricular haemmorhage, subdural haemmorhage, seizure, or sepsis between the caesarean delivery and vaginal delivery groups. Caesarean delivery compared with vaginal delivery was associated with increased odds of respiratory distress syndrome (38). The authors concluded that ceasarean delivery was not associated with improved neonatal outcomes in preterm SGA newborns.
>
> This echoed findings of an earlier Cochrane review on randomized trials comparing a policy of planned immediate caesarean delivery versus planned vaginal delivery for preterm birth [39]. This included only 4 studies of 116 women and results showed that there was no significant difference between planned immediate caesarean section and planned vaginal delivery with respect to infant morbidity or mortality. Furthermore, mothers were more likely to experience major maternal postpartum complications in the group allocated to planned immediate caesarean section compared with the group randomized to vaginal delivery (RR 7.21, 95% CI 1.37–38.08; 4 trials, 116 women).

> ❝ **Expert comment**
>
> When a woman is in spontaneous preterm labour, it is essential for her and the obstetrician to discuss and clarify the optimal mode of delivery, in terms of her future well-being and that of the baby. This remains a difficult and controversial subject; current clinical guidelines state that prematurity is not an indication in itself for caesarean section. Mode of delivery and a decision regarding intrapartum monitoring should ideally be clearly documented in her plan of care to ensure continuity with on-call teams overnight or on weekends. The potential for a scarred uterus (possibly even classical), and survival with long-term handicap, must also be considered when proceeding with aggressive intervention in extremely preterm pregnancies.

The baby was born in good condition with Apgars of 10 at 1 minute and 10 at 5 minutes. The umbilical cord venous pH was 7.34, with base excess –4.9. Sadly, the baby died 14 days later. A postmortem did not reveal any specific cause, although the placental histology showed uteroplacental underperfusion with infarcted villi.

> ✪ **Learning point** Antibiotics in labour for Group B strep prophylaxis
>
> - Early-onset group B streptococcus (EOGBS) disease is the leading cause of serious neonatal sepsis in developed countries, affecting 0.5–3 babies per 1000 live births.
> - GBS is a common inhabitant of the bowel, from which it ascends from the perineum to the vagina. Carriage rates are around 38% of sexually active women. As a commensal, it rarely causes disease in healthy adults, but if transmitted to the baby during labour, it can lead to invasive disease.
> - The risk of developing EOGBS during labour among infants born to colonized mothers is around 12 per 100 births, with a fatality rate of between 8% and 15% [40].
> - Prematurity (<34 weeks) is the greatest risk factor for death from GBS [40]. In these women the organism acts as a pathogen causing both maternal puerperal sepsis and neonatal septicaemia, either of which may lead to death.
> - The optimal screening method for identifying and treating at-risk women with GBS remains a controversial subject. Whilst the USA and Australia have written guidelines encouraging screening
>
> (continued)

> ➕ **Clinical tip** GBS prophylaxis
>
> The RCOG recommend prophylaxis in the presence of one or more of [45]:
>
> - a previous baby affected by GBS.
> - GBS bacteriuria in the current pregnancy.
> - preterm labour (and preterm rupture of membranes in established labour).
> - prolonged rupture of membranes.
> - pyrexia in labour.

[41], the UK remains hesitant to introduce population screening on the basis of lack of randomized controlled trials on the subject.
- The available studies on screening and treating have not demonstrated a reduction in all causes of neonatal mortality [42] and concerns exist about theoretical risks for the mother and baby including anaphylaxis and infection with resistant organisms.
- It is not possible to eradicate GBS, therefore therapy is aimed at those who are known to be carriers at the time of greatest risk (i.e. during delivery). There is evidence that prophylaxis started early in labour will prevent 75% of early-onset infection in the neonate [43, 44].

⭐ **Learning point** Magnesium sulphate to reduce risk of cerebral palsy

Antenatal maternal administration of magnesium sulphate has been shown to significantly reduce the incidence of cerebral palsy in premature neonates [46]. Magnesium sulphate is widely used in the prevention of eclampsia. It crosses the placenta and demonstrates neuro-protection in experimental studies. As an anti-oxidant it reduces pro-inflammatory cytokines and increases cerebral blood flow and prevents large fluctuations in blood pressure. A systematic review of five RCTs including 6145 babies showed that antenatal administration of magnesium sulphate before delivery under 34 weeks' gestation reduced the risk of cerebral palsy and gross motor dysfunction (RR 0.68; 95% (CI) 0.54–0.87) [46]. The impact of the neuroprotective effect was similar to that seen of steroids on mortality and intraventricular haemorrhage. (See Chapter 8 for more details on antenatal steroids). The largest trial to-date found no evidence of increasing risk of death with increasing dose. Magnesium sulphate can be given immediately before delivery. The number of women needed to treat in order to prevent one case of cerebral palsy is 63. The optimal mode of dosing and administration is not yet defined; the American College of Obstetricians and Gynecologists (ACOG) recommend a protocol based on available published data, and draft Australian College guidelines provide more detailed dosage recommendations. Recommended gestation for treatment is also yet to be confirmed; Australian National Clinical Practice Guidelines recommended MgSO4 only at <30 weeks' gestation, whereas the ACOG gave no official opinion was regarding a gestational age cut-off [47].

Discussion

Patient history has an accuracy of 90% for the diagnosis of PPROM so should not be ignored. The presence of fluid pooling at the os is usually diagnostic, but commercial tests are available for less clear cases. Subclinical intra-uterine infection has been implicated as a major aetiological factor in the pathogenesis of PPROM and the associated maternal and neonatal morbidity which may follow. Amniotic fluid infection is closely associated with fetal inflammation, and newborn and infant adverse events are intimately linked to this fetal inflammatory process. Clinical chorioamnionitis is present on admission in 1–2% of women who present with PPROM and subsequently develops in 3–8% of women. In the majority of cases amniotic fluid infection in the setting of PPROM does not produce the signs and symptoms traditionally used as diagnostic criteria for clinical chorioamnionitis.

The management aims of PPROM are to ensure a reduction in neonatal morbidity with attention to maternal well-being. Therapies are designed to prolong pregnancy and reduce neonatal morbidity without impacting upon maternal morbidity. Expectant management, use of erythromycin, antenatal corticosteroids, and maternal and fetal surveillance are currently suggested. Intra-uterine infection is an indication for delivery and a contraindication to expectant management. The benefits of intrapartum antibiotic prophylaxis for the prevention of early-onset group B streptococcal infection of the neonate are well established. Although robust evidence supports the use of antenatal magnesium sulphate for neuroprotection of the fetus prior to very preterm birth,

---

💬 **Expert comment**

It is almost impossible to conduct large prospective trials with rare neurological outcomes. The question is, is there sufficient evidence to routinely introduce this to all women likely to deliver seriously preterm. Once this has occurred, there will be no going back. One option would be to introduce the intervention nationally, on a regional basis, and audit its impact comparing those areas which have adopted its use, with those who have not. The NHS has a unique governance structure which will allow this.

💬 **Guest expert comment (neonatology)**

Although further trials on MgSO4 now seem unlikely, there remain unanswered questions including dose and target group. The NNT comes down significantly as the gestational age for inclusion gets more severe, because the rate of cerebral palsy increases with decreasing gestation. We also need to know whether the effect persists out into childhood. The developmental studies so far have stopped at two years, but one might anticipate that improved cognitive outcomes are likely in parallel to the reduction in prevalence of cerebral palsy.

there have been no published trials comparing different treatment regimens. Research still needs to be conducted to evaluate comparisons of different dosages and other variations in regimens, evaluating both maternal and infant outcomes [48]. Difficulty arises regarding the optimum gestational age for delivery, but delivery should occur when the risks of continuing with the pregnancy outweigh risk of immaturity.

A Final Word from the Expert

Infection and inflammation play a large part in the causal pathway to preterm delivery. However, strategies to prevent or treat this infection to prolong pregnancy or reduce morbidity in the baby have proved elusive.

Trials of antibiotics have proved valuable in the face of ruptured membranes and probably in the reduction of risk of group B streptococcal infection after birth, where acute infection is the target.

Spontaneous preterm labour without ruptured membranes seems to pose a real dilemma. ORACLE showed that this might be associated with increased prevalence of disability and cerebral palsy among survivors, possibly mediated through prolonging pregnancy in the face of ongoing infection/inflammation, which leads onto brain injury in the baby. Clearly this is an important consideration and leads to the conclusion that not all prolongation of pregnancy may be in the baby's best interests.

References

1. Maxwell GL. Preterm premature rupture of membranes. *Obstet Gynecol Surv* 1993;48:576–83.
2. Merenstein GB, Weisman LE. Premature rupture of the membranes: neonatal consequences. *Semin Perinatol* 1996;20:375–80.
3. Douvas SG, Brewer JM, McKay ML, Rhodes PG, Kahlstorf JH, Morrison JC. Treatment of premature rupture of the membranes. *J Reprod Med* 1984;29:741–4.
4. Test G, Levy A, Wiznitzer A, Mazor M, Holcberg G, Zlotnik A, Sheiner E. Factors affecting the latency period in patients with preterm premature rupture of membranes. *Arch Gynecol Obstet* 2011 Apr; 283(4):707–10.
5. Broekhuizen FF, Gilman M, Hamilton PR. Amniocentesis for gram stain and culture in preterm premature rupture of the membranes. *Obstet Gynecol* 1985;66:316–21.
6. Cotton DB, Hill LM, Strassner HT, Platt LD, Ledger WJ. Use of amniocentesis in preterm gestation with ruptured membranes. *Obstet Gynecol* 1984;63:38–43.
7. Ismail MA, Zinaman MJ, Lowensohn RI, Moawad AH. The significance of C-reactive protein levels in women with premature rupture of membranes. *Am J Obstet Gynecol* 1985;151:541–4.
8. Romem Y, Artal R. C-reactive protein as a predictor for chorioamnionitis in cases of premature rupture of the membranes. *Am J Obstet Gynecol* 1984;150:546–50.
9. Watts DH, Krohn MA, Hillier SL, Wener MH, Kiviat NB, Eschenbach DA. Characteristics of women in preterm labour associated with elevated C-reactive protein levels. *Obstet Gynecol* 1993;82:509–14.
10. Carroll SG, Papaioannou S, Ntumazah IL, Philpott-Howard J, Nicolaides KH. Lower genital tract swabs in the prediction of intrauterine infection in preterm prelabour rupture of the membranes. *Br J Obstet Gynaecol* 1996;103:54–9.

11. Carroll SG, Papiaoannou S, Nicolaides KH. Assessment of fetal activity and amniotic fluid volume in the prediction of intrauterine infection in preterm prelabor amniorrhexis. *Am J Obstet Gynecol* 1995;172:1427–35.

12. Ferguson MG, Rhodes PG, Morrison JC, Puckett CM. Clinical amniotic fluid infection and its effect on the neonate. *Am J Obstet Gynecol* 1995;151:1058–61.

13. Friedman ML, McElin TW. Diagnosis of ruptured fetal membranes, Clinical study and review of the literature. *Am J Obstet Gynecol* 1969;104:544–50.

14. Cousins LM, Smok DP, Lovett SM, Poelter DM. AmniSure placental alpha microglobulin-1 rapid immunoassay versus standard diagnostic methods for detection of rupture of membranes. *Am J Perinatol* 2005;22:317–20.

15. Rutanen EM, Kärkkäinen TH, Lehtovirta J, Uotila JT, Hinkula MK, Hartikainen AL. Evaluation of a rapid strip test for insulin-like growth factor binding protein-1 in the diagnosis of ruptured fetal membranes. *Clin Chim Acta* 1996 Sep 30; 253(1-2):91–101.

16. Tagore S, Kwek K. Comparative analysis of insulin-like growth factor binding protein-1 (IGFBP-1), placental alpha-microglobulin-1 (PAMG-1) and nitrazine test to diagnose premature rupture of membranes in pregnancy. *J Perinat Med* 2010 Nov; 38(6):609–12.

17. Mulhair L, Carter J, Poston L, Seed P, Briley A. Prospective cohort study investigating the reliability of the AmnioSense method for detection of spontaneous rupture of membranes. *BJOG* 2009 Jan; 116(2):313–8.

18. Birkenmaier A, Ries JJ, Lapaire O, Hösli I. Methods for the diagnosis of rupture of the fetal membranes in equivocal cases. *Eur J Obstet Gynecol Reprod Biol* 2012 Mar; 161(1):115–16.

19. Weissmann-Brenner A, O'Reilly-Green C, Ferber A, Divon MY. Values of amniotic fluid index in cases of preterm premature rupture of membranes. *J Perinat Med* 2009;37(3):232–5.

20. Lewis DF, Major CA, Towers CV, Asrat T, Harding JA, Garite TJ. Effects of digital vaginal examination on latency period inpreterm premature rupture of membranes. *Obstet Gynecol* 1992;80:630–4.

21. Kenyon SL, Taylor DJ, Tarnow-Mordi W; ORACLE Collaborative Group. Broad-spectrum antibiotics for preterm, prelabour rupture of fetal membranes: the ORACLE I randomised trial. *Lancet* 2001 Mar 31; 357(9261):979–88.

22. Royal College of Obstetricians and Gynaecologisrs. Green-top Guideline No. 44. Preterm Prelabour Rupture of Membranes. *October* 2010.

23. Kenyon SL, Taylor DJ, Tarnow-Mordi W; ORACLE Collaborative Group. Broad-spectrum antibiotics for spontaneous preterm labour: the ORACLE II randomised trial. ORACLE Collaborative Group. *Lancet* 2001 Mar 31; 357(9261):989–94.

24. Kenyon S, Pike K, Jones DR, Brocklehurst P, Marlow N, Salt A, *et al.* Childhood outcomes after prescription of antibiotics to pregnant women with spontaneous preterm labour: 7-year follow-up of the ORACLE II trial. *Lancet* 2008 Oct 11; 372(9646):1319–27.

25. Simcox R, Sin WA, Seed PT, Briley A, Shennan AH. Prophylactic antibiotics for the prevention of preterm birth in women at risk: a meta-analysis. *Aust N Z J Obstet Gynaecol* 2007;47:368–77.

26. Bedford Russell AR, Murch SH. Could peripartum antibiotics have delayed health consequences for the infant? *BJOG* 2006;113:758–65.

27. Turner MA, Jacqz-Aigrain E, Kotecha S. Azithromycin, Ureaplasma and chronic lung disease of prematurity: a case study for neonatal drug development. *Archives of disease in childhood* 2012;97(6):573–7.

28. DiGiulio DB, Romero R, Kusanovic JP, Gómez R, Kim CJ, Seok KS, *et al.* Prevalence and diversity of microbes in the amniotic fluid, the fetal inflammatory response, and pregnancy outcome in women with preterm pre-labor rupture of membranes. *Am J Reprod Immunol* 2010 Jul 1;64(1):38–57.

29. Nygren P, Fu R, Freeman M, Bougatsos C, Klebanoff M, Guise JM; US 10 Preventative Services Task Force. Evidence on the benefits and harms of screening and treating

pregnant women who are asymptomatic for bacterial vaginosis: an update review for the US Preventative Task Force. *Ann Intern Med* 2008;148:220–33.

30. National Institute for Health and Clinical Excellence. Antenatal care: routine care for the healthy pregnant woman. 2008. < http://www.nice.org.uk/Guidance/CG62 >

31. Mercer BM, Crocker LG, Boe NM, Sibai BM. Induction versus expectant management in premature rupture of the membranes with mature amniotic fluid at 32 to 36 weeks: a randomized trial. *Am J Obstet Gynecol* 1993 Oct; 169(4):775–82.

32. Cox SM, Leveno KJ. Intentional delivery versus expectant management with preterm ruptured membranes at 30-34 weeks' gestation. *Obstet Gynecol* 1995 Dec; 86(6):875–9.

33. Naef RW 3rd, Allbert JR, Ross EL, Weber BM, Martin RW, Morrison JC. Premature rupture of membranes at 34 to 37 weeks' gestation: aggressive versus conservative management. *Am J Obstet Gynecol* 1998 Jan; 178(1 Pt 1):126–30.

34. NICE Induction of Labour guidelines July 2008 < http://www.nice.org.uk/nicemedia/ live/12012/41255/41255.pdf >

35. Van der Ham DP, Vijgen SM, Nijhuis JG, van Beek JJ, Opmeer BC, Mulder AL, *et al*; on behalf of the PPROMEXIL trial group. Induction of Labor versus Expectant Management in Women with Preterm Prelabor Rupture of Membranes between 34 and 37 Weeks: A Randomized Controlled Trial. *PLoS Med* 2012 Apr; 9(4):e1001208.

36. Buchanan SL, Crowther CA, Levett KM, Middleton P, Morris J. Planned early birth versus expectant management for women with preterm prelabour rupture of membranes prior to 37 weeks' gestation for improving pregnancy outcome. *Cochrane Database Syst Rev* 2010 Mar 17;(3):CD004735.

37. Tita AT, Andrews WW. Diagnosis and management of clinical chorioamnionitis. *Clin Perinatol* 2010 Jun; 37(2):339–54.

38. Werner EF, Savitz DA, Janevic TM, Ehsanipoor RM, Thung SF, Funai EF, Lipkind. HS. Mode of delivery and neonatal outcomes in preterm, small-for-gestational-age newborns. *Obstet Gynecol* 2012 Sep; 120(3):560–4.

39. Alfirevic Z, Milan SJ, Livio S. Caesarean section versus vaginal delivery for preterm birth in singletons. *Cochrane Database Syst Rev* 2012 Jun 13;6:CD000078. doi: 10.1002/14651858. CD000078.pub2.

40. Kaambwa B, Bryan S, Gray J, Milner P, Daniels J, Khan KS, Roberts TE. Cost-effectiveness of rapid tests and other existing strategies for screening and management of early-onset group B streptococcus during labour. *BJOG* 2010 Dec; 117(13):1616–27.

41. Baker CJ, Byington CL, Polin RA. Committee on Infectious Diseases; Committee on Fetus and Newborn, Policy statement—Recommendations for the prevention of perinatal group B streptococcal (GBS) disease. *Pediatrics* 2011 Sep; 128(3):611–16.

42. Smaill F. Intrapartum antibiotics for group B streptococcal colonisation. *Cochrane Database Syst Rev* 2000;(2):CD000115.

43. Boyer KM, Gotoff SP. Prevention of early onset neonatal group B streptococcal disease with intrapartum chemoprophylaxis. *N Engl J Med* 1986;314:1665–9

44. Davies HD, Adair CE, Schuhcat A, Low DE, Sauve RS, McGeer A. Physician's prevention programme and incidence of neonatal group B streptococcal disease in 2 Canadian regions. *CMAJ* 2001;185

45. RCOG Greentop guidelines No. 36. Prevention of early onset neonatal Group B Streptococcus Infection. July 2012

46. Doyle LW, Crowther CA, Middleton P, Marret S, Rouse D. Magnesium sulphate for women at risk of preterm birth for neuroprotection of the fetus. *Cochrane Database Syst Rev* 2009 Jan 21;(1):CD004661.

47. Magee L, Sawchuck D, Synnes A, von Dadelszen P. SOGC Clinical Practice Guideline. Magnesium sulphate for fetal neuroprotection. *J Obstet Gynaecol Can* 2011 May; 33(5):516–29.

48. Bain E, Middleton P, Crowther CA. Different magnesium sulphate regimens for neuroprotection of the fetus for women at risk of preterm birth. *Cochrane Database Syst Rev* 2012, Feb 15.

Pulmonary hypertension in pregnancy

Ruth Curry

❶ **Expert Commentary** Philip Steer
❶ **Guest Expert** Lorna Swan

Case history

A 28-year-old nulliparous woman attended her local hospital at 10 weeks' gestation for her initial antenatal check in a midwife-led clinic. She was once told, at a school medical aged 12 years -old, that she had a heart murmur, but this had never been investigated. Prior to pregnancy she had been fit and well, although she had never enjoyed sports. She was not on any regular medication and had no family history of any medical problems. Because of her history, the midwife referred her to the consultant obstetrician who saw her at 16 weeks' gestation.

On auscultation of the heart she had an ejection systolic murmur; examination was otherwise unremarkable and a routine echocardiogram was requested. Because the echo was not requested urgently, it was not performed until 22 weeks' of gestation. It revealed a large atrioventricular septal defect (AVSD) with a large atrial component, a common atrioventricular valve and pulmonary hypertension (PH). She was subsequently referred urgently to the combined cardiac obstetric service at her local tertiary centre.

> ✪ **Learning point** Cardiac disease and pregnancy
>
> The incidence of heart disease during pregnancy in the UK has remained constant at 0.9% over several decades [1]. However, the recent UK Confidential Enquiries into Maternal and Child Health identified cardiac disease as the commonest cause of maternal death, with a maternal mortality rate in the triennium 2006–2008 of 23.1 per million maternities (up from 7.6 per million in the 1987–1990 enquiry) [2].
>
> There has been a progressive decline in deaths related to congenital cardiac disease (Table 11.1), with acquired cardiac diseases such as myocardial infarction, cardiomyopathy, and aortic dissection leading as the major cardiac causes of maternal death. Additionally, the 2003–2005 enquiry saw the first two deaths in the UK from rheumatic heart disease since the 1991–1993 triennium; both occurred in recent immigrants.

> ❝ **Expert comment**
>
> When unaccompanied by any other abnormality, an ejection systolic murmur is an entirely normal finding in pregnancy. It typically varies with posture and reflects increased stroke output.

Table 11.1 Pregnancy-related risks for women with congenital heart disease by specific lesion (Adapted from Uebing, *et al.,* 2006) [3]

Lesion	Exclude before pregnancy	Potential hazards	Recommended treatment during pregnancy and peripartum
Low-risk lesions			
Ventricular septal defects	Pulmonary hypertension	Arrhythmias Endocarditis (unoperated or residual defect)	
Atrial septal defects (unoperated)	Pulmonary hypertension Right heart failure	Arrhythmias Thromboembolic events	Thromboprophylaxis if bed-rest is required Consider low-dose aspirin during pregnancy
Coarctation (repaired)	Re-coarctation Aneurysm formation at site of repair (MRI) Associated lesion such as bicuspid aortic valve (with or without aortic stenosis or aortic regurgitation), ascending aortopathy Systemic hypertension Ventricular dysfunction	Pre-eclampsia (CoA is the only congenital heart lesion known as an independent predictor of pre-eclampsia) Aortic dissection Congestive heart failure Endarteritis	β-blockers if necessary to control systemic blood pressure Spontaneous vaginal delivery is usually recommended for these women but consider elective caesarean section before term in case of aortic aneurysm formation or uncontrollable systemic hypertension
Tetralogy of Fallot (repaired)	Residual right ventricular outflow tract obstruction Severe pulmonary regurgitation Right ventricular dysfunction Di George syndrome	Arrhythmias Right ventricular failure Endocarditis	Consider preterm delivery in the rare case of right ventricular failure
Moderate-risk lesions			
Mitral stenosis	Severe stenosis Pulmonary venous hypertension	Atrial fibrillation Thromboembolic events Pulmonary oedema	May require β-blockers Low-dose aspirin Consider bed-rest during third trimester with additional thromboprophylaxis
Aortic stenosis	Severe stenosis (peak pressure gradient on Doppler ultrasonography > 80 mmHg, ST segment depression, symptoms) Left ventricular hypertrophy or dysfunction	Arrhythmias Angina Endocarditis Left ventricular failure	Bed-rest during third trimester with thromboprophylaxis Consider balloon aortic valvotomy (for severe symptomatic valvar stenosis) or preterm caesarean section if cardiac decompensation ensues (bypass surgery carries 20% risk of fetal death)

Lesion	Exclude before pregnancy	Potential hazards	Recommended treatment during pregnancy and peripartum
Low-risk lesions			
Systemic right ventricle (TGA after atrial switch procedure, ccTGA)	Ventricular dysfunction Severe systemic atrioventricular valve regurgitation Bradyarrhythmias and tachyarrhythmias Heart failure (NYHA > II) Obstruction of venous pathways after atrial switch as venous blood flow significantly increases during pregnancy	Right ventricular dysfunction (potentially persisting after pregnancy) Heart failure Arrhythmias Thromboembolic events Endocarditis	Regular monitoring of heart rhythm Restore sinus rhythm in case of atrial flutter (cardioversion usually effective and safe) Alter afterload reduction therapy (stop ACE inhibitors; consider β-blockers) Low-dose aspirin (75 mg)
Cyanotic lesions without pulmonary hypertension	Ventricular dysfunction Other end-organ involvement	Haemorrhage (bleeding diathesis) Thromboembolic events Increased cyanosis Heart failure Endocarditis	Consider bed-rest and oxygen supplementation to maintain oxygen saturation and promote oxygen tissue delivery Thromboprophylaxis with low molecular weight heparin
Fontan-type circulation	Ventricular dysfunction Arrhythmias Heart failure (NYHA > II) Intra-cardiac clots	Heart failure Arrhythmias Thromboembolic complications Endocarditis Increasing cyanosis	Consider anticoagulation with low molecular weight heparin and aspirin throughout pregnancy Maintain sufficient filling pressures and avoid dehydration during delivery
High-risk lesions			
Marfan syndrome (unoperated)	Aortic root dilatation > 4 cm Severe mitral regurgitation Other aortic aneurysms	Dissection of aorta Heart failure	β-blockers in all patients Consider elective caesarean section when aortic root > 45 mm
Eisenmenger syndrome; other pulmonary hypertension	Ventricular dysfunction Arrhythmias	30–50% risk of death related to pregnancy Arrhythmia Heart failure Thromboembolic complications	Therapeutic termination should be offered If pregnancy continues, aggressive medical therapy with pulmonary dilator therapy, anticoagulation and supplementary oxygen should be considered Close monitoring necessary for > 10 days postpartum

✪ Learning point Cardiovascular changes in pregnancy

Pregnancy is associated with substantial physiological changes in the cardiovascular system which are poorly tolerated in women with PH (Figure 11.1). Systemic vascular resistance (SVR) falls to 70% of non-pregnant levels by eight weeks' gestation, secondary to a marked peripheral vasodilatation induced by both endocrine and local factors [4]. This state of relative vascular underfill is associated with a 50% increase in cardiac output (CO) and blood volume. Despite the increase in CO, a reduction in pulmonary vascular resistance (PVR) prevents any rise in pulmonary arterial pressure (PAP) [5].

In labour contractions, increase venous return by up to 500 ml as uterine blood returns to the circulating pool [6], with a consequent rise in CO by up to 20% [7]. A further rise in CO of 60–80% has been reported immediately after delivery [6], despite the concomitant blood loss, this rise being due to a sudden increase in venous return following relief of aorto-caval compression and from additional blood moving from the retracting uterus back into the systemic circulation. This can result in a substantial rise in ventricular filling pressures and stroke volume, and may lead to clinical deterioration in women with severe cardiac disease.

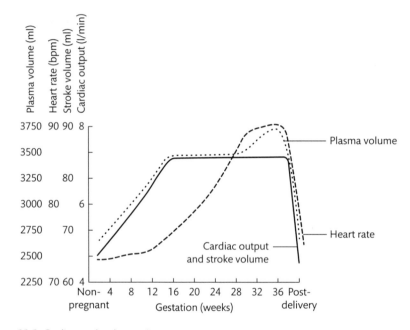

Figure 11.1 Cardiovascular changes in pregnancy.

Reproduced from *Heart*, Pregnancy in heart disease, SA Thorne, Vol. 90, No. 4 2004, with permission from BMJ Publishing Group Ltd.

✪ Learning point Planning antenatal care

- Any woman with a history of heart disease should be referred as soon as possible to a joint clinic attended by a consultant cardiologist, obstetrician, and anaesthetist with experience of caring for such patients in pregnancy.
- Risk assessment of the particular lesion must be performed and antenatal care planned accordingly, with low-risk women being returned to routine care.
- Poor functional class (NYHA III and IV), left heart obstruction, cyanosis, and presence of PH are associated with higher rates of maternal and fetal complications [8].

(continued)

- Higher-risk women should be seen regularly by an appropriately trained consultant obstetrician: the frequency of the visits and of further investigations (e.g. repeat echocardiography or Holter monitors) will be determined by the severity of the disease and the patient's symptoms.
- All women should have a baseline ECG and echocardiogram.
- Women with congenital heart disease should be referred for fetal echocardiography to screen for fetal cardiac anomalies. Serial fetal growth scans may be indicated in women with severe heart disease or cyanosis, or for those taking β-blockers.

➕ Clinical tip Assessment of the pregnant woman with cardiac disease

- At each visit the patient should be asked about breathlessness and the presence of palpitations or chest pain.
- Blood pressure should be measured manually with a sphygmomanometer, according to the guidelines of the British Hypertension Society [9].
- Measurement of the heart rate is best done by auscultation over the heart as the radial pulse is often difficult to detect, particularly in the presence of an arrhythmia; a rising pulse rate may be one of the first signs of cardiac decompensation.
- Auscultation of the heart sounds is important; a careful categorization of any murmurs present at the beginning of pregnancy is essential so that any changes can be evaluated appropriately.
- Auscultation of the lungs should be routine to check for any signs of pulmonary oedema.
- Cyanotic women should have their oxygen saturations checked with pulse oximetry.

➕ Clinical tip BP measurement

- The woman should be seated comfortably, relaxed against the back of her chair with her arm at the level of the left atrium.
- She should not be talking during measurement of the blood pressure as this may substantially elevate BP.
- At least 5 minutes should be allowed between entering the consultation room and taking the blood pressure, to allow a raised blood pressure due to exercise to settle.
- The obstetrician should be aware of the importance of the five Korotkoff sounds.
  - K5 (disappearance) rather than K4 (muffling) is now accepted as the most appropriate estimation of diastolic BP in pregnancy.
  - In pregnancy K5 may be much lower than K4, or even zero, in which case both K4 and K5 should be recorded separately.
  - BP should be measured to the nearest 2 mmHg, which means that the sphygmomanometer cuff pressure should only be reduced by 2 mmHg with each heartbeat.

⭐ Learning point Pulmonary hypertension (PH)

- PH is defined at cardiac catheterization as a mean pulmonary artery pressure (PAP) of greater than 25 mmHg at rest [10]. The causes are multifactorial (see Learning point: Classification of PH).
- In very large left-to-right shunts (e.g. ventricular septal defects), excess pulmonary blood flow may lead to progressive maladaptation in the pulmonary circulation and an increase in PVR.
- In its extreme form, pulmonary pressures equal or even exceed systemic pressures (Eisenmenger physiology) which may have a detrimental effect on right ventricular function (Figure 11.2).
- Women with PH with an already pressure-overloaded right ventricle may struggle to cope with the additional cardiovascular demands of pregnancy, and the fall in SVR may worsen the right to left shunt seen in Eisenmenger syndrome (Figure 11.2). The hormonal and haematological consequences of pregnancy are thought to be additional insults to the pulmonary circulation.
- Patients with PH tolerate pregnancy poorly, with the rate of functional deterioration increasing from the second trimester onwards, and the majority of deaths occurring within the first postnatal month, usually as a result of right heart failure.

(continued)

💬 Expert comment

A useful tip is for the obstetrician to collect the patient personally from the waiting area, and accompany her to the consultation room. This way, the obstetrician can observe how fast the woman can walk, and assess her pulse rate and respiratory frequency immediately upon sitting down in the consultation room (i.e. assess the effect of exercise). This emphasizes the importance of continuity of care, because even subtle changes in the woman's ability to walk comfortably can be detected provided that the same clinician is seeing her at each visit.

💬 Expert comment

The importance of taking accurate BP measurement cannot be over-emphasized. Detection of even small systematic changes in pressure, especially in the third trimester, is vital for the early detection of pre-eclampsia (which can have devastating consequences in women with severe cardiac disease), and for the detection of cardiac decompensation, especially if associated with a rising heart rate.

➕ Clinical tip Auscultation of the heart

- Heart sounds should be auscultated at each visit.
- Attention should be paid to the loudness and type of murmur (systolic or diastolic).
- The loudness of the murmur will often increase by up to one grade during pregnancy as a result of the increasing cardiac output.
- A sudden increase in volume may indicate pathology, e.g. the onset of bacterial endocarditis or the development of valve incompetence.
- Development of a new murmur, or significant changes from baseline, should be investigated further with urgent echocardiography.

⭐ **Learning point** Eisenmenger syndrome

Eisenmenger syndrome occurs when the pulmonary vascular resistance exceeds the systemic resistance and leads to reversal of a left to right shunt (usually an ASD or VSD), allowing deoxygenated blood to flow directly into the systemic circulation, with the result that the patient becomes hypoxic (Figure 11.2).

✚ **Clinical tip** Symptoms and signs of PH

- The major symptoms of PH are fatigue and breathlessness; these are initially mild but usually progress.
- Syncope and pre-syncope are ominous symptoms.
- Chest pain may occur due to RV ischaemia but is rare.
- There are usually few clinical signs in mild disease; a loud second heart sound may be present.
- Overt right heart failure with ankle oedema or ascites only occurs very late.
- Advanced PH is associated with tachycardia, elevated jugular venous pressure (JVP), right ventricular heave, tricuspid regurgitation, loud pulmonary component of the second heart sound, pulmonary regurgitation, hepatomegaly, ascites, and peripheral oedema.

💬 **Expert comment**

Women with long-established PH may have adjusted their lifestyle to cope with their limited exercise tolerance, and so history taking must be specific. If asked 'do you get short of breath climbing stairs', the woman may reply 'no', because she avoids stairs entirely. The correct question is 'how many steps can you climb without stopping because of breathlessness?'

- The increase in venous return at delivery may trigger severe pulmonary vasoconstriction, reducing the venous return to the left side of the heart still further and resulting in a fall in systemic blood pressure, which may be fatal despite vigorous attempts at resuscitation [11].

Unrestrictive VSD

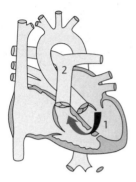 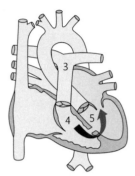

1. Large shunt from LV to RV
2. Excessive pulmonary blood flow

3. Progressive "damage" to pulmonary vasculature
4. Elevation of pulmonary artery & RV pressures
5. Pressure equalisation & reversal of shunt leading to desaturation

Figure 11.2 Diagram illustrating the progressive reversal of a left to right shunt and Eisenmenger syndrome.

The patient was reviewed the following week in the multidisciplinary clinic. Functionally she was well with no symptoms of shortness of breath, palpitations, chest pain, pre-syncope or syncope. Examination revealed a BP of 92/50 and pulse rate of 90 bpm. She had a soft systolic murmur and loud second heart sound. She had mild peripheral cyanosis but had no finger clubbing. Resting oxygen saturations were 92% in air.

⭐ **Learning point** Classification of PH

The World Health Organisation (WHO) updated the classification of PH in 2009 [12] as follows:

1. Pulmonary Arterial Hypertension (PAH)

   - Idiopathic (IPAH)

   - Heritable (HPAH)

   - Associated with connective tissue disorder (e.g. scleroderma), congenital heart disease (including Eisenmenger physiology), portal hypertension, HIV, drugs/toxins, persistent PH, or the newborn, among others

2. Pulmonary veno-occlusive disease (PVOD) or pulmonary capillary haemangiomatosis (PCH)

3. PH associated with left heart disease

4. PH associated with lung disease and/or hypoxaemia

5. PH due to chronic thrombotic and/or embolic disease (CTEPH)

6. PH with unclear multifactorial mechanisms—including sarcoidosis, splenectomy, vasculitis, neurofibromatosis among others

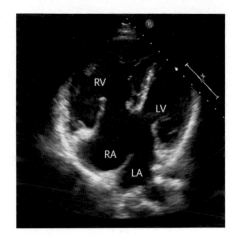

Figure 11.3 Echocardiogram demonstrating complete atrioventricular septal defect (AVSD) with common AV valve and large primum ASD, dilated right atrium, and right ventricle

(RA—right atrium; RV—right ventricle; LA—left atrium; LV—left ventricle).

⭐ **Learning point** NYHA classification of cardiovascular disease

The New York Heart Association (NYHA) classification of cardiovascular disease is one way of categorizing functional status in both pregnant and non-pregnant patients with cardiovascular disease:

Class I: Patients who are not limited by cardiac disease in their physical activity. Ordinary physical activity does not precipitate occurrence of symptoms such as fatigue, palpitations, dyspnoea, and angina.

Class II: Patients in whom the cardiac disease causes a slight limitation in physical activity. These patients are comfortable at rest, but ordinary physical activity will precipitate symptoms.

Class III: Patients in whom the cardiac disease results in a marked limitation of physical activity. They are comfortable at rest, but less than ordinary physical activity will precipitate symptoms.

Class IV: Patients in whom the cardiac disease results in an inability to carry on physical activity without discomfort. Symptoms may be present even at rest, and discomfort is increased by any physical activity.

It could be argued that many pregnant women fall into NYHA Class II, with symptoms such as mild exertional dyspnoea and palpitations being common in pregnancy.

❝ **Guest expert comment (cardiology)**

In the initial stages of PH, many patients are misdiagnosed as having asthma. A low threshold for requesting specialist echocardiography is therefore necessary if a woman complains of persistent breathlessness, especially if there is no wheeze on auscultation.

Repeat echocardiography by an expert in congenital heart disease confirmed the diagnosis of an atrioventricular septal defect with a large atrial component (ostium primum ASD) with a bidirectional shunt (Figure 11.3). Right ventricular systolic pressure (RVSP) was estimated at 90 mmHg. The right ventricle (RV) was significantly dilated but with preserved systolic function, and moderate right atrioventricular valve (RAVV) regurgitation. The main pulmonary artery (MPA) was dilated. Left ventricular (LV) function was good with only mild left atrioventricular valve (LAVV) regurgitation. The patient had a 6-minute walk test (6MWT) distance of 395 m, during which time her oxygen saturations fell from 91% to 76% in air.

❝ **Guest expert comment (cardiology)**

An echocardiogram and an ECG are usually sufficient to diagnose and follow cardiac patients during pregnancy. Other imaging modalities are easily accessible and are adjuvants in particular circumstances. For example, MRI is an excellent modality for imaging the aorta. However, for the

(continued)

majority of patients echocardiography provides a sufficiently full anatomical and physiological assessment.

Echocardiography during pregnancy is a particular skill and requires further specialist knowledge/training. The normal cardiovascular changes of pregnancy need to be fully understood and considered when describing echocardiographic appearances at varying gestations. Patients with complex congenital heart disease lesions are outwith the normal scanning repertoire of most imaging departments.

High-risk patients may require serial imaging. This has logistic implications in terms of ensuring continuity in terms of the expert echocardiographer and the equipment used. The most difficult and key component of echocardiography in these patients is the assessment of biventricular function and of pulmonary artery pressures.

Following review by three consultants (cardiology, obstetrics, and anaesthetics) in the combined cardiac obstetric clinic, the patient was quoted a 25–30% risk of maternal mortality or significant maternal morbidity during the pregnancy. The major risks were deemed to be of right heart failure, pulmonary hypertension crisis, significant thrombosis, and arrhythmia. The additional fetal risks were predominately related to prematurity and exposure to hypoxia. There would be a small but increased risk of congenital heart disease in the fetus (3–5% compared with the background UK incidence of 0.8% [3]). The option of terminating the pregnancy was discussed with the patient. However, this was not acceptable to her due to the relatively late gestation (now 23 weeks), and she elected to continue with the pregnancy despite a good understanding of the maternal and fetal risks described.

❝ Guest expert comment (cardiology)

Recent case series suggest that the outcomes of pregnancies in women with pulmonary hypertension are improving. This may be due to the widespread use of sildenafil to improve the function of the pulmonary vasculature, and the use of prostanoids such as Iloprost, and intravenous prostacyclin, as vasodilators.

❝ Guest expert comment (cardiology)

A patient with significant cyanotic congenital heart disease will usually have an elevated haemoglobin level as a compensatory mechanism for chronic hypoxia. This patient should have a haemoglobin of about 18 g/dL given her oxygen levels. The most common reason for not having an appropriately high haemoglobin is to have an incidental iron deficiency which limits erythropoesis.

⊘ Evidence base Maternal mortality in PH

Series studied in the 1990s reported a maternal mortality of 30–56% [13], probably due to the limited ability of women with PH to adapt to the cardiovascular changes of pregnancy. However, more recent data from a systematic review [11] and two case series [14,15] suggest that maternal mortality may in fact be lower, with reported rates of 10–25%. The time of highest risk appears to be in the early postnatal period [13], with refractory right heart failure reported as the commonest cause of death [11]. Current guidelines continue to recommend discouraging pregnancy, with use of maximally effective contraception and early termination should pregnancy occur [16, 17].

⊘ Evidence base Fetal outcomes in PH

Poor fetal outcomes have been well documented with high rates of preterm delivery (PTD) (85–100%), fetal growth restriction (FGR) (3–33%), and fetal/neonatal loss (7–13%) [11, 13, 17]. Cyanotic congenital cardiac disease is associated with a higher incidence of low birthweight infants compared to acyanotic congenital heart disease [18–20]. Maternal oxygen saturations below 85% are predictive of poor pregnancy outcome with a live birth rate of only 12% [21]. As a result of this hypoxaemia, there is a compensatory erythrocytosis which is independently related to birthweight below the fiftieth centile [21]. The fetal effects of cyanosis may be further exacerbated by the inability of the cardiac output to increase during pregnancy. The risks for both mother and baby are highest for those women in NYHA classes III and IV pre-pregnancy [8].

The patient was commenced on targeted pulmonary vasodilator therapy with sildenafil 20 mg tds. Ferrous sulphate 200 mg daily was prescribed because she had a significant anaemia with an Hb of 9.6 g/dL secondary to iron deficiency. Therapeutic low molecular weight heparin (enoxaparin 40 mg bd) was added due to the risks of paradoxical embolism, arrhythmia and the increased risk of thrombosis in pregnancy.

> ⭐ **Learning point** Treatment of PH
>
> Increasing understanding of the pathophysiology of PH has led to the introduction of advanced treatments for this condition including sildenafil, bosentan, and inhaled or infused prostacyclin analogues. All have produced symptomatic and functional benefit in non-pregnant patients. Moreover there is only a limited evidence base for the use of these therapies during pregnancy, although it is tempting to attribute the recent reduction in maternal mortality to their use [11].
>
> - *Sildenafil:* inhibits cGMP-specific phosphodiesterase type 5, decreasing the degradation of cGMP and leading to local release of nitric oxide and vasodilatation.
> - *Bosentan:* competitive antagonist of endothelin-1 at endothelin-A and endothelin-B receptors. It reduces pulmonary vascular resistance by blocking the action of endothelin-1 (which causes pulmonary vasoconstriction) at these receptors. Animal models have shown that bosentan has teratogenic effects and it is therefore contraindicated in pregnancy.
> - *Prostacyclins:* bind to endothelial prostacyclin receptors, increasing cAMP which activates protein kinase A (PKA), leading ultimately to smooth muscle relaxation and vasodilatation.

> ⭐ **Learning point** Thromboprophylaxis in PH
>
> Idiopathic pulmonary hypertension (iPH) is characterized by hypertrophy, vasoconstriction, and thrombus formation in the pulmonary microvasculature. Additionally, pregnancy is associated with a sixfold increase in thrombosis risk compared with age-matched non-pregnant controls (a risk which is doubled again in the immediate puerperium), which is further increased in Eisenmenger patients. There is also a risk of paradoxical embolism due to the right-to-left shunt and significant arrhythmias in these patients. Thus, thromboprophylaxis for these patients must be considered [11,22].

The patient was reviewed weekly by an obstetric consultant with experience of supervising women with heart disease in the antenatal clinic, and every other week by a cardiologist in the combined cardiac obstetric clinic. The patient's clinical progress was tracked by symptoms review, assessments of resting saturations and detailed assessment of ventricular function by regular echocardiography. Fetal echocardiography and anomaly scans were normal. Serial fetal growth scans demonstrated low growth velocity with abdominal circumference consistently between the fifth and tenth centile, but normal amniotic fluid volume and umbilical artery velocimetry. Screening for gestational diabetes showed normoglycaemia. The patient's anticoagulation was monitored with anti-Xa levels.

> 💬 **Expert comment**
>
> There is no evidence regarding the optimal anticoagulant regimens in Eisenmenger patients and uncertainty continues, especially in Eisenmenger patients in whom a balance must be struck between their thrombotic risk and an increased tendency to bleeding, particularly pulmonary haemorrhage.

> ⭐ **Learning point** Planning the delivery
>
> - Repeat multidisciplinary review should occur at 32–34 weeks' gestation to establish a plan of management for the delivery. This will include which personnel should be involved, the type of analgesia to be used, the mode of delivery, and if vaginal birth is to be attempted, the appropriate length of the active second stage.
> - Prophylaxis against postpartum haemorrhage should be discussed.
> - Postpartum management such as need for thromboprophylaxis, change in medications, high-dependency monitoring, and length of stay required in hospital, together with any immediate post-partum investigations such as echocardiography and the timing of postnatal cardiac and obstetric review will be decided.
> - These decisions should be recorded clearly in the medical notes.

As the pregnancy continued, the patient became progressively more breathless; by 29 weeks' gestation she could only just manage to walk up one flight of stairs and her resting oxygen saturations had fallen to 86 % on air. She was discussed at the weekly multidisciplinary team meeting, and plans were made for delivery at 34 weeks' gestation by elective caesarean section.

> **✪ Learning point** Mode of delivery
>
> The ideal mode of delivery for patients with PH continues to be uncertain [23, 24]. Vaginal delivery is in general associated with smaller haemodynamic changes and less risk of haemorrhage, infection, and venous thromboembolism than delivery by elective caesarean section [25]. Nevertheless, caesarean section may become necessary for a variety of reasons, both fetal (there is a high risk of fetal growth restriction with consequent poor tolerance of labour) and maternal (increasing respiratory difficulty or heart failure), and when performed in labour, may be associated with increased blood loss and rates of infection [25].
>
> Preterm induction of labour is often prolonged and is associated with a higher rate of emergency caesarean delivery than induction of labour at term. Elective caesarean section therefore offers the advantage of timing the delivery to ensure optimal conditions, not least in terms of making sure that senior and experienced staff are present at the birth, and that an ITU bed is available post-operatively.
>
> If a trial of vaginal delivery is considered appropriate, labour should not be induced unless for specific obstetric reasons or signs of cardiovascular decompensation (e.g. deterioration in symptoms, rising heart rate, deterioration of cardiac function on echocardiography), as spontaneous labour is generally more successful than induced labour. A prolonged active second stage of labour should be avoided, with a low threshold for assisted delivery and the length of active second stage determined by the individual patient's condition. The patient's gestation and previous obstetric history will influence the likelihood of a successful vaginal delivery and therefore the decision-making process regarding mode of delivery.

> **✪ Learning point** Pain relief in labour
>
> Haemodynamics are altered substantially during labour and delivery secondary to pain, anxiety and uterine contractions. Basal CO has been reported to increase by about 12% during labour with a further rise during contractions of up to 20% [26]. The magnitude of increase in CO during contractions increases as labour progresses. Pain and anxiety have a significant effect on both HR and blood pressure (BP). Both systolic and diastolic BP increase markedly during contractions, with even greater augmentation during the second stage of labour.
>
> These haemodynamic changes are greatly influenced by anaesthesia and analgesia. The painful stimulus during delivery can be effectively interrupted by blocking the T10 to L1 nerve roots before their entrance into the spinal cord (caudal, low epidural, or low subarachnoid blocks). Reduction of pain by epidural anaesthesia may limit the haemodynamic changes and the progressive rise in CO seen between contractions. Carefully administered, regional anaesthesia is probably safe in patients with severe cardiac disease, although the optimum mode of employment is not conclusively established.

> **❖ Expert comment**
>
> An advantage of general anaesthesia is that it allows the intra-operative monitoring of cardiac function with trans-oesophageal echocardiography (TOE). However, recent experience [11] suggests that slow incremental regional block may be preferable as it avoids the deleterious effects of positive pressure ventilation on post-operative respiratory function.

The patient underwent an uncomplicated lower segment caesarean section at 34 weeks under general anaesthesia. As the patient was deemed to be at particular risk this was performed in a cardiac centre, with both a cardiac and an obstetric anaesthetist, and access to advanced care (such as nitric oxide, assist devices, and extracorporeal membrane oxygenation ECMO) should it be required.

A female infant weighing 1484 g (fifth centile, gender-adjusted weight for gestational age) was delivered, with Apgar scores of 3 at 1 minute, and 6 at 5 minutes. The baby was subsequently transferred to neonatal intensive care (NICU). The uterus was atonic and so 2 Hayman uterine compression sutures were inserted, resulting in a much reduced rate of uterine bleeding. She was also given a low-dose syntocinon infusion of 10 mU/min over four hours. Total blood loss was 1000 ml and she was transfused three units of blood.

> ⊕ **Clinical tip** Management of the third stage
> - In normal pregnancy, uterotonics have been shown to significantly reduce the risk of postpartum haemorrhage (PPH) by up to 50% [27]. However, they have significant haemodynamic effects, which may make them potentially hazardous in women with cardiac disease.
> - Ergometrine causes vasoconstriction (especially in the coronary arteries) and hypertension.
> - Bolus doses of oxytocin cause an increase in pulmonary vascular resistance, and a reduction in systemic vascular resistance causing hypotension and tachycardia [28].
> - Two recent randomized controlled trials have suggested ECG changes suggestive of myocardial ischaemia associated with oxytocin administration in healthy women undergoing elective caesarean section with regional anaesthesia [29, 30].
> - Recent advice from the RCOG recommends a low-dose (12–40 mU/min) syntocinon infusion for up to four hours (longer if necessary), and consideration of the use of uterine compression sutures, as in this case [31].

The patient recovered well on the intensive care unit. Her postnatal course was uneventful and at two weeks she was feeling almost back to her pre-pregnancy health. She was advised about the need for maximally effective contraception. Her daughter needed ventilatory support with continuous positive airways pressure for the first two days of life, and at six days had bowel dilatation suggestive of early necrotizing enterocolitis. Fortunately this settled with intravenous nutrition and the baby was allowed home five weeks after birth, her weight having exceeded 2000 g.

At her six month follow-up the patient remained symptomatically stable without significant deterioration in her cardiac parameters.

Discussion

Pregnancy in women with pulmonary hypertension (PH) is rare, with an estimated incidence of 1.1 per 100 000 maternities [32], but it is associated with significant maternal and fetal morbidity and mortality. Use of advanced therapies has revolutionized the treatment of PH outside of pregnancy, and although data on their use in pregnancy are limited, the safety of PGI_2 (prostacyclin) analogues and sildenafil during pregnancy is now supported by numerous case reports and several small series in the literature. However, the risk of maternal mortality remains high, so early and effective counselling about effective contraceptive options and pregnancy risks should continue to play a major role in the management of such patients when they reach reproductive maturity.

The importance of managing all such patients in tertiary referral centres by experienced multidisciplinary teams cannot be over-emphasized [14, 15]. In the event of a pregnancy (either planned or unplanned) established pathways need to be in place to review the patient promptly and to discuss the options for ongoing care. When patients present with a new diagnosis, time is of the essence. This patient was not referred to the specialist centre until she was 22 weeks, therefore limiting her options regarding the pregnancy and optimal care. Every obstetric unit and cardiac centre should be aware of its local referral pathway for high-risk cardiac patients.

A Final Word from the Expert

Despite an encouraging trend towards improved outcome, patients with Pulmonary Hypertension are still amongst some of those at highest risk during pregnancy. It is therefore imperative that all patients are fully counselled about the risks of pregnancy from a young age. They should be given expert advice and support to have the most effective and safe form of contraception. Such counselling is outwith the expertise of the average adult or paediatric cardiologist, and therefore an obstetrician/gynaecologist with appropriate experience should always be included. Ideally, the consultation should be with the cardiologist and obstetrician both present at the same time, to ensure that their advice is fully coordinated.

References

1. Steer PJ. Pregnancy and Contraception. In Gatzoulis MA, Swan L, Therrien J, Pantely GA, (eds). *Adult Congenital Heart Disease: a practical guide*. Malden, MA: Blackwell Publishing, 2005
2. Lewis G. (ed.). Saving Mothers' Lives: Reviewing maternal deaths to make motherhood safer—2006-08. The Eighth Report of the Confidential Enquiries into Maternal Deaths in the United Kingdom. *BJOG* 2011 Mar 118 Suppl 1: 1–203.
3. Uebing A, Steer PJ, Yentis SM, Gatzoulis MA. Pregnancy and congenital heart disease. *BMJ* Feb 2006;332:401–6.
4. Gelson E, *et al*. Cardiovascular changes in normal pregnancy. In: *Heart Disease and Pregnancy*. London: RCOG Press, 2006, 29–44.
5. Hunter S, Robson SC. Adaptation of the maternal heart in pregnancy. *Br Heart J* 1992;86:540–43.
6. Ueland K, Hansen JM. Maternal Cardiovascular Dynamics. 3. Labour and delivery under local and caudal analgesia. *Am J Obstet Gynecol* 1969;103:8–18.
7. Robson SC, Dunlop W, Boys RJ, Hunter S. Cardiac output during labour. *BMJ* 1987;295:1169–72.
8. Siu SC, Sermer M, *et al*. Risk and predictors for pregnancy-related complications in women with heart disease. *Circulation* 1997;96:2789–94.
9. British Hypertension Society: How to measure blood pressure. http://www.bhsoc.org/how_to_measure_blood_pressure.stm
10. McLaughlan VV, Archer SL, Badesch DB, Barst RJ, Farber HW, Lindner JR, *et al*. ACCF/AHA 2009 Expert Consensus Document on Pulmonary Hypertension: A Report of the American College of Cardiology Foundation Task Force on Expert Consensus Documents and the American Heart Association Developed in Collaboration With the American College of Chest Physicians; American Thoracic Society, Inc; and the Pulmonary Hypertension Association. *J Am Coll Cardiol* 2009;53:1573–1619.
11. Bédard E, Dimopoulos K, Gatzoulis MA. Has there been any progress made on pregnancy outcomes among women with pulmonary arterial hypertension? *Eur Heart J* 2009;30:256–65.
12. Simmoneau G, Robbins IM, Beghetti M, Channick RN, Delcroix M, Denton CP, *et al*. Updated clinical classification of pulmonary hypertension. *J Am Coll Cardiol* 2009;54:543–54.
13. Weiss BM, Zemp L, Seifert B, Hess OM. Outcome of pulmonary vascular disease in pregnancy: a systematic overview from 1978 through 1996. *J Am Coll Cardiol* 1998;31:1650–7.
14. Kiely DG, Condliffe R, Webster V, Mills GH, Wrench I, Gandhi SV, *et al*. Improved survival un pregnancy and pulmonary hypertension using a multidisciplinary approach, *BJOG* 2010 Apr; 117(5): 565–74.

15. Curry RA, Fletcher C, Gelson E, Gatzoulis MA, Woolnough M, Richards N, *et al.* Pulmonary hypertension and pregnancy: a review of 12 pregnancies in nine women. *BJOG* 2012 May; 119(6): 752–61. doi: 10.1111/j. 1471-0528.2012.03295.x. Epub 2012 Mar 6.

16. Galiè N, Hoeper MM, Humbert M, Torbicki A, Vachiery JL, Barbera JA, *et al.* ESC Committee for Practice Guidelines (CPG). *Eur Heart J* 2009;30:2493–537.

17. Yentis SM, Steer PJ, Plaat F. Eisenmenger's syndrome in pregnancy: maternal and fetal mortality in the 1990s. *Br J Obstet Gynaecol* 1998 Aug; 105(8): 921–2.

18. Presbitero P, Somerville J, Stone S, Aruta E, Spiegalhalter D, Rabajoli F. Pregnancy in cyanotic heart disease. *Circulation* 1994;89:2673–6.

19. Chia P, Raman S, Tham SW. The pregnancy outcome of acyanotic heart disease. *J Obstet Gynaecol Res* 1998 Aug; 24(4): 267–73

20. Sawney H, Suri V, Vashishta K, Gupta N, Devi K, Grover A. Pregnancy and congenital heart disease—maternal and fetal outcome. *Aust NZJ Obstet Gynaecol* 1998 Aug; 38(3): 266–71.

21. Whittemore R, Hobbins JC, Engle MA. Pregnancy and its outcome in women with and without surgical treatment of congenital heart disease. *Am J Cardiol* 1982;50:641–51.

22. Bonnin M, Mercier FJ, Sitbon O, Roger-Christoph S, Jais X, Humbert M, *et al.* Severe pulmonary hypertension in pregnancy: mode of delivery and anaesthetic management of 15 consecutive cases. *Anaesthesiology* 2005 Jun; 102(6): 1133–7; discussion 5A–6A.

23. Curry R, Swan L, Ster PJ. Cardiac disease in pregnancy. *Curr Opin Obstet Gynecol.* 2009 Dec; 21(6): 508–13.

24. Daliento L, Somerville J, Presbitero P, Menti L, Prach-Prever S, Rizzoli G, *et al.* Eisenmenger syndrome. Factors relating to deterioration and death. *Eur Heart J* 1998 (Dec); 19(12): 1845–55.

25. NICE Clinical Guidance: Caesarean Section, 2004. http://www.nice.org.uk/nicemedia/pdf/CG13NICEguidance.pdf

26. Robson SC, Dunlop W, Boys RJ, Hunter S. Cardiac output during labour. *BMJ* 1987;295:1169–72.

27. NICE Clinical Guidance: Intrapartum Care, 2008. http://www.nice.org.uk/nicemedia/pdf/CG55NICEguidance.pdf

28. Price LC, Forrest P, Sodhi V, Adamson DL, Nelson-Piercy C, Lucey M, *et al.* Use of vasopressin after caesarean section in idiopathic pulmonary arterial hypertension. *Br J Anaesthesia* 2007;99:552–5.

29. Jonsson M, Hanson U, Lidell C, Norden-Lindeberg. ST depression at caesarean section and the relation to oxytocin dose. A randomized controlled trial. *BJOG* 2009;117:76–83.

30. Svanstrom MC, Biber B, Hanes M, Johansson G, Naslund U, Balfors EM. Signs of myocardial ischaemia after injection of oxytocin: a randomized controlled double-blind comparison of oxytocin and methylergometrine during caesarean section under spinal anaesthesia. *Br J Anaesthesia* 2008;100:683–9.

31. RCOG Good Practice No 13. Cardiac disease in Pregnancy.

32. Knight M, Kurinczuk JJ, Spark P, Brocklehurst P. United Kingdom Obstetrics Surveillance System (UKOSS) Annual Report 2007. Oxford: National Perinatal Epidemiology Unit.

12 The challenges and controversies of pregnancy and diabetes

Parag K. Thaware and Matthew Cauldwell

ⓘ Expert Commentary David R McCance

Case history

A 35-year-old woman, of Indian descent, was referred to the local joint antenatal diabetes clinic by her GP at eight weeks' gestation. This was her second pregnancy, conceived through IVF. Her past obstetric history included the birth of baby girl (spontaneous conception) at 38 weeks' gestation by caesarean section. During that pregnancy she developed gestational diabetes and had required subcutaneous insulin from 28 weeks' gestation. The patient had found it difficult to monitor her capillary blood glucose levels regularly despite close supervision and support from the specialist diabetes team. She was induced at 38 weeks' gestation but required an emergency caesarean section for failure to progress at 3 cm. Her baby daughter weighed 3.9 kg and had normal Agpars at delivery. Postnatally, her blood sugars remained above target, and she was commenced on Metformin, but in addition, insulin therapy was required for glycaemic control within a year. She was encouraged to lose weight but with limited success.

⊘ Landmark trial The Hyperglycaemia and Adverse Pregnancy Outcome [HAPO] study [1]

For decades, the entity of GDM has been an issue of controversy. Long-standing differences exist with respect to the diagnostic method, glycaemic thresholds for diagnosis, and the strategy for screening women at risk (Table 12.1). Against this background, the Hyperglycaemia and Pregnancy Outcome (HAPO) study was designed specifically to examine the relevance of minor degrees of hyperglycaemia during pregnancy, short of diabetes, for maternal/fetal outcome.

- A large multicentre, multicultural observational study involving 23 000 pregnant women
- Subjects underwent a 75 g oral glucose tolerance test at 24–32 weeks' gestation
- The results (Figure 12.1) showed a continuous association between maternal glycaemic levels during pregnancy and each of the primary outcomes (macrosomia, clinical neonatal hypoglycaemia, primary caesarean section, and cord c-peptide levels)
- Each 0.4 mmol/l increase in the fasting plasma glucose was associated with an:
  ○ odds ratio of 1.38 (95 % CI 1.32–1.44) for birthweight > ninetieth percentile
  ○ odds ratio of 1.11 (95 % CI 1.06–1.15) for primary caesarean section
  ○ odds ratio of 1.08 (95 % CI 0.98–1.19) for neonatal hypoglycaemia

In the absence of a threshold, these data were central to informing consensus recommendations for diagnosis and screening of GDM by the International Association of the Diabetes and Pregnancy Study Groups (IADPSG) [2]. To-date, the new criteria have been adopted by some countries but in others remain under review (Table 12.2).

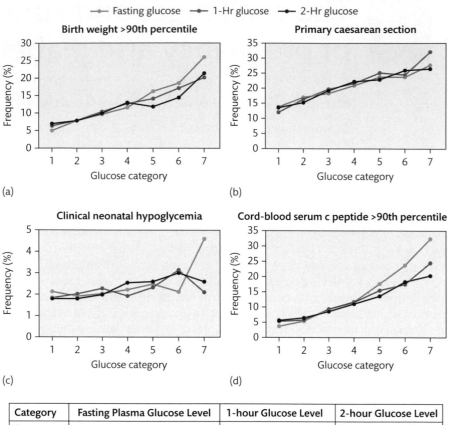

Figure 12.1 Frequency of primary outcomes across maternal glucose categories in the HAPO study.

From the New England Journal of Medicine, The HAPO Study Cooperative Research Group, Hyperglycemia and Adverse Pregnancy Outcomes, Vol 358 No 19 Copyright 2008 Massachusetts Medical Society. Reprinted with permission from Massachusetts Medical Society.

After 3 years of secondary sub-fertility, the patient and her partner again sought help from fertility services in India. She had had a successful single embryo transfer on her second cycle of IVF and travelled back to the UK where they intended to deliver.

At the first antenatal clinic visit at 10 weeks, the patient was on a basal bolus insulin regimen of Insulin Aspart (a fast-acting insulin analogue), 10–14 units pre meals and 26 units of Insulin Detemir (a long acting insulin analogue) at bedtime. Given the planned nature of the pregnancy, she had been taking folic acid 5 mgs

> ⊗ **Learning point** Gestational diabetes mellitus and type 2 diabetes
>
> Beginning in early pregnancy and progressing through to the third trimester, the contribution of increased maternal adiposity and elaboration of hormones from the placenta (including human placental growth hormone and TNF-α) play a major role in inducing maternal insulin resistance and relative glucose intolerance. If maternal pancreatic insulin secretion is unable to compensate, and levels of maternal hyperglycaemia cross a predefined diagnostic threshold, gestational diabetes mellitus (GDM) or hyperglycaemia in pregnancy is diagnosed. The rapid correction of glucose levels after delivery of the placenta highlights the significant contribution of placental hormones to hyperglycaemia in pregnancy. All patients with GDM should be offered glucose testing around 6 weeks after delivery to ensure reversion to normal glucose tolerance unless there is clear evidence of persisting hyperglycaemia postnatally.
>
> Compared to women with normal glucose tolerance during pregnancy, women with gestational diabetes mellitus have significantly decreased insulin sensitivity both before and during pregnancy despite matching for weight [10]. However, both groups have a similar percent decrease in insulin sensitivity through pregnancy. Overweight and obese women have decreased insulin sensitivity compared with lean or average weight women, although both groups have a similar 50% decrease over the period of gestation [11]. These data are consistent with the underlying pathophysiology of GDM resulting in a 50–60% increase in type 2 diabetes in the 10–15 years after diagnosis of GDM [12]. A systematic review (including over 20 cohort studies and > 30000 women with GDM pregnancies) found that these women had at least a sevenfold increase in the risk of developing future type 2 diabetes compared with women who had normoglycaemic pregnancies [13]. It is likely that a significant proportion of women who develop type 2 diabetes after GDM had pre-existing but undiagnosed type 2 diabetes.
>
> The relevance of ethnicity, obesity and family history to GDM and type 2 diabetes, together with the frequent association of GDM with other components of the metabolic syndrome, and the recognized risk of type 2 diabetes after GDM, point to a similar pathophysiology of both disorders.

Table 12.1 Diagnostic criteria and screening strategies for gestational diabetes prior to IADPSG recommendations

	Recommended diagnostic test	Diagnostic thresholds (mmol/L)				No. of abnormal values needed	Recommended screening strategy
		Fasting	1 hour	2 hour	3 hour		
WHO 1999 [3]	75 g OGTT	≥ 7.0	-	≥ 7.8	-	1	No specific recommendations
NICE 2008 [4]	75 g OGTT	≥ 7.0	-	≥ 7.8	-	1	Diagnostic testing at 24–28 wk gestation if risk factors present
ADA (before 2011) and ACOG 2011 [5,6]	100 g OGTT Carpenter and Coustan criteria*	≥ 5.3	≥ 10.0	≥ 8.6	≥ 7.8	at least 2	Diagnostic testing at 24–28 wk gestation if risk factors present or a screening 1 hr 50 g OGTT abnormal
	100 g OGTT National Diabetes Data Group criteria*	≥ 5.8	≥ 10.6	≥ 9.2	≥ 8.0		

IADPSG—International Association of Diabetes in Pregnancy Study Groups; WHO—World Health Organisation; NICE—National Institute for Health and Clinical Excellence; SIGN—Scottish Intercollegiate Guidelines Network; ADA—American Diabetes Association; ACOG—American College of Obstetricians and Gynecologists; FPG—fasting plasma glucose; OGTT—oral glucose tolerance test
*recommendations were that either of the two criteria could be used

Table 12.2 2010 IADPSG recommendations* for diagnosis and screening of GDM

Recommended diagnostic test	Diagnostic thresholds (mmol/L)				No. of abnormal values needed	Recommended screening strategy
	Fasting	1 hour	2 hour	3 hour		
75 g OGTT	≥ 5.1 or	≥ 10.0 or	≥ 8.5	-	1	FPG/HbA1c in early gestation; if normal, 2 hr 75 g OGTT at 24-28 wks

* Adopted by ADA [7], in part by SIGN [8], and most recently by the WHO [9]

daily for some months prior to conception, although her HbA1c was very poor at 80 mmol/mol (DCCT aligned units 9.5 %). Mild background diabetic retinopathy was noted on retinal screening 6 months previously, and microalbuminuria had been documented in the preconception period. She reported that she regularly rotated her injection sites. She had stopped Ramipril 5 mg, as advised by her GP, on discovery of pregnancy.

Since her successful IVF treatment, the patient stated that she was more motivated to improve her diabetes control. Her capillary glucose readings, which she had been monitoring four times a day, were reportedly in the range 6–9 mmol/L pre-breakfast, 6–8 mmol/L pre-lunch, and 9–13 mmol/L pre-evening meal and before bed. Her average capillary glucose in the preceding month, on the basis of four to five readings per day, was 9.5 mmol/L. She possessed the necessary equipment to test for urinary ketones but had not needed to use it. The patient reported two hypoglycaemic episodes during the preceding week at a time when she was eating poorly due to nausea. There was no other history of hypoglycaemia or episodes needing

✪ Learning point Preconception counselling

While this was a planned pregnancy, and the patient had been advised to start high-dose folic acid by her fertility unit in India prior to undertaking IVF, she had never received any formal support or advice that could have been interpreted as preconception counselling and HbA1c at booking was very poor. NICE has developed guidance [2], which seeks to empower women with diabetes so they are not only aware of the adverse risks associated with diabetes in pregnancy (as listed), but they also realize that they have a contribution to make to reduce these risks.

Although all mothers should be aware of the need for near normal blood sugar levels prior to pregnancy, it is important to emphasize that any reduction in HbA1c will reduce the risk for an individual patient, and that the outcome for the majority of women with pregnancy and diabetes is good.

Key elements of preconception counselling include [14]:

- Discussion about future pregnancy plans
- Education about the importance of pre-pregnancy care and how this can improve pregnancy outcomes
- Education about the increased risks of poor pregnancy outcome with poor glycaemic control before and during early pregnancy
- Advice about how to access pre-pregnancy care, including contact details for self referral
- Education of women with type 2 diabetes about revision of treatment to optimize control before conception, including the possible need for insulin before and/or during pregnancy
- Documentation about use and provision of contraception and advice about contraception
- Education about necessity for commencement of folic acid supplements before pregnancy
- Education about avoidance of teratogenic drugs during pregnancy
- Discussion about how diabetic complications may affect any future pregnancy
- Information about the importance of urgent referral should an unplanned pregnancy occur

⭐ **Learning point** Screening and surveillance for diabetes-related complications during pregnancy

- All pregnant women with diabetes preceding pregnancy should receive retinal assessment by digital imaging following their first antenatal clinic appointment and again at 28 weeks if the first assessment is normal. In the presence of diabetic retinopathy, an additional retinal assessment should be performed at 16–20 weeks [2].
- If pre-proliferative diabetic retinopathy is found during pregnancy, ophthalmological follow-up is recommended for at least 6 months following the birth of the baby.
- Diabetic retinopathy should not be considered a contraindication to rapid optimization of glycaemic control in women who present with a high HbA1c in early pregnancy. Diabetic retinopathy should not be considered a contraindication to vaginal birth.
- All pregnant women with diabetes preceding pregnancy should receive testing for renal disease in the form of an early morning urinary albumin-to-creatinine ratio (ACR) and serum electrolyte levels (if not done in the preceding 12 months). If proteinuria is greater than 1+, urinalysis should be checked at each antenatal visit.
- Pregnant women with diabetic nephropathy should receive input from a specialist renal physician if serum creatinine is greater than 120 micromol/L or if total 24-hour urinary protein excretion is greater than 2 g.

💬 **Expert comment**

In the presence of significant proteinuria, consider thromboprophylaxis if 24-hour urinary protein level is greater than 5 g, and aspirin 75 mg daily if level below 5 g [2].

⭐ **Learning point** Pregnancy and diabetes-related complications

- Diabetic retinopathy
  - Pregnancy may result in progression of retinopathy in patients with diabetes [15,16].
  - Risk factors for progression are pre-existing retinopathy, poor pre-conception glycaemic control, longer duration of diabetes, rapid improvement in glycaemia during the first trimester, and previous or pregnancy-induced hypertension.
  - Rapid optimization of glycaemia is not contraindicated in pregnant women with diabetic retinopathy, but regular retinal assessments are recommended.

- Diabetic nephropathy
  - There is an increased risk of progression of nephropathy in women with type 1 diabetes and impaired renal function [17].
  - Diabetic nephropathy, including microalbuminuria without renal impairment, is associated with an increased risk for pre-eclampsia and preterm delivery [18,19].
  - Overt diabetic nephropathy is associated with intra-uterine growth retardation and fetal distress [18].
  - Specialist nephrology input and optimal management of blood pressure are recommended for such women.

- Diabetic ketoacidosis during pregnancy
  - Diabetic ketoacidosis during pregnancy is often related to vomiting of pregnancy, but also to other causes including the use of betamimetic drugs, failure to continue regular insulin therapy, and infection.
  - Patients should be reminded of the sick-day rules and of emergency contact numbers. In those who are unwell with reduced oral intake/vomiting with hyperglycaemia and ketonuria, urgent advice should be sought and admission arranged especially if adequate hydration cannot be maintained.

⊕ **Clinical tip** Glycaemic targets during pregnancy

- Self-monitoring of capillary blood glucose is recommended in management of diabetes during pregnancy (before meals, one hour after meals, and before bed)
- There is a significant risk of hypoglycaemia with insulin therapy, especially during the first trimester, and glycaemic targets should be individualized
- If safe, the recommended target capillary glucose levels are: fasting or before meals, between 3.5 and 5.9 mmol/L, and 1 hour after meals, less than 7.8 mmol/L [2]
- Adjusting treatment to postprandial blood glucose is associated with better outcomes in women with type 1 and gestational diabetes

✪ **Learning point** Hypoglycaemia in pregnancy

- There is an increased risk of hypoglycaemia (including severe hypoglycaemia) in women with insulin-treated diabetes during pregnancy, compounded by the need for intensification of insulin therapy.
- The risk is highest during the first trimester when insulin sensitivity improves and pregnancy-related nausea and vomiting occur. Other mechanisms include impairment of counter-regulatory hormone response to hypoglycaemia and diminished hypoglycaemia awareness.
- Education regarding the management of hypoglycaemia and precautions during driving should be reiterated at the first opportunity during pregnancy. Each woman should be given glucagon for administration by a partner or family member in the case of emergency.
- Frequent hypoglycaemia with a rapid fall in insulin requirements in later pregnancy in insulin-treated patients should arouse suspicion of placental insufficiency and merits urgent assessment of fetal well-being.
- The UK medical standards for fitness to drive with respect to hypoglycaemia have recently changed, with no more than one episode of hypoglycaemia requiring external assistance now being permissible in the preceding 12 months [20].

✪ **Learning point** Hypoglycaemic agents and pregnancy

- Insulin therapies commonly used during pregnancy:
  - Rapid-acting analogue insulins are frequently used as they are less prone to cause hypoglycaemia and can be taken immediately prior to meals—e.g. Insulin Aspart (*Novorapid*), Lispro (*Humalog*), and Glulisine (*Apidra*). Insulin Aspart and Lispro are licensed for use during pregnancy (FDA category B- and EMA-approved); Glulisine is FDA category C.
  - Basal insulins include human NPH insulin, and the long-acting insulin analogues Insulin Detemir (*Levemir*) and Insulin Glargine (*Lantus*). Recent RCT data in women with type 1 diabetes suggest that Insulin Detemir is as effective as human NPH and is safe for use during pregnancy [21]; this drug has recently been approved by the FDA (category B) and the EMA for use in pregnancy.

- Oral hypoglycaemic agents during pregnancy:
  - Metformin and Glibenclamide can be used during pregnancy in patients with type 2 diabetes or gestational diabetes [2].
  - Other agents are not routinely used during pregnancy.

third-party help. She had a car driving license and regularly drove to work. She was a non-smoker and did not drink alcohol.

On examination, her BMI was 35 kg/m². Blood pressure was 124/72 mmHg. The rest of the examination was normal. Insulin injection sites were unremarkable. Fundoscopy revealed mild bilateral background diabetic retinopathy but without involvement of the macula. Peripheral sensation was normal with monofilament testing 5/5 in each foot and the feet appeared healthy. Her HbA1c was 80 mmol/mol (DCCT-aligned units 9.5 %), Hb 12.3 g/dl, platelets 229 × 10^9/l, urea 3.6 mmol/l, and creatinine 55 μmol/l. Liver function tests were normal. A spot urine albumin-to-creatinine ratio was elevated at 10 mg/mmol (normal range < 3).

Management of her antenatal care was conducted fortnightly at the joint antenatal metabolic clinic by a multidisciplinary team including an obstetrician, diabetologist, diabetes specialist nurse, dietician, and diabetes specialist midwife. She was referred to the dietitian for lifestyle advice and encouragement to adhere to her diabetic diet. The patient received counselling regarding fetal and maternal complications associated with diabetes, the importance of good diabetes control during pregnancy including glycaemic targets, the management of hypoglycaemia, and of precautions to be taken while driving. She was asked to monitor her capillary blood glucose on a daily basis before and one hour after meals, and at

> **★ Learning point** Dietary advice and exercise
>
> - The main aim of structured dietary advice for women with diabetes is to optimize glycaemic control and so help them to avoid large variations in their blood glucose levels. In women who are on insulin therapy (primarily type 1), it is particularly important to educate them about the dangers of developing ketosis as well as hypoglycaemia.
> - Diabetic women should be provided with dietary education to allow them to understand what are the healthy nutritional requirements for normal fetal growth, and to try and avoid accelerated fetal growth patterns.
> - While low glycaemic index (GI) diets may assist in reducing postprandial hyperglycaemia, there are no large, adequately powered trials, and a recent Cochrane review did not find any significant benefits on maternal and infant health outcomes among GDM women [22].

> **❻ Expert comment**
>
> A healthy lifestyle of moderate physical activity and a well-balanced diet should be encouraged for all women during pregnancy. For women with type 2 diabetes or GDM, many of whom will have been previously unfit, realistic and appropriate exercise for pregnancy should be advocated. Encouraging 20 minutes of walking once or twice a day after meals is easily achievable and can lower postprandial blood glucose values. For women with GDM, combining exercise with a dietary program improves glycaemic control and reduces the need for insulin treatment.

> **★ Learning point** Adverse outcomes in pregnancy with pre-existing diabetes [4, 23–25]
>
> **Fetal**
>
> - Stillbirth
> - Increased perinatal mortality
> - Preterm delivery
> - Macrosomia
> - Shoulder dystocia and birth injuries
> - Congenital anomalies, e.g. neural tube defects and congenital heart disease
> - Respiratory distress syndrome
> - Neonatal metabolic derangements: hypoglycaemia, neonatal jaundice, hypocalcaemia, hypomagnesaemia, polycythaemia, and hyperviscosity
>
> **Maternal**
>
> - Miscarriage
> - Accelerated diabetic retinopathy and nephropathy
> - Increased frequency of hypoglycaemia and hypoglycaemia unawareness
> - Diabetic ketoacidosis
> - Pre-eclampsia
> - Infection
> - Increased operative delivery rates

> **⊘ Evidence base** Pre-existing diabetes and fetal outcome
>
> The Confidential Enquiry into Maternal and Child Health (CEMACH) [23] involving over 3000 women with type 1 and type 2 diabetes in England, Wales and Northern Ireland during 2002–2003 showed that women with diabetes preceding pregnancy had:
>
> - Four times higher perinatal mortality
> - Threefold increase in neonatal congenital anomalies
> - Two times higher rate for macrosomia
> - More than 2.5 times higher rate of shoulder dystocia
> - Ten times higher rate of Erb's palsy, and
> - Two times higher spontaneous preterm delivery rate

bedtime. In light of the history of background retinopathy, she was referred to an ophthalmologist.

At follow-up two weeks later, she reported several further episodes of hypoglycaemia however none of these needed external assistance and hypoglycaemia became less problematic as pregnancy proceeded. HbA1c improved to 61 mmol/mol (7.7 %) by the end of the first trimester.

Her twentieth-week anomaly scan, including cardiac ultrasound, was normal, with fetal abdominal circumference at the seventy-fifth percentile. Subsequent

---

🕻 Expert comment

The increasing prevalence rates of type 2 diabetes in the general population are being translated into pregnancy. Observational data and meta analyses have clearly shown that the risk of adverse outcome in type 2 diabetes is similar to that of type 1 diabetes. In addition, these women are less likely to plan their pregnancy. As the majority of women with type 2 diabetes will be managed in the community, it is critical that they receive appropriate education in primary care. The important message is that both type 1 and type 2 diabetes require careful pregnancy planning and close maternal fetal/surveillance.

✔ Evidence base Optimal glycaemic control can reduce adverse pregnancy outcomes

- **Optimal glycaemic control during conception and first trimester can reduce rates of fetal major congenital anomalies in women with pre-gestational diabetes.**
  - o Randomized controlled trials are understandably difficult to design in order to examine this question directly; as a consequence evidence is largely available from non-randomized trials and retrospective cohort studies.
  - o Epidemiological data have shown a direct association between peri-conception glycaemic control and the risk of fetal malformations in type 1 and type 2 diabetes [26].
  - o A meta-analysis of eight prospective and eight retrospective studies reported a lower pooled rate of major congenital anomalies in those with preconception care (2.1 %) versus those without (6.5 %) [27].
  - o Good glycaemic control in women has been associated with spontaneous miscarriage and congenital anomaly rates similar to those of the general population [28].
  - o In women with type 1 diabetes, glycaemic management with glucose targets in the normal reference range resulted in none of the neonates being born with macrosomia [29].

- **Optimal glycaemic control during pregnancy can reduce rates of fetal macrosomia in pregnant women with gestational diabetes.**
  - o A randomized controlled trial in women requiring insulin therapy for gestational diabetes (predominantly Hispanic) showed that targeting the postprandial glucose level, compared to preprandial, reduced the risk of macrosomia (9 % versus 36 %, respectively) [30].
  - o Two large randomized controlled trials demonstrated that treatment of women with gestational diabetes mellitus resulted in a reduced rate of large for gestational age neonates compared with control women (14.5–22 %) [31,32].

- **Impact of optimal glycaemic control during pregnancy on other pregnancy outcomes in gestational diabetes mellitus.**
  - o The ACHOIS trial showed a reduction in a composite primary outcome consisting of neonatal death, shoulder dystocia, bone fracture, and nerve palsy in women treated for glucose intolerance during pregnancy (1 %) compared with control women (4 %) [31].
  - o Monitoring postprandial versus preprandial glucose levels in women with gestational diabetes was shown to reduce rates of caesarean section for cephalopelvic disproportion (12 % versus 36 %), neonatal hypoglycaemia (3 % versus 21 %), shoulder dystocia (3 % versus 18 %), and third- or fourth-degree perineal lacerations (9 % versus 24 %) [30].
  - o Studies have reported a reduction in incidence of pre-eclampsia with treatment of milder glucose intolerance during pregnancy (2.5 % versus 5.5 % in those without treatment) [32], and with targeting of postprandial compared with preprandial glucose monitoring in women with type 1 diabetes (3 % versus 21 %, respectively) [33].
  - o In women needing insulin during pregnancy, a more intensive regimen (4 times a day) was shown to result in lower rates of neonatal hypoglycaemia and hyperbilirubinaemia compared with twice-daily insulin [34].

> **✪ Learning point** Fetal monitoring and care in pregnant women with diabetes
>
> Fetal monitoring in women with diabetes is as per routine antenatal care, and includes a twentieth-week fetal anomaly scan and a fetal cardiac scan (as described). In addition, the following aspects should also be noted:
>
> - Regular ultrasound monitoring of fetal growth (using estimated fetal weight and abdominal circumference) and amniotic fluid volume should commence from the 28th week and continue at four-weekly intervals
> - Before 38 weeks' gestation, monitoring of fetal well-being using Doppler assessment, liquor volume, and cardiotocograh should be considered in women with certain complications, e.g. fetal intra-uterine growth restriction, nephropathy, pre-eclampsia, known macrovascular disease. The frequency of monitoring is decided on an individual basis by a senior obstetrician, and it takes into account the mother's own obstetric risk factors as well as information from scans and blood/urine tests
> - Umbilical artery ultrasound has been shown to be a better predictor of fetal outcomes in women with diabetes compared with cardiotocography or biophysical profile [35]
> - A fetal cardiology scan should be undertaken for women with both type 1 and type 2 diabetes as there is a strong correlation in early pregnancy between HbA1c and the risk of congenital malformations. Large retrospective case studies have shown the relative risk of a diabetic mother having a baby with a cardiac abnormality is up to three times greater than the background rate even when HbA1c is in an acceptable range (5.6–6.8%) [36,37]

growth scans estimated fetal weight to be just below the ninetieth percentile for gestational age with normal liquor volumes and Doppler ultrasound measurements.

The patient requested an early appointment with her obstetrician at 26 weeks to discuss mode of delivery. She was very keen to attempt vaginal delivery; however, after counselling regarding the risks and benefits, it was agreed to defer a final decision regarding delivery until her antenatal visit around 36 weeks.

The patient continued to be reviewed at fortnightly intervals during pregnancy. From around 26 weeks, there was a progressive increase in her capillary blood glucose levels, necessitating frequent adjustment of her insulin doses as guided by frequent telephone contact with diabetic specialist nursing staff. Serial monitoring of fetal abdominal circumference showed the baby's growth to be between the fiftieth and ninety-fifth centile. Her previous obstetric notes were reviewed. She was still keen to proceed with vaginal birth, but abdominal palpation revealed the baby to be breech and this was confirmed on a portable bedside scan. In discussion with the consultant obstetrician, it was decided to repeat the fetal assessment scan one week later to see if the baby had spontaneously verted. Unfortunately, this was not the case and after explanation of the options, she consented to external cephalic version which was arranged for the following week, preceded by a repeat scan.

Unfortunately, attempted ECV on two occasions was unsuccessful. She was booked for an elective caesarean at 38 weeks and a decision was made to give antenatal steroids to reduce the risk of transient tachypnoea of the newborn. The patient was admitted to the delivery suite the evening of her failed ECV and received two doses of dexamethasone 12 mg, 24 hours apart. She received supplementary insulin to cover the steroid treatment according to the unit's local algorithm.

The patient was admitted early on the morning of her planned caesarean section. She was reviewed by the anaesthetist and by the obstetric registrar who verified the consent form. She underwent a routine low segment caesarean section (LSCS) and delivered a healthy baby girl who weighed 3.7 kg. Soluble insulin was commenced just before starting the procedure in the form of an intravenous insulin and

> **❝ Expert comment**
>
> Patients require admission to hospital for careful monitoring of blood glucose during steroid therapy. The decision to use steroids is made after careful obstetric consideration and is indicated particularly when early delivery may be necessary.

➕ **Clinical tip** Glycaemic management with systemic steroid therapy for fetal lung maturation

Use of systemic steroids for fetal lung maturity is not contraindicated in women with diabetes. There is, however, a need for close monitoring of capillary blood glucose levels during this time, given the significant increase in insulin requirements. Some obstetric units have developed a pregnancy algorithm such as the one which follows, which can obviate the need for a variable dose insulin infusion when administering steroids for fetal lung maturation.

An algorithm to guide glycaemic management during systemic betamethasone therapy [40]:

- Day 0: (1st dose betamethasone at 1600 h): 30% increase in bed-time insulin
- Day 1: (2nd dose betamethasone 24 hours later): 50% increase in all (pre steroid) insulin doses
- Day 2: 50% increase in all (pre steroid) insulin doses
- Day 3: 30% increase in all (pre steroid) insulin doses
- Day 4: 20% increase in all (pre steroid) insulin doses
- Day 5: gradual reduction to pre steroid insulin doses

⭐ **Learning point** Care of the newborn of a diabetic mother

Apart from routine neonatal assessment and care, the following should be offered:

- Blood glucose measurement at two hours post birth.
- Blood sampling for hyperbilirubinaemia, polycythaemia, hypocalcaemia, and hypomagnesaemia, as dictated by clinical examination.
- Neonatal echocardiogram in the presence of a heart murmur or if there are symptoms and/or signs of congenital heart disease.
- Neonatal intensive care should be considered for symptomatic hypoglycaemia, jaundice, respiratory distress, cardiac failure, preterm birth, and when there is need for intravenous fluid therapy, tube feeding, or exchange transfusion for polycythaemia.
- All neonates should receive feeding as soon as possible to minimize the risk of hypoglycaemia.

💬 **Expert comment**

Certain comorbidities can increase anaesthetic risks in women with diabetes, e.g. autonomic neuropathy, nephropathy, and obesity, and anaesthetic assessment should be considered. Close glycaemic monitoring is required in diabetic women during general anaesthesia.

💬 **Expert comment**

Maintenance of blood glucose levels between 4 and 7 mmol/l during labour has been shown to reduce neonatal hypoglycaemia and distress [41,42], and is recommended by NICE Guidelines [4].

💬 **Expert comment**

The significant fall in insulin requirements in the postpartum period, particularly during breastfeeding may require additional carbohydrate intake or further reductions in insulin dosing to reduce the risk of hypoglycaemia.

⭐ **Learning point** Glycaemic management in the peri-partum period and follow-up

- In women with type 1 and insulin-treated type 2 and gestational diabetes, commence insulin/ dextrose infusion at onset of labour with hourly monitoring of capillary glucose during labour and delivery, aiming for a target glucose of 4–7 mmol/l [41,42].
- In other types of diabetes, monitor capillary blood glucose at hourly intervals and consider intravenous insulin if target glycaemia is not maintained.
- In women with type 1 diabetes prior to pregnancy, the insulin dose is reduced approximately to 50% of the pre-pregnancy dose in the immediate postpartum period, followed by subsequent active dose titration.
- Women on Metformin or Glibenclamide for diabetes before pregnancy can continue to take these drugs in the postpartum period while breastfeeding but each case should be reviewed on an individual basis. Women with gestational diabetes should stop insulin and/or oral hypoglycaemic agents after delivery but continue preprandial glucose monitoring for 24 hours to ensure that these return to normal.
- Arrangements should be made for all women with diabetes prior to pregnancy to be referred back to their physician after pregnancy for ongoing follow-up. They should be advised regarding the need for careful planning of any future pregnancy and provided with emergency contact numbers. Women with gestational diabetes should have a fasting glucose or oral glucose tolerance test after a minimum of 6 weeks postnatally, followed by a fasting glucose on an annual basis They should also receive lifestyle advice to reduce the risk of future type 2 diabetes, and recurrence of gestational diabetes in subsequent pregnancies.

dextrose infusion with hourly monitoring of capillary blood glucose as per local agreed policy, to maintain glucose levels between 4 and 7 mmol/L. There was no neonatal hypoglycaemia.

Her further glycaemic management followed liaison with the local specialist diabetes team. The patient wished to breastfeed and this was commenced within 30 minutes of birth. Her insulin therapy was reduced to approximately half that which she was taking before pregnancy while her metformin was continued. Her blood glucose targets were relaxed to those prior to pregnancy (4–7 mmol/l per meals). Her post-operative recovery was uneventful and she was fit for discharge by day 3. She was again encouraged regarding dietary compliance and given general lifestyle advice. Early midwifery community follow-up was arranged, and postnatal diabetes review was organized for six weeks.

Discussion

The care of pregnant women with diabetes can be challenging for both patient and clinician. In this case the key areas in the management of such pregnancies have been highlighted.

Diabetes preceding pregnancy (type 1 and type 2) and gestational diabetes mellitus (GDM) are 2 distinct clinically relevant forms of diabetes associated with pregnancy. It has been estimated that 0.3–0.4 % of all child births in England, Wales, and Northern Ireland occur in women with type 1 and type 2 diabetes [23]. By contrast, GDM is defined as carbohydrate intolerance of variable severity with onset or first recognition during pregnancy with prevalence rates of 9.3–25.5 % depending on ethnicity and diagnostic criteria [43].

Both diabetes preceding pregnancy and GDM are associated with adverse pregnancy outcomes, but the increased risk of miscarriage and congenital malformations is more specific to women with the former. Women with diabetes preceding pregnancy may experience a 1.4–1.6-times higher risk for progression of pre existing diabetic retinopathy, particularly in the context of poor glycaemic control [15,16]. Published studies have not shown significant worsening of microalbuminuria or mild diabetic nephropathy with pregnancy [15,44]. However, with moderate to severe renal impairment up to 45 % women may experience a permanent decline in renal function with pregnancy [17]. As highlighted, there is an increased risk of severe hypoglycaemia in women with type 1 diabetes on insulin therapy, particularly in the first trimester. Other complications include an increased incidence of diabetic ketoacidosis which is associated with significant morbidity and mortality.

Optimizing glycaemic control remains central to the management of pregnant women with diabetes in order to reduce the risk of adverse outcomes. In patients with diabetes preceding pregnancy, this has been shown to reduce the risk of congenital anomalies [27,28]. In all types of diabetes, including GDM, improving glucose control has been associated with a reduction in the risk of macrosomia and other adverse outcomes [30–33]. However, intensification of glycaemic control must always be individualized and balanced against the risks of hypoglycaemia.

If fetal macrosmia is suspected, there is an increased risk for shoulder dystocia and stillbirth. In such situations, careful obstetric supervision is vital with the mode of delivery being based on consideration of the relevant factors. Post-term pregnancy beyond 38–39 weeks' gestation in women with diabetes is associated with increased risk of fetal macrosomia and shoulder dystocia [45]. It is recommended that women with diabetes should be offered elective induction of labour or delivery by caesarean section after 38 completed weeks' gestation [4]. Ideally, childbirth should be conducted in a centre where emergency advanced neonatal resuscitation and care are available.

A Final Word from the Expert

The outlook for women with diabetes has greatly improved since the discovery of insulin. However, the goal of the 1989 St Vincent Declaration, that the outcome of diabetic pregnancy should approximate that of non-diabetic pregnancy, has yet to be realized. Mortality and malformation rates remain several times higher in women with diabetes than in the background population. The last few years have seen the publication of a number of landmark observational studies and randomized trials, which have the potential to alter the diagnostic and therapeutic landscape considerably, but the translation of some of these data into clinical practice has proved difficult. In addition, the changing epidemiology of diabetes in pregnancy, an expanding therapeutic arsenal, and increasing awareness of the long-term implications of diabetic pregnancy for both mother and baby, all present new challenges for clinical care, scientific research, and public health. Practically, the management of diabetes in pregnancy remains demanding for both the patient and clinician. A multidisciplinary model of care is now accepted as the ideal but the diverse backgrounds of the stakeholders have contributed to the difficulty in achieving a uniform approach to the management of these patients.

Despite these limitations, the outcome of pregnancy for most women with diabetes is good, and this undoubtedly reflects improved obstetric surveillance and better management of maternal hyperglycaemia over the last several decades. The aim is, through education and maternal empowerment, to optimize blood glucose control both before and during pregnancy, so that pregnancy may proceed as normally as possible and result in the birth of a normal baby at near term.

References

1. Hyperglycemia and Adverse Pregnancy Outcomes *N Engl J Med* 2008;358:1991–2002.
2. International Association of Diabetes and Pregnancy Study Groups Recommendations on the Diagnosis and Classification of Hyperglycemia in Pregnancy. *Diabetes Care* 2010;33:676–82.
3. World Health Organization and Department of Non-communicable Disease Surveillance Definition, diagnosis and classification of diabetes mellitus and its complications. Report of a WHO consultation. Part 1: diagnosis and classification of diabetes mellitus. Geneva: World Health Organisation. 1999.
4. National Institute for Health and Clinical Excellence National Collaborating Centre for Women's and Children's Health. *Diabetes in pregnancy: management of diabetes and its complications from preconception to the postnatal period*. 2008. http://www.nice.org.uk/cg63
5. American Diabetes Association Standards of Medical Care in Diabetes-2010. *Diabetes Care* 2009;33:S11–S61.
6. Committee Opinion No. 504: Screening and diagnosis of gestational diabetes mellitus. *Obstet Gynecol* 2011;118:751–3.

7. American Diabetes Association Standards of Medical Care in Diabetes—2011. *Diabetes Care* 2010;34:S11–L S61.

8. Scottish Intercollegiate Guidelines. *Network Management of diabetes. A national clinical guideline.* 2010. http://www.sign.ac.uk/pdf/sign116.pdf

9. Diagnostic Criteria and Classification of Hyperglycaemia First Detected in Pregnancy. WHO/NMH/MND/13.2. 2013.

10. Catalano PM, Houston L, Amini SB, Kalhan SC. Longitudinal changes in glucose metabolism during pregnancy in obese women with normal glucose tolerance and gestational diabetes mellitus. *Am J Obstet Gynecol* 1999;180:903–16.

11. Catalano PM, Ehrenberg HM. The short and long term implications of maternal obesity on the mother and her offspring. *BJOG* 2006;113:1126–33.

12. Kim C, Newton KM, Knopp RH. Gestational diabetes and the incidence of Type 2 diabetes: a systematic review. *Diabetes Care* 2002;25:1862–8.

13. Bellamy L, Casas JP, Hingorani AD, Williams D. Type 2 diabetes after gestational diabetes: a systematic review and meta analysis. *Lancet* 1999;373:1773–9.

14. Temple RC. Pre pregnancy care for Type 1 and Type 2 diabetes. In: *A Practical Manual of Diabetes in Pregnancy.* McCance DR, Maresh M, Sacks D. Oxford: Blackwell-Wiley, 77–87 (2010).

15. The Diabetes Control and Complications Trial Research Group. Effect of pregnancy on microvascular complications in the diabetes control and complications trial. *Diabetes Care* 2000;23:1084–91.

16. Klein BE, Moss SE, Klein R. Effect of pregnancy on progression of diabetic retinopathy. *Diabetes Care* 1990;13:34–40.

17. Purdy LP, Hantsch C, Molitch ME, Metzger BE, Phelps RL, Dolley SL, *et al.* Effect of pregnancy on renal function in patients with moderate-to-severe diabetic renal insufficiency. *Diabetes Care* 1996;19:1067–74.

18. Dunne FP, Chowdhury TA, Hartland A, Smith T, Brydon PA, McConkey C, *et al.* Pregnancy outcome in women with insulin-dependent diabetes mellitus complicated by nephropathy. *QJM* 1999;92:451–4.

19. Ekbom P, Damm P, Feldt-Rasmussen B, Feldt-Rasmussen U, Mølvig J, *et al.* Pregnancy Outcome in Type 1 Diabetic Women with microalbuminuria. *Diabetes Care* 2001;24:1739–44.

20. Drivers Medical Group. *At a glance guide to the current medical standards of fitness to drive.* DVLA: Swansea, 2011. http://www.dft.gov.uk/dvla/medical/ataglance.aspx

21. Mathiesen ER, Hod M, Ivanisevic M, Garcia SD, Brøndsted L, Jovanovič L, et al. on behalf of the Detemir in Pregnancy Study Group. Maternal Efficacy and Safety Outcomes in a Randomized, Controlled Trial Comparing Insulin Detemir With NPH Insulin in 310 Pregnant Women With Type 1 Diabetes. Diabetes Care 2012;35(10):2012–17.

22. Hans S, Crowther CA, Middleton P, Heatley E. Different types of dietary advice for women with gestational diabetes mellitus. *Cochrane Database Syst Rev* March 28:CD009275. doi:10.1002/14651858.CD009275.pub2. 2013.

23. *Confidential Enquiry into Maternal and Child Health: Pregnancy in Women with Type 1 and Type 2 Diabetes in 2002-03, England, Wales and Northern Ireland.* London: CEMACH. (2005).

24. Persson M, Norman M, Hanson U. Obstetric and perinatal outcomes in type 1 diabetic pregnancies: A large, population-based study. *Diabetes Care* 2009;32:2005.

25. McCance, D, Maresh M, Sacks D. *A Practical Manual of Diabetes in Pregnancy.* Chichester: John Wiley & Sons, 2010.

26. Bell R, Glinianaia S, Tennant P, Bilous RRankin J. Peri-conception hyperglycaemia and nephropathy are associated with risk of congenital anomaly in women with pre-existing diabetes: a population-based cohort study. *Diabetologia* 2012;55:936–47.

27. Ray JG, O'Brien TE, Chan WS. Preconception care and the risk of congenital anomalies in the offspring of women with diabetes mellitus: a meta-analysis. *QJM* 2001;4:435–44.

28. The Diabetes Control Complications Trial Research Group. Pregnancy outcomes in the Diabetes Control and Complications Trial. *Am J Obstet Gynecol* 1996;174:1343–53.

29. Jovanovic L, Druzin M, Peterson CM. Effect of euglycemia on the outcome of pregnancy in insulin-dependent diabetic women as compared with normal control subjects. *Am J Med* 1981;71:921–7.

30. de Veciana M, Major CA, Morgan MA, Asrat T, Toohey JS, Lien JM, *et al.* Postprandial versus preprandial blood glucose monitoring in women with gestational diabetes mellitus requiring insulin therapy. *N Engl J Med* 1995;333:1237–41.

31. Crowther CA, Hiller JE, MosJ JR, McPhee AJ, Jeffries WS, Robinson JS, *et al.* Effect of treatment of gestational diabetes mellitus on pregnancy outcomes. *N Engl J Med* 2005;352:2477–86.

32. Landon MB, Spong CY, Thom E, Carpenter MW, Ramin SM, Casey B, *et al.* A multicenter, randomized trial of treatment for mild gestational diabetes. *N Engl J Med* 2009;361:1339–48.

33. Manderson JG, Patterson CC, Hadden DR, Traub AI, Ennis C, McCance DR. Preprandial versus postprandial blood glucose monitoring in type 1 diabetic pregnancy: a randomized controlled clinical trial. *Am J Obstet Gynecol* 2003;189:507–12.

34. Nachum Z, Ben-Shlomo I, Weiner E, Shalev E. Twice daily versus four times daily insulin dose regimens for diabetes in pregnancy: randomised controlled trial. *BMJ* 1999;319:1223–7.

35. racero LA. Comparison of umbilical Doppler velocimetry, nonstress testing, and biophysical profile in pregnancies complicated by diabetes. *J Ultrasound Med* 1996;15:301–8.

36. Suhonen L, Hiilesmaa V, Teramo K. Glycaemic control during early pregnancy and fetal malformations in women with type 1 diabetes mellitus. *Diabetologia* 2000;43(1):79–82.

37. Bell R, Glinianaia SV, Tennant PWG, Bilious RW, Rankin J. Peri-conception hyperglycaemia and nephropathy are associated with risk of congenital anomaly in women with pre-existing diabetes: a population-based cohort study. *Diabetologia* 2012;55:936–47.

38. Landon MB, Leindecker S, Spong CY, Hauth JC, Bloom S, Varner MW, *et al.* The MFMU Caesarean Registry: factors affecting the success of trial of labour after previous caesarean delivery. *Am J Obstet Gynecol* 2005;193:1016–23.

39. deMeeus JB, Ellia F, Magnin G. External cephalic version after previous caesarean section: a series of 38 cases. *Eur J Obstet Gynecol Reprod Biol* 1998;81:65–8.

40. Kennedy A, Hadden DR, Ritchie CM, Gray O, McCance DR. Insulin algorithm for glycaemic control following corticosteroid therapy in Type 1 diabetic pregnancy. *Diabetic Medicine* 2003;20:81.

41. Curet LB, Izquierdo LA, Gilson GJ, Schneider JM, Perelman R, Converse J. Relative effects of antepartum and intrapartum maternal blood glucose levels on incidence of neonatal hypoglycemia. *J Perinatol* 1997;17:113–15.

42. Mimouni F, Miodovnik M, Siddiqi TA, Khoury J, Tsang RC. Perinatal asphyxia in infants of insulin-dependent diabetic mothers. *Journal of Pediatrics* 1988;113:345–53.

43. Sacks DA, *et al.* Frequency of gestational diabetes mellitus at collaborating centers based on IADPSG consensus panel-recommended criteria: the Hyperglycemia and Adverse Pregnancy Outcome (HAPO) Study. *Diabetes Care* 2012;35;526–8.

44. Vérier-Mine O, Chaturvedi N, Webb D, Fuller JH. Is pregnancy a risk factor for microvascular complications? The EURODIAB Prospective Complications Study. *Diabetic Med* 2005;22:1503–9.

45. Kjos SL, Henry OA, Montoro M, Buchanan TA, Mestman JH. Insulin-requiring diabetes in pregnancy: a randomized trial of active induction of labor and expectant management. *Am J Obstet Gynecol* 1993;169:611–15.

HIV in pregnancy: the dilemmas of management

Shreelata Datta and Martina Toby

Ⓒ **Expert Commentary** Kate Harding
Ⓒ **Guest Expert** Annemiek de Ruiter

Case history

A 31-year-old primiparous African woman was seen by her midwife at 10 weeks' gestation for an initial booking assessment. She had been diagnosed HIV-positive four years previously and was under follow up with the local HIV physician. As she had been well with a CD4 count of >400×cells/mm³ no treatment had been required. Her last cervical smear had been 6 months earlier and was normal. BMI was 23 and booking BP was 104/80. This was a planned pregnancy with her HIV-negative partner, having decided to omit condom usage during her fertile period. She was counselled on the need for routine antenatal screening including for rubella, hepatitis B, and syphilis serology. She consented to the full screen which was negative and confirmed rubella immunity.

> ✪ **Learning point** What is HIV and how common is HIV in pregnancy in the UK?
>
> HIV is a retrovirus which can be transmitted through sexual intercourse, blood transfusion, intravenous drug use, from mother to child during pregnancy and during breastfeeding. The HIV virus can be divided into two major sub-types: HIV1 and HIV2. HIV1 is responsible for the majority of infection and leads to chronic viral infection.
>
> Infection with the HIV virus leads to RNA transcription predominantly within CD4 lymphocytes, impairing cellular immunity, causing immunosuppression, and eventually leading to Acquired Immunodeficiency Syndrome (AIDS). The first cases of AIDS were reported in homosexual males in 1981.
>
> According to a Public Health England report in 2010 [1] there were 91 500 people living with HIV in the UK, of whom 30 000 were women. The prevalence of HIV infection in women giving birth in the UK has increased annually for over 20 years. In 2009, unlinked serosurveillance testing residual bloodspots for routine neonatal screening showed a prevalence of HIV infection of 2.2 per 1000 pregnant women. HIV prevalence among women giving birth remained highest in London (3.9 per 1000), and has been stable since 2004. The prevalence in the rest of England has increased fivefold over the past decade, to reach 1.43 per 1000 in 2009. Among UK-born pregnant women in 2009, HIV prevalence was 0.46 per 1000. Worldwide, the WHO estimates that there are 1.4 million HIV-infected women in developing countries alone in 2010, with only 48% of these women receiving antiretroviral therapy (ART). Over 90% of pregnant women with HIV reside in sub-Saharan Africa.

Her viral load at booking was 6081 copies/mL, with a CD4 count of 456×cells/mm³ (normal range 500–1200 cells/mm³). Booking bloods—including LFTs, toxoplasmosis screen, and hepatitis serology—were all normal. A first trimester ultrasound at 12 weeks' gestation confirmed the estimated due date, excluded a multiple pregnancy, and she was screened as low risk for trisomy. Her midwife referred her to the multidisciplinary HIV-in-pregnancy team.

⊗ **Learning point** Antenatal HIV screening and management

- All pregnant women should have screening for hepatitis B, HIV infection, syphilis, and rubella at booking in every pregnancy as part of the Infectious Diseases in Pregnancy Screening Programme [2].
- Fourth-generation laboratory assays are recommended for the first-line HIV test for antenatal screening. Diagnosis relies on a positive screening ELISA (enzyme-linked immunosorbent assay), together with a confirmatory Western blot. Rapid testing has a minimum sensitivity of 95 % [3].
- Health professionals should ensure that the HIV result is clearly documented, but should also explore the patient's wishes for confidentiality at the time of diagnosis and during antenatal care.
- If a patient declines an HIV test, this should be documented clearly in the maternity notes and her reasons should be carefully explored. Screening can be offered again at 28 weeks, particularly in high-risk patients; rapid HIV tests can be used to deliver results within 20 minutes of the sample being taken.
- All patients newly diagnosed as HIV-positive should have their social circumstances reviewed as there may be significant emotional, relationship, legal, and financial issues which arise from the diagnosis of HIV.
- There is often little time for the woman to come to terms with the implications of HIV on her health and pregnancy, and to develop a rapport with the health care professionals treating her.
- Each maternity unit should have a named respondent who informs the National Study of HIV in Pregnancy and Childhood of all HIV-positive pregnancies [4].

⊕ **Clinical tip** Booking blood tests in HIV-positive patients

As well as routine antenatal screening tests, blood tests at booking for HIV-positive patients should include lymphocyte subsets, quantitative RNA PCR measurements of viral load, genotypic resistance test, and liver function tests. The plasma viral load should be monitored in conjunction with the HIV physicians [5].

Where HIV positive women are taking highly active retroviral therapy (HAART) at the time of booking, the RCOG Green-top Guidelines [5] recommend screening for gestational diabetes. Genital infection screening should take place at both booking and at 28 weeks, and any infection detected should be treated.

❝ **Expert comment**

Combined first trimester screening with nuchal translucency, HCG and PAPP-A, and maternal age are estimated to be as reliable in women with HIV as in the HIV-negative population [6]. Invasive testing should be avoided where possible due to the theoretical risk of transmission. Although older studies (in the pre-HAART era) showed increase transmission rates in women who had had an amniocentesis, more recent studies of women on HAART have reported no transmissions in over 100 amniocenteses [7]. It is prudent for all those performing prenatal diagnosis to ascertain the HIV status of their patient before doing the test and delaying the test if possible until viral load (VL) < 50 copies/mL. If they are HIV-positive with a detectable VL, treatment with HAART for four weeks is likely to reduce the risk of transmission [8]. If not on treatment and the invasive diagnostic test procedure cannot be delayed until viral suppression is complete, it is important to consult with the HIV team. If there are no contraindications and no baseline genotypic resistance, it is usually recommended that women should commence HAART to include Raltegravir and be given a single dose of Nevirapine 2–4 hours before the procedure.

> ✪ **Learning point** Pregnancy complications associated with HIV infection
>
> | Maternal complications | Fetal complications |
> | --- | --- |
> | Increased risk of: | Increased risk of: |
> | Chorioamnionitis | Preterm delivery |
> | Postpartum endometritis | |
> | Wound infection | |

> ❝ **Guest expert comment (HIV Physician)**
>
> Untreated HIV is associated with an increased risk of spontaneous preterm birth (sPTB). There also appears to be an association of sPTB with the use of HAART in pregnancy, an association not seen with Zidovudine monotherapy. It has been suggested that this association is attributable to protease inhibitors, or Ritonavir-boosted protease inhibitors; however, a large study in the UK and Ireland [9] demonstrated increased risk of sPTB with HAART compared to mono or dual therapy, and did not show an increase when comparing protease inhibitors with non- nucleoside reverse transcriptase inhibitors within the HAART group. The large prospective randomized PROMISE (Promoting Maternal Infant Survival Everywhere) study (>6000 pregnant women with HIV infection) hopes to address some of the questions that remain with regard to HIV, HAART, and sPTB [10].

> ✪ **Learning point** The perinatal HIV multidisciplinary team
>
> All pregnant women with HIV should be reviewed and managed by a multidisciplinary team. The HIV perinatal team includes an HIV physician, midwife, HIV-specialist nurse, HIV pharmacist, obstetrician, and an infectious disease paediatrician, who will support women in understanding the whole package of HIV care, in particular for those who are finding the diagnosis hard to accept and are reluctant to accept treatment. Early referral to the paediatric team can help women come to terms decisions around breastfeeding. It may be necessary to involve social workers, psychiatrists, counsellors, interpreters, and health visitors [8].

20 weeks

After a normal 20-week anomaly scan, she was seen by the obstetric team to discuss treatment (Table 13.1) and mode of delivery. The option of taking HAART to achieve a viral load of <50 copies/ml and a planned vaginal delivery, or taking Zidovudine monotherapy and having a planned caesarean section at 38 weeks' gestation was discussed. She opted for HAART (which was started at 22 weeks') with the plan for a vaginal delivery.

> ✪ **Learning point** When to initiate antiretroviral therapy?
>
> Although pregnancy has no clear effect on HIV progression, all pregnant HIV-positive women should be advised to take antiretroviral therapy. Without treatment, HIV is vertically transmitted in approximately 25 % of cases [11]. In the non-pregnant patient, HAART is usually commenced when CD4 count drops below 350. Additional consideration is needed in the pregnant patient. All pregnant HAART-naïve woman should have commenced antiretrovirals by week 24 of pregnancy at the latest, regardless of CD4 count.
>
> Clinician choice of HAART is dependent on the viral load of the mother, her individual preferences, resistance pattern of the virus, and whether the treatment is simply for prevention of mother-to-child transmission (MTCT) (temporary HAART), or lifelong treatment for the mother (Table 13.1).

Table 13.1 Initiation of antiretroviral therapy in pregnancy

Patient	Advice
HAART prior to conception	Continue prescribed regimen throughout pregnancy and postpartum.
Asymptomatic, CD4<350* Symptomatic HIV disease or opportunistic infection Untreated, presenting >28 weeks	Start HAART as soon as possible
Asymptomatic, CD4>350, VL<30 000	Start temporary HAART by 24 weeks at the latest gestation if opting for SVD
Asymptomatic, CD4>350, VL>30 000	Start HAART at the start of the second trimester
Untreated, in labour	Give Nevirapine 200 mg immediately, with four drugs to include Raltegravir, and include intravenous Zidovudine
Asymptomatic, CD4>350, VL<10 000	Offer Zidovudine monotherapy if opting for a CS

*If the patient is experiencing pregnancy-related vomiting and nausea, starting HAART at the start of the second trimester is reasonable.

✪ **Learning point** Choice of drug therapy

- The three classes of antiretroviral drug most commonly used in pregnancy are nucleoside reverse transcriptase inhibitors (NRTI), non-nucleoside reverse transcriptase inhibitors (NNRTI) and protease inhibitors (PI). The most common regimens include a combination of two NRTIs, and a PI or an NNRTI. Treatment protocols are individualized for each patient. The safety and efficacy of the most common HAART regimens have not been studied in pregnancy [12]. The BHIVA 2012 guidelines recommend Zidovudine with Lamivudine, Tenofovir, and Emtricitabine, or Abacavir and Lamivudine as backbone (see Table 13.2).
- A longer duration of HAART is associated with reduced mother-to-child transmission; each week of HAART reduces the odds of transmission.
- Although there are over 20 different types of medication used to treat HIV, the most appropriate HAART regimen is generally determined by the HIV physicians. Drug resistance is detected on genotype/phenotype.

❝ **Guest expert comment (HIV physician)**

Raltegravir is an integrase inhibitor which is included in a four-drug regimen for women presenting untreated in labour as it lowers the viral load very rapidly. Single-dose Nevirapine is also included in this situation as it also lowers the viral load rapidly, and crosses the placenta efficiently this providing additional protection to the fetus.

❝ **Guest expert comment (HIV physician)**

Women who start HAART in pregnancy with the aim of a vaginal delivery should ideally achieve an undetectable viral load (<50 c/ml) by 36 weeks, at which point delivery decisions are made. A recent study in the UK showed that many women were currently starting HAART too late and were not achieving the necessary viral load drop, resulting in a caesarean section [13]. A more detailed analysis showed that a starting viral load of around 30 000 c/ml was a critical cut-off and as a result women with a starting viral load of >30 000 c/ml are advised to commence HAART at the start of the second trimester, whereas in women with a lower viral load, treatment can commence slightly later. It is important to have achieved a degree of viral load suppression by the time of fetal viability, therefore all women should have commenced HAART by 24 weeks at the latest.

➕ **Clinical tip** Using Nevirapine at delivery

Nevirapine has a long half-life and a low barrier to the development of resistance. If it is used around delivery, it is important to liaise with the HIV team so that antiretroviral drugs can be discontinued in such a manner to minimize the development of maternal drug resistance.

➕ **Clinical tip** Side effects of HAART

HAART regimens are commonly associated with gastrointestinal disturbances when first used, and can cause hepatotoxicity. Rarely, nucleoside analogue drugs can cause neuropathy, cardiomyopathy, myopathy, pancreatitis, hepatic steatosis, and lactic acidosis which may be confused with HELLP (haemolysis, elevated liver enzymes, low platelet) syndrome. Non-nucleoside reverse transcriptase inhibitors can cause rash and hepatotoxicity, so transaminase levels should be monitored throughout pregnancy.

Table 13.2 Common drug classes used to treat HIV in pregnancy

Drug class	Examples
Nucleoside reverse transcriptase inhibitor (NRTI)	Zidovudine (AZT)
	Lamivudine (3TC)
	Tenofovir (TDF)
	Abacavir (ABC)
Non-nucleoside reverse transcriptase inhibitor (NNRTI)	Nevirapine (NVP)
	Efavirenz (EFV)
Protease inhibitor (PI)	Darunavir (DRV)
	Atazanavir*(ATV)
	Lopinavir (LPV)

N.B. Atazanavir causes a rise in maternal serum bilirubin. This is as a result of inhibition of UDP-glucuronosyl transferase leading to a rise in unconjugated bilirubin. This is to be expected in all women on Atazanavir.

⊕ Clinical tip Zidovudine (AZT) monotherapy

AZT is a nucleoside reverse transcriptase inhibitor which can be used as monotherapy in women with a relatively low viral load (<10 000 c/ml) and a good CD4 count (>350) who plan to undergo an elective caesarean section. It should be initiated between 20 and 24 weeks' gestation. It is given orally twice daily, intravenously at delivery according to weight, and discontinued immediately thereafter [4].

⊕ Clinical tip Pneumocystis carinii pneumonia (PCP)

If the CD 4 count falls below 200 cells/mm², co-trimoxazole should be prescribed for PCP prophylaxis. This should be supplemented with folic acid 5 mg daily to counteract the anti-folate action of trimethoprim.

⓬ Expert comment

For those who wish to start triple therapy with HAART, early initiation not only allows for adequate time to achieve an undetectable viral load, but also gives time for the woman to become accustomed to the treatment, adjust to any early side effects (such as nausea and vomiting), and time for the team to assess not only tolerance, but response to the medication.

⊘ Evidence base Prevention of mother-to-child transmission of HIV

In the absence of breastfeeding, 75 % of transmission events occur during the intrapartum period, and 25 % occur during the antenatal period [15]. It was previously thought that significant risk factors for vertical transmission of HIV include prolonged labour, amniotic membrane rupture beyond 4 hours, a high viral load at delivery, chorioamnionitis, and prematurity [16]. Current evidence would suggest that the most important predictor of vertical transmission is viral load at delivery, which directly correlates to the risk of transmission [11, 17].

A key paper in our progress to virtual elimination of mother-to-child transmission of HIV was published in the New England Journal of Medicine in 1994 [18]. This showed a reduction in transmission following treatment of 67 % (from 25.5–8.3 %) in women who were treated with Zidovudine during pregnancy and intravenous Zidovudine intrapartum. Following this, treatment became widespread and current transmission rates are quoted as low as 0.1 % in women on HAART who avoid breastfeeding [19].

✪ Learning point Mode of delivery

A decision about the mode of delivery should be made by 36 weeks' gestation and is influenced by the woman's viral load. The aim of treatment must therefore be to reduce this as far as possible (in most cases it is possible to reduce it to <50 copies/ml). With a viral load of <50 copies/ml, mode of delivery has little if any influence on the risk of transmission, and vaginal delivery (without Zidovudine infusion) can be recommended [8]. In addition, for this cohort, women with uncomplicated breech presentation, external cephalic version can be offered beyond 36 weeks' gestation, as can vaginal birth after caesarean section.

Delivery by elective lower segment caesarean section (LSCS) at 38 weeks to prevent labour is recommended for women [8]:

- Taking Zidovudine monotherapy.
- On HAART with a viral load >400 copies/mL.

For women with a viral load of 50–399 copies/mL, mode of delivery can be discussed. If they are on HAART and the viral load is falling it is unlikely that the mode of delivery will have a significant effect on the risk of MTCT, although the data are unclear.

> **✓ Evidence base** Risk of mother-to-child transmission (MTCT) of HIV and mode of delivery
>
> In 1999, a randomized study showed a reduced risk of MTCT in women having planned lower segment caesarean section (LSCS) compared with those having planned vaginal delivery [20]. This prompted widespread use of elective LSCS in women with HIV. All of these women were treated with Zidovudine monotherapy (both antenatally and in labour). This would not have brought viral loads down to the levels seen today.
>
> In 2008, two papers again changed management for women with HIV in pregnancy. The UK database of 5151 deliveries in the UK and Ireland showed the overall risk of MTCT of 1.2%. This was reduced to 0.8% in women who had had at least 14 days of HAART. Among those on HAART, the risk of MTCT for women who had a planned vaginal delivery versus planned caesarean section, the rate of transmission was the same in both groups (0.7%). For those who had an emergency LSCS, it was 1.7% [21]. These findings were echoed by a study in France [22] and Europe in 2010 [23].

> **✚ Clinical tip** Viral load monitoring
>
> Viral load is an important determinant of transmission. Plasma viral load, liver function, and full blood count (as measures of drug toxicity) should be monitored:
>
> • At least every three months and at week 36 in women on long-term ART. In women who commence HAART in pregnancy, viral load should be measured two to four weeks after commencing HAART, a minimum of once every trimester as well as at week 36 and delivery.
> • Two weeks after starting or changing therapy.
> • At delivery.
> • As directed by HIV physicians.

26 weeks

At 26 weeks she was tolerating the treatment well, did not complain of nausea or vomiting, and had a normal blood profile

28 weeks

At 28 weeks' gestation she was seen in the pregnancy day assessment unit with flu-like symptoms, a cough, vomiting, and a temperature of 37.9 °C. Her heart rate was noted to be 116 beats per minute, with a blood pressure of 115/66. On examination, chest was clear and urine dipstick was negative. Blood cultures and bloods were sent, and she was admitted and commenced on intravenous (IV) Cefuroxime (for suspected pneumonia), and Oseltamivir phosphate (for atypical influenza H1N1). She was nursed in isolation. The following morning she appeared to be clinically improving, with a temperature of 37.1 °C and her chest was clear; IV antibiotics were converted to oral therapy. Blood results are shown in Table 13.3.

An ALT of 82 units/L (normal range 7–41units/L) raised the differential diagnosis of obstetric cholestasis (despite the lack of itching). She was discharged home with antenatal clinic follow up.

At her antenatal follow-up appointment, bile acids were normal (excluding obstetric cholestasis), as was a liver ultrasound. Swabs confirmed that the patient had contracted an enterovirus, but her ALT continued to rise to 117–units/L (Figure 13.1).

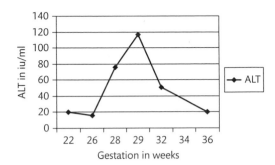

Figure 13.1 ALT level trend between 22 and 36 weeks.

Table 13.3 Blood results

Parameter	Result	Parameter	Result
Hb	10.7	ALP	78
WCC	11	**ALT**	**82**
Lymphocytes	0.8	Albumin	29
Platelets	244	Bile acids	6
Sodium	136	Hepatitis A	Previous infection evident
Potassium	4.2	Hepatitis B	Not detected
Creatinine	78	Hepatitis C	Not detected
Urea	3.2	H1N1 swab	Negative

32 weeks

At 32 weeks, she remained clinically well though her ALT was still elevated at 51 (Figure 13.1). Bile acids were consistently normal, as was her blood pressure, with no protein in the urine. Ultrasound scans at 32 and 36 weeks showed normal growth velocity and liquor volume.

36 weeks

At her 36-week antenatal appointment, her liver function normalized (Figure 13.1) and a definitive diagnosis of post-viral mild hepatitis was made.

⊗ **Learning point** Abnormal liver function in pregnancy

Abnormalities of liver function tests are common in pregnant women on HAART.

Differential diagnosis includes:

- Obstetric cholestasis.
- Pre-eclampsia (with HELLP syndrome).
- Acute viral hepatitis and reaction to antiretroviral treatment.

In addition, pregnant women with late-stage HIV have a higher risk of opportunistic infections such as PCP. Having excluded PET, acute viral hepatitis A, B, C, and CMV, attention was turned to obstetric cholestasis (a clinical diagnosis of exclusion), and drug reaction. Consultation with the HIV physician is helpful but occasionally only observant anticipation will reveal the correct diagnosis (as in this case). Had her ALT continued to rise and had she developed pruritis, the diagnosis would have changed to obstetric cholestasis and treatment with ursodeoxycholic acid plus consideration of delivery at 38 weeks.

⟨⟨ **Guest expert comment (HIV physician)**

A rise in ALT can occur as a result of antiretroviral toxicity. Communication between the HIV and obstetric teams is crucial to inform on necessary investigations. If HAART toxicity is suspected, it may be necessary to change the HAART regimen.

Mode of delivery was again discussed and she agreed that a vaginal delivery was suitable as her viral load had responded well to treatment and had remained <50 c/ml for some weeks. She was also informed that unless deemed necessary by the obstetric team during labour, fetal scalp electrode monitoring, fetal blood sampling, and ventouse delivery were best avoided. She was aware that an ARM would be performed only if clinically indicated. The midwifery team counselled her on the importance of avoiding breastfeeding. Carbegoline 1 mg orally was to be given within the first 24 hours post delivery to suppress milk production.

41 weeks

At 41+3 weeks, she underwent a membrane sweep by her midwife, and the possibility of an induction of labour was discussed if she did not present in spontaneous labour. Within 24 hours of the sweep, she presented in early labour at 2 cm. She was managed as a 'normal' pregnancy with intermittent auscultation and elected to have Entonox for analgesia.

She initially progressed well but progress slowed at 9 cm dilatation. After 2 hours with no further progress, an amniotomy was performed. Three hours later she was still 9 cm with the baby in an occipito-transverse position. She agreed to Syntocinon infusion (after an epidural) and was fully dilated 2 hours later with the head 1 cm below the ischial spines, and a direct occipito-anterior position. One hour was allowed for head descent. This was followed by 1 hour of active pushing. As delivery was still not imminent despite an hour of active pushing and an hour of involuntary pushing, a forceps delivery was discussed. While this was being set up the patient

---

⭐ **Learning point** Management of labour

There is no evidence to suggest that labour in women with HIV on HAART with a viral load of <50 c/ml should be managed differently to other women. Principles of management are generally based on minimizing the exposure of the fetus to maternal fluids (although infants are not thought to be at significantly higher risk with longer duration of ruptured membranes, as shown in the evidence base). In general, the BHIVA guidelines recommend management should follow the NICE guideline for intrapartum care [24].

- Induction of labour can be considered; there is no contraindication to the use of prostaglandins or membrane sweep in patients on HAART with a viral load <50 copies/mL.
- In women with previous caesarean sections, a trial of scar can be considered where the viral load is <50 copies/mL.
- Intrapartum intravenous Zidovudine infusion is recommended in women if the VL >10 000 copies/mL, regardless of the mode of delivery. Untreated women with an unknown VL should also be given intravenous Zidovudine in labour.
- There is a theoretical concern that if amniotomy is performed with the membranes close to the fetal scalp, the fetal skin could be broken which could increase risk of transmission.
- Invasive procedures such as fetal blood sampling and fetal scalp electrodes are best avoided. However, the BHIVA 2012 writing group have concluded that it is unlikely that the use of fetal scalp electrodes and fetal blood sampling increases the risk of transmission in women taking HAART with an undetectable viral load.
- Although forceps are associated with less fetal trauma than vacuum delivery, if the VL is <50 copies/mL, it is unlikely that the type of instrument used will affect the MTCT. There is no increase in the risk of mother-to-child transmission associated with episiotomy.

(continued)

- Where caesarean section is indicated, the RCOG recommend that blood loss should be minimized throughout and the membranes should be ruptured only when the head is delivered through the uterine incision. There is no evidence to recommend timing of cord clamping. As delayed cord clamping increases the neonatal haemoglobin by a placenta-to-fetal transfusion, there is little to suggest that this would increase MTCT, therefore delayed cord clamping can be considered.
- Maternal plasma viral load and CD4 lymphocyte count should be taken at delivery.

✔ Evidence base Ruptured membranes

Whilst initial studies suggested that ruptured membranes at term in an HIV infected pregnant woman was associated with an increase in risk of vertical HIV transmission of 2% per hour of membrane rupture, this was mistakenly believed to mean that the risk of transmission after 24 hours would be of the order of 50%. In fact, the increase in risk reported was a 2% increase of the background risk. Thus if the risk was of the order of 1% transmission at 24 hours, the risk would have been 1% plus 0.5% (2% of 1% being 0.02%) [25]. This evidence informed recommendations to initiate delivery as soon as possible after rupture of membranes in HIV-positive pregnant women at term. A recent study [17] has shown that the risk of transmission is related to viral load, not length of ruptured membranes, with similar rates of transmission with membrane rupture of more or less than six hours.

The BHIVA 2012 guidelines recommend expediting delivery in all cases of term, pre-labour spontaneous rupture of the membranes. The mode of delivery is influenced by maternal viral load:

- VL < 50 copies/mL—immediate induction of labour
- VL 50–999 copies/mL consider LSCS
- VL > 1000 copies/mL—immediate LSCS

✪ Learning point Preterm rupture of membranes

In women with preterm pre-labour ruptured membranes there is concern that prolonged ruptured membranes can lead to chorioamnionitis, and this can increase the risk of vertical transmission. The BHIVA 2012 current recommendation is that for women with (PPROM) < 28 weeks, steroids should be given for fetal lung maturation and decision for delivery made by the joint HIV–perinatal team. At > 34 weeks' gestation, infection is a greater risk for the baby than prematurity, and therefore labour should be initiated without delaying for steroids. In women who are 28–34 weeks' gestation steroids should be given and labour initiated once they are effective (i.e. 48 hours after the first dose). Broad-spectrum antibiotics should be given if there is evidence of chorioamnionitis.

---

managed to achieve a spontaneous vaginal delivery (with second-degree tear) of a healthy female infant with Apgars 9 and 10, weighing 3.86 kg.

After delivery, the baby was not bathed immediately (due to concern regarding neonatal hypothermia without reduction of risk of MTCT). The baby was reviewed by the neonatology team, blood was taken for HIV RNA and she was prescribed Zidovudine for four weeks (the first dose was given two hours after delivery). HAART was stopped in the mother. The mother was given 1 mg of Cabergoline four hours after delivery, and agreed not to breastfeed.

At follow-up, both mother and baby were well. The baby remained HIV-negative at two years of age. Initial infant bloods would have been positive for HIV antibody as these are maternally derived. The patient was counselled on the merits of condom usage to protect her partner, and other contraception (e.g. Mirena intra-uterine System (IUS) to prevent conception), and annual cervical cytology.

✚ Clinical tip Stopping ART postpartum

- Continue ART in women with a CD4 cell count < 350 cells/mm², with an AIDS defining illness or in women with a CD4 cell count between 350–500 cells/mm² with hepatitis B or C co-infection.
- Discontinue ART if CD4 cell count is above 500 cells/mm².

○ **Learning point** Managing the neonate

● **Infant feeding**

All HIV-positive women in the UK are advised not to breastfeed. Cabergoline (1 mg) can be used to suppress lactation to aid mothers who agree not to breastfeed. Those who deliver a very preterm baby may wish to use donated breast milk to give their infant the benefit of breast milk without the risk of HIV. There is no evidence that pasteurization of breast milk prevents transmission. Denying HIV-positive women the ability to breastfeed their infant can be one the hardest things for them to accept, and is best achieved with careful counselling and support.

● **Infant post-exposure prophylaxis (PEP)**

All neonates should be treated with antiretroviral therapy within four hours of birth. Neonates should be treated with Zidovudine monotherapy if maternal VL is <50 copies/mL at 36 weeks' gestation, but in all other cases, HAART should be used. The choice of drugs given to the baby also depends on the mother's treatment, and prophylaxis should be continued for four weeks.

Establishing a diagnosis of HIV infection in the neonate is complicated by transplacentally acquired maternal antibodies, which can take up to 18 months to clear. HIV-1 DNA PCR assay to detect pro-viral DNA (or RNA) in peripheral blood mononuclear cells is the primary mechanism to diagnose HIV. It is important to test the mother for HIV DNA by PCR prior to delivery to ensure that the primers used to detect infant HIV DNA are appropriate. Infants should be tested during the first 48 hours prior to hospital discharge, six weeks (two weeks post infant prophylaxis), and 12 weeks of age. A final HIV antibody test can be performed at 18 months [2]. If there are additional risks (e.g. breastfeeding), monthly testing of the mother is also recommended, and infant testing needs to continue until 18 months after cessation of feeding. Although some units advocate immediate infant bathing, there is no clear evidence to suggest that there is any benefit in early bathing.

⊘ **Evidence base** Infant feeding and MTCT

For many women, the advice not to breastfeed is one of the most difficult aspects of preventing MTCT, and has the potential to stigmatize her within her community or family. Early studies (in the pre-HAART era) showed a doubling of the risk of transmission with breastfeeding (5–10% risk) [26]. In the UK this led to child protection action being taken in a number of cases where the mother either insisted on breastfeeding or covertly breastfed, resulting in a number of infants taken into care to prevent MTCT.

More recent studies [27] have demonstrated transmission rates of 0–3% after six months' exclusive breastfeeding if the mother is treated with Nevirapine. On the basis of these studies, the WHO has published new infant feeding guidelines applicable to resource-poor regions where bottle feeding is not acceptable, feasible, affordable, or safe [19]. If breastfeeding is to be pursued, WHO recommends the use of postpartum antiretroviral therapy (either maternal HAART or infant Nevirapine) to reduce the risk of HIV transmission during the period of breastfeeding. Although infant Nevirapine is cheaper, it exposes the infant to a greater dose of antiretrovirals.

In the UK, where bottle-feeding is safe, sustainable, and feasible, breastfeeding is discouraged. Carbegoline 1 mg (for the mother) is recommended within 24 hours of delivery to suppress lactation. There are a number of routes to access financial support for the purchase of infant milk in the UK both for women entitled to benefits and those who are not (e.g. illegal immigrants and those declined refugee status). For further information, consult the British HIV Association (BHIVA) and Children's HIV Association (CHIVA) Position Statement on Infant Feeding in the UK (November 2010) [28].

○ **Learning point** HIV and cervical cytology

All women newly diagnosed with HIV should have cervical surveillance performed annually; cytology with an initial colposcopy examination where possible. The screening age recommendations follow those for HIV-negative women.

(continued)

Despite the higher cervical treatment failure rate, high-grade cervical intraepithelial neoplasia (CIN should be managed according to national guidelines. HAART reduces HIV viral load, and may reduce HPV viral load, so the prevalence and incidence of cervical abnormality may also fall with antiretroviral therapy. A higher incidence of CIN and recurrence following treatment is thought to be due to reduced immune activity against HPV. Even cohorts using HAART are at increased risk of abnormal cytology, although HAART may increase the regression of low-grade lesions [29].

Psychosocial and legal considerations

At the time of admission, the patient's main concern was regarding non-disclosure of her HIV status. She had not informed her partner or any member of her family or social group of her HIV status. The team supported the patient's needs and wishes both medically and socially, and reassured her that her confidentiality would be maintained. The importance of ensuring that the general practitioner was informed was emphasized (so that if the baby became unwell he would know what to look for). Like many women, she had some concerns about this because he was a member of her community, but after discussion with her HIV physician she became convinced that it was in her best interest for the GP to be made aware, and she consented to communication with the GP.

She had several discussions with the HIV health adviser, and a plan with time-lines was made regarding when she would disclose her HIV status to her partner once the baby was born. This plan was discussed with the rest of the team. Her desire for confidentiality was passed on to the rest of the team to ensure that her diagnosis was not mentioned in the presence of any companions, and strategies for her to use when discussing the fact that she was not breastfeeding were highlighted.

❻ Expert comment

Although disclosure is encouraged in all cases, this may take some time. Women should be given supportive guidance, relevant to their circumstances, social, or cultural issues. Reasons for refusing disclosure should be explored and may include fear of domestic violence or relationship breakdown. This can create a conflict between the doctor's duty of confidentiality to the patient and a duty to prevent harm to others. Breaking confidentiality to inform a sexual partner is sanctioned as a 'last resort' by the World Health Organisation, General Medical Council, and the British Medical Association. Difficult disclosure cases should be managed by the multidisciplinary team, with a low threshold for legal advice. Accurate documentation of discussions and a disclosure strategy are essential. Reassurance about confidentiality is vital, particularly around family members and friends who may not know the diagnosis but who are involved in the care of the pregnancy. Women from communities with high levels of HIV awareness may be concerned about HIV disclosure when discussing interventions such as medication during pregnancy, and avoiding breastfeeding. At the same time, women should be informed of the benefits of safer sex practices and the use of condoms to prevent HIV and other sexually transmitted infections. Forced disclosure may have a negative uptake on HIV testing and result in the patient losing trust in the healthcare team.

Discussion

HIV is one of the most important infectious diseases in the world. Its prevalence in women giving birth in the UK has increased annually for over 20 years. Reducing mother to child transmission depends on minimizing the maternal viral load which in turn depends on identifying all women with HIV either prior to pregnancy or in early pregnancy. The introduction of 'opt-out' screening for HIV in early pregnancy has dramatically reduced the number women delivering with HIV who do not know their status.

In women who are known to have HIV prior to pregnancy, pre-conceptual counselling includes screening for and treating STIs, checking immunizations, optimizing maternal nutritional status, and reviewing therapy. In some cases, methods of conception which minimize transmission to her partner should also be discussed.

Actual treatment regimen in pregnancy is influenced by maternal choice and takes into account mode of delivery, drug resistance, and treatment prior to pregnancy (in those with a pre-existing diagnosis). The multidisciplinary team is of vital importance as many of these women have a complex social background with 'fragile' immigration status, concern about the stigma' of the disease, and in some cases, a long history of interaction with the HIV team.

With the appropriate support, women with HIV remain engaged with the clinicians, thus giving themselves and their children the best chance of normal or near-normal life expectancy.

Key Management Points

- All pregnant women should be tested for HIV in the first trimester or as soon as possible if they present for antenatal care later in pregnancy. If they are high risk, a repeat test can be advocated. HIV test results should be clearly documented in the maternity notes. HIV-positive women must be reassured of confidentiality, and although informing their partner is encouraged, their decision must be supported. The minimum composition of the antenatal multidisciplinary team includes an obstetrician, specialist midwife, HIV specialist, and paediatrician.
- In women with a new diagnosis of HIV, effective ART should be commenced by 24 weeks' gestation, wherever possible. Viral load is an important determinant of transmission and should be quantified regularly throughout the pregnancy.
- In the investigation of any illness in a pregnant woman with HIV, both her obstetric condition and complications from HIV or her medication should be considered. The planned mode of delivery should be formalized by 36 weeks' gestation. Vaginal delivery is recommended for women with a viral load <50 copies/ml.
- Breastfeeding should be avoided wherever possible, as this increases transmission by at least 3 % even in those whose viral load is suppressed. Cabergoline 1 mg orally within 24 hours of birth should be administered to suppress breast-milk production.
- Neonatal ART therapy should be administered within four hours of delivery, with HIV testing at day 1, 6 weeks, and 12 weeks post birth with a final test at 18 months of age.
- Follow-up advice includes measures for family planning with safer sex, annual cervical cytology, and optimizing viral load prior to a further pregnancy. Long-term planning is essential to ensure that the woman maintains contact with her healthcare team.

A Final Word from the Expert

While it is recognized that it is important that it is clearly stated in the notes that the patient is HIV positive to allow those caring for her to give her the appropriate treatment (especially when she is admitted in labour), this can lead to inadvertent disclosure when using hand-held notes. In this case, confidentiality was maintained through careful handover between members of the team (especially in labour and on the postnatal ward).

Care should be taken to avoid inadvertent disclosure to a woman's partner or family members, as they may be unaware of her HIV diagnosis, even though they may attend antenatal clinic with her and be present during the delivery. As most women in the UK carry their own notes and members of their family often read them, confidentiality may be difficult to maintain. Clues such as 'VL< 20', or 'viral infection' may alert the healthcare workers without alarming the woman or informing her family. Whilst women should be encouraged to disclose their HIV status to their partner, the patient's wishes should be respected. The HIV team are very experienced with this issue and should be involved. The HIV health adviser will work with the patient to plan for controlled disclosure of her status, at the same time ensuring that any unaware partner is not put at risk. Advice should be given about the use of condoms and safe sex practices, to prevent transmission of HIV and other sexually transmitted infections to an uninfected partner. Where necessary, legal advice and multidisciplinary support can be sought.

Rarely, women may refuse any intervention during pregnancy or declare their intention to breastfeed the baby against advice. These cases should be discussed with social services pre-delivery so that a strategy can be developed. If the mother's VL is undetectable and she is on effective HAART, a referral to child-protection teams is not usually necessary. Both mother and baby should be under review with monthly maternal viral loads, and HAART should be continued for a minimum of 1 week after breastfeeding has stopped.

References

1. Health Protection Agency. *HIV in the United Kingdom:2010 Report*. HPA: London, 2010. <:http://www.hpa.org.uk/webc/HPAwebFile/HPAweb_C/1287145367237>
2. IDPS Programme Standards 2010. <http://infectiousdiseases.screening.nhs.uk/standards
3. National Institute of Clinical Excellence. *Antenatal Care: Routine care for the healthy pregnant woman*. NICE: London, 2008. <http://www.nice.org.uk/nicemedia/live/11947/40115/40115.pdf>
4. National Study of HIV in pregnancy and childhood. UCL:London. <http://www.ucl.ac.uk/nshpc>
5. Royal College of Obstetricians and Gynaecologists. *Management of HIV in pregnancy*. Green-top Guideline 39. 2010. London, RCOG.
6. Savvidou MD, Samuel I, Syngelaki A, Poulton M, Nicolaides KH. First-trimester markers of aneuploidy in women positive for HIV. *BJOG* 2011;118(7):844–8.
7. Mandlebrot L, Jasseron C, Ekoukou D, Batallan A, Bongain A, Pannier E, *et al*.AT ANRS French Perinatal Cohort (EPF). Amniocentesis and mother to child human immunodeficiency virus transmission in the Agence Nationale de Recherches sur le SIDA et les Hepatites Virales French Perinatal Cohort. *Am J Obs Gynaecol* 2009;200:160. E1–9.
8. BHIVA and CHIVA. Guidelines for the management of HIV infection in pregnant women. BHIVA: Bristol, 2012. <http://www.bhiva.org>

9. Townsend CL, Cortina-Borja M, Peckham CS, Tookey PA. Antiretroviral therapy and premature delivery in diagnosed HIV-infected women in the United Kingdom and Ireland. *AIDS* 2007;21:1019–26.

10. NIAID: Bethesda, MD, 2010. <http://www.niaid.nih.gov/news/newsreleases/2010/pages/promise.aspx>

11. Senise J, Bonafe S, Castelo A. The management of HIV infected pregnant women. *Curr Opin Obstet Gynaecol* 2012;24:395–401.

12. Sturt AS, Dokubo EK, Sint TT. Antiretroviral therapy (ART) for treating HIV infection in ART-eligible pregnant women. *Cochrane Database Syst Rev* 2010 Mar 17;(3): C D008440.

13. Read PJ, Mandalia S, Khan P, Harrisson U, Naftalin C, Gilleece Y, *et al.* London HIV Perinatal Research Group. When should HAART be initiated in pregnancy to achieve an undetectable HIV viral load by delivery? *AIDS* 2012;26:1095–103.

14. The European Mode of Delivery Collaboration. Elective caesarean-section versus vaginal delivery in prevention of vertical HIV-1 transmission: a randomised clinical trial. *Lancet* 1999;353:1035–9.

15. Mock PA, Shaffer N, Bhadrakom C, Siriwasin W, Chotpitayasunondh T, Chearskul S, *et al.* Maternal viral load and timing of mother-to-child HIV transmission, Bangkok, Thailand. Bangkok Collaborative mother-to-child HIV transmission Study Group. *AIDS* 1999C; 13;407-14.

16. Mofensen LM, Lambert JS, Stiehm ER, Bethel J, Meyer WA 3rd, Whitehouse J, *et al.* Risk factors for perinatal transmission of human immunodeficiency virus type 1 in women treated with zidovudine. Pediatric AIDS Clinical Trials Group Study 185 Team. *N Engl J Med* 1999;341:385-93.

17. Haile-Selassie H, Masters J, de Ruiter A, Tookey P. Duration of ruptured membranes and vertical transmission of HIV: data from national surveillance in the UK and Ireland. 5th Annual Conference of the Children's HIV Association. CHIVA: Bristol, 2011. <http://www.chiva.org.uk/professionals/health/events/previous/conference11/index.html>

18. Connor EM, Sperling RS, Gelber R, Kiselev P, Scott G, O'Sullivan MJ, *et al.* Reduction of maternal-infant transmission of human immunodeficiency virus type 1 with zidovudine treatment. Pediatric AIDS Clinical Trials Group Protocol 076 Study Group. *N Engl J Med* 1994;331(18):1173–80.

19. World Health Organisation. Guidelines on HIV and Infant Feeding 2010: Principles and recommendations for infant feeding in the context of HIV and a summary of evidence. Geneva: WHO, 2010 (FAAST).

20. Beckerman K, Morris AB, Stek A. Mode of delivery and the risk of vertical transmission of HIV-1. *N Engl J Med* 1999;341:205–6.

21. Townsend CL, Cortina-Borja M, Peckham CS, de Ruiter A, Lyall H, Tookey PA. Low rates of mother-to-child transmission of HIV following effective pregnancy interventions in the United Kingdom and Ireland, 2000–2006. *AIDS* 2008;22 (8):973–81.

22. Warszawaski J, Tubiana R, Le Chenadec J, Blanche S, Teglas JP, Dollfus C, *et al.* Mother-to-child HIV transmission despite antiretroviral therapy in the ANRS French Perinatal Cohort. *AIDS* 2008;22:289–99

23. Boer K, England K, Godfried MH, Thorne C. Mode of delivery in HIV-infected pregnant women and prevention of mother-to-child transmission: changing practices in Western Europe. *HIV Med* 2010;11(6):368–78.

24. NICE Guideline Number 57: Intrapartum Care. NICE: London, 2007.

25. The International Perinatal *HIV Group. Duration of ruptured membranes and vertical transmission of HIV-1: a meta-analysis from 15 prospective cohort studies. AIDS* 2001;15(3):357–68.

26. Dunn D, Newell ML, Ades A, Peckham C. Risk of Human Immunodeficiency virus type 1 transmission through breastfeeding. *Lancet* 1992;240:585–8.

27. Shapiro RL, Hughes MD, Ogwu A, Kitch D, Lockman S, Moffat C, *et al.* Antiretroviral regimens in pregnancy and breast-feeding in Botswana. *N Engl J Med* 2010;362:2282–94.

28. British HIV Association (BHIVA) and Children's HIV Association (CHIVA) Position Statement on Infant Feeding in the UK. BHIVA: London, November 2010. <http://www.bhiva.org/documents/Publications/InfantFeeding10.pdf>

29. BSCCP Guidelines for the NHS Cervical Screening Programme, 2nd edn. BSCCP: Birmingham, 2010. <https://www.bsccp.org.uk/resources/colposcopy-and-programme-management>

14 SLE in pregnancy: lupus nephritis flare or pre-eclampsia—a diagnostic challenge

Gabriella Gray

⑥ Expert Commentary Catherine Nelson-Piercy

Case history

A 34-year-old patient presented for pre-pregnancy counselling referred by her rheumatologist. Two years previously she was diagnosed with systemic lupus erythematosus (SLE) and lupus nephritis. There was no other significant medical or family history and her BMI was 22. She had one healthy child who was born six years previously. That pregnancy was complicated by spontaneous rupture of the membranes at 33 + 4 weeks' gestation, and the delivery of a 2.2 kg infant occurred 48 hours later. Placental histology showed mild, focal acute chorioamnionitis.

Her diagnosis of SLE had been made following a period of illness 2 years previously. She experienced symptoms including joint pain and swelling, fatigue, and facial oedema. At the time she had a mild malar rash, mouth ulcers, and synovitis of the knee. She was noted to be hypertensive with a blood pressure (BP) of 160/90 with associated proteinuria quantified as 0.7 g/24 hours. Blood tests showed the presence of anti-nuclear and anti-double stranded DNA antibodies and anticardiolipin (IgG) antibodies (18 GPL IU/mL) and a serum creatinine of 150 micromol/L. She underwent a renal biopsy, which showed class III and V nephritis (Figure 14.1 and Table 14.1).

> **⑥ Expert comment**
>
> Histological class guides both treatment and prognosis of lupus nephritis.

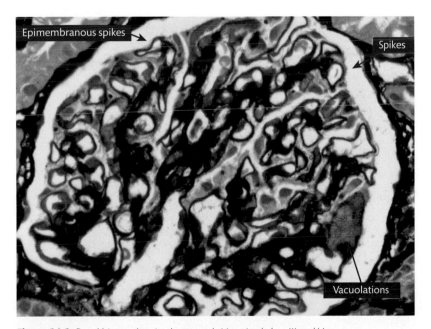

Figure 14.1 Renal biopsy showing lupus nephritis, mixed class III and V.

> ✪ **Learning point** Systemic lupus erythematous (SLE)
>
> SLE is an autoimmune disorder, which affects 0.05% of the population. Its peak incidence is in the group aged 15–40 with a 9:1 female to male ratio, therefore affecting mainly women of childbearing age. It is diagnosed through a combination of signs and symptoms.
>
> The American College of Rheumatologists (ACR) revised criteria for SLE [1].
>
> At least 4 out of 11 must be present:
>
> - malar rash
> - discoid lupus
> - photosensitive rash
> - mouth ulcers
> - arthritis
> - serositis
>   - pericarditis OR
>   - pleurisy
> - nephritis
>   - proteinuria ≥ 3 + or ≥ 0.5 g/24 hours OR
>   - cellular casts in urine
> - CNS lupus
>   - seizures OR
>   - psychosis
> - haematological abnormalities
>   - leukopenia/lymphopenia OR
>   - haemolytic anaemia OR
>   - thrombocytopenia
> - positive ANA
> - presence of other antibodies
>   - anti double stranded DNA
>   - anti La
>   - anti Ro
>   - Sm
>   - lupus anticoagulant/anticardiolipin antibodies

Table 14.1 Histological classification of lupus nephritis [2]

WHO (histological) class	Description
I	Minimal mesangial lupus nephritis
II	Mesangial proliferative lupus nephritis
III	Focal (proliferative) lupus nephritis
IV	Diffuse (proliferative) lupus nephritis
V	Membranous lupus nephritis
VI	Advanced sclerosing lupus nephritis

> ✪ **Learning point** Fertility and conception in SLE
>
> - Fertility is not affected [3] and pregnancy occurs at the same rate even with active disease [4]except for rare cases of end stage renal failure requiring renal replacement therapy.
> - Women who conceive during a flare are more likely to flare again during pregnancy [5].
> - Women who conceive during periods of high disease activity have poorer obstetric outcomes, pregnancy-induced hypertension (PIH), pre-eclampsia, and low birthweight than those who conceive when in remission [5].

> ✪ **Learning point** Pre-pregnancy counselling
>
> Pre-pregnancy counselling should be offered to all patients with SLE, especially those with renal involvement.
>
> The aim of pre-pregnancy management is to ensure conception occurs following at least a six-month period of disease remission and to optimize treatment with non-teratogenic medication. It also enables clinicians to inform women of the likelihood of a successful pregnancy and of the likelihood of complications.
>
> The counselling should be conducted by a renal physician with experience in looking after pregnant women, an obstetrician with experience in renal and connective tissue disease in pregnancy, and an obstetric physician if available. Women should seek advice six to 12 months prior to the planned conception.
>
> At the pre-pregnancy visit, the history and diagnosis should be reviewed [6]. Specific points to be covered are symptoms of active disease, previous thromboembolic events, previous pregnancies and their outcomes. Drug history is important; it should encompass duration of therapy, response to treatment, and potential teratogenicity. Patients should be informed of pregnancy risks and potential complications.
>
> End organ damage should be assessed [6]. A physical examination should be undertaken including measurement of blood pressure (BP) and urinalysis. Further investigations, which are pertinent to counselling and management, should be performed: FBC, antiphospholipid antibodies (APL) (anticardiolipin antibodies, lupus anticoagulant), renal function and liver function, 24-hour urine protein quantification, or urinary protein-to-creatinine ratio (PCR), ANA (antinuclear antibodies), and anti-double stranded DNA (anti-dsDNA), anti-Ro and anti-La antibodies, complement C3, C4 levels, rubella antibodies. The results of these investigations allow assessment of disease activity and specific counselling concerning the risk of complications.

> ✚ **Clinical tip** Baseline investigations
>
> - Evaluation of the renal function (creatinine) will give an indication of the severity of kidney damage and will help with counselling regarding outcome (Table 14.4).
> - The quantification of urine protein serves as a baseline investigation. It is in part reflective of severity of existing damage, and subsequent trends in pregnancy may help with diagnosing pre-eclampsia in pregnancy.
> - Antiphospolipid antibodies are valuable in the clinical context of obstetric or thrombotic history. A diagnosis of antiphospholipid syndrome (APS) will guide management including need for thromboprophylaxis (Table 14.2).
> - Anti-Ro and anti-La antibodies influence fetal outcome (they are associated with neonatal lupus syndromes, including congenital heart block and neonatal cutaneous lupus).
> - Anti-double stranded DNA antibody titre rise and complement (C3, C4) levels fall with disease activity and are useful for assessing this.

ⓒ Expert comment

30% of patients with SLE have APL antibodies [7]. These can be associated with both thromboembolic and obstetric complications, in which case it is termed antiphospholipid *syndrome* (APS) [8]. The prognosis of APS is worse, as both thrombotic and obstetric complications: fetal loss, fetal growth restriction (FGR), and pre-eclampsia are more common than with APL alone. In addition, many of these complications can be prevented by anticoagulant prophylaxis with aspirin and LMWH started early [9]. The differentiation between the APL and APS is very important [7], determines the management, and is based on strict criteria [10].

ⓒ Expert comment

This patient had a previous preterm delivery and was known to have antiphospholipid antibodies (anti-cardiolipin). On careful history-taking, however, there were no indications that this was due to placental insufficiency. Spontaneous preterm rupture of membranes followed by delivery is indicative of chorioamnionitis, which was supported by placental histology. There was no indication of pre-eclampsia and the baby was appropriately grown. Therefore, although the patient had a preterm delivery and had APL antibodies, the diagnostic criteria for APS are not fulfilled [7].

Table 14.2 Criteria for the diagnosis of antiphospholipid syndrome [10]

Vascular thrombosis: ≥ 1 clinical episode of arterial, venous, or small vessel thrombosis. Thrombosis must be objectively confirmed. For histopathological confirmation, thrombosis must be present without inflammation of the vessel wall.

Pregnancy morbidity:

a. ≥1 unexplained deaths of a morphologically normal fetus ≥10 weeks' of gestation.

b. ≥1 premature delivery of a morphologically normal fetus <34 weeks' gestation because of:

   (i) severe pre-eclampsia or eclampsia defined according to standard definitions.

   (ii) recognized features of placental insufficiency.

c. ≥ 3 unexplained consecutive miscarriages <10 weeks' gestation, with maternal and paternal factors (anatomic, hormonal, or chromosomal abnormalities) excluded.

Laboratory criteria: The presence of antiphospholipid antibodies (aPL), on two or more occasions at least 12 weeks' apart and no more than five years prior to clinical manifestations, as demonstrated by ≥ one of the following.

a. Presence of lupus anticoagulant in plasma

b. Medium- to high-titre anticardiolipin antibodies (>40 GPL or MPL, or >ninety-ninth percentile) of IgG or IgM isoforms

c. anti-β_2 glycoprotein-I antibody (anti-β_2GP I) of IgG or IgM present in plasma.

Upon diagnosis of her SLE, treatment was instituted with mycophenolate mofetil and high-dose steroids (prednisolone 1 mg/kg/day) and lisinopril. The steroid dose was progressively reduced as the clinical condition improved and then discontinued. The patient was relatively well over the next 18 months, with one or two episodes of joint pains and swelling, with the most recent attack being two months previously. The BP and renal function remained stable, albeit with mild proteinuria.

✪ Learning point Medication for lupus nephritis

Medication for lupus nephritis should only be started, modified, and stopped by renal physicians with expertise. The role of the obstetrician is to be conversant with the possible effects of the drugs on the fetus and the pregnancy and the implications of possible effects (e.g. what a certain cardiac defect means, how is it detected and treated), and with the implications of stopping a drug (lupus flare, active maternal disease leading to growth restriction, preterm labour, fetal demise). It is also the role of the obstetrician to explain the implications of prematurity and potential obstetric complications such as

(continued)

pre-eclampsia. A list of the main drugs used to treat lupus nephritis and relevant clinical information is included here.

Immunosuppressants

Azathioprine and hydroxychloroquine are safe in pregnancy. Clinicians should explain that a flare of the disease poses a higher risk to maternal and fetal health than the medication itself. Tacrolimus and cyclosporine are also safe.

Mycophenolate mofetil is now one of the first line agents in treatment of lupus nephritis. There is good evidence that exposure in pregnancy causes congenital malformations including hypoplastic nails, shortened fifth fingers, diaphragmatic hernia, microtia (ear deformity,) micrognathia, cleft lip and palate, and congenital heart defects [11] in up to 22% of exposed cases. In cases where the patient has been stable, this agent can be switched to azathioprine. On rare occasions, the medication needs to be continued (for example, if the disease is active in pregnancy); in this case, the risks and benefits of the drug to both mother and fetus should be carefully explained.

Rituximab carries a risk of transient neonatal B cell depletion and severe immunosuppression.

Antihypertensives

Angiotensin-converting enzyme (ACE) inhibitors are used to control proteinuria and hypertension in renal disease and also to treat hypertension in general. However, within the fetus they can cause anomalies of the cardiovascular system, central nervous system (CNS), and kidneys with resulting growth restriction, anhydramnios secondary to renal failure, anuria, and fetal death [12, 13]. They should be discontinued usually prior to pregnancy, unless they are being used for control of heavy proteinuria in nephrotic patients, in which case they can be discontinued at confirmation of pregnancy. For those that require BP control, amlodipine which is also given once a day, is well tolerated and a safe alternative.

Anti-inflammatory drugs

Caution should be exercised with NSAIDs and COX2 inhibitors (these cause luteinized unruptured follicle-anovulation and premature closure of ductus arteriosus if given after 28 weeks). Long-term high-dose steroids have the potential to cause osteopenia and adrenal suppression. There is a possible very small risk of cleft lip +/- palate when used in the first trimester of pregnancy [14].

✚ Clinical tip ACE inhibitors

When to stop or change an ACE inhibitor to an alternative safe in pregnancy will depend on several factors. If used for treatment of hypertension, they should be stopped at the time of discontinuation of contraception. In women in whom pregnancy may take longer to achieve (advanced age, subfertility) and in those in whom it is used to treat heavy proteinuria (> 1 g/24 hours), it should be continued while trying to get pregnant, as a long period without treatment results in loss of renoprotection. The patient should be advised to perform regular pregnancy tests and stop the ACE inhibitor as soon as she has a positive pregnancy test since the risk of teratogenicity starts at 6 weeks.

At the pre-pregnancy clinic visit, physical examination showed a very mild facial rash, no mouth ulcers, minimal soft tissue swelling around the left knee, and no peripheral oedema. BP was 120/80 and 1 + proteinuria was seen on dipstick. Blood results are shown in Table 14.3.

Table 14.3 Baseline (pre-pregancy) investigations (abnormal in bold)

WBC: 6×10^9/L	Albumin: 36 g/L
Hb: 10.1 g/L	ALP: 70 IU/L
Plt: 98×10^9/L	ALT: 23 IU/L
Na: 140 mmol/L	PCR: 80 mg/mmol
K: 4.5 mmol/L	**24 h protein: 0.89 g/save**
Creatinine: 100 micromol/L	**anti-Ro: positive**
	anti-La: positive
Lupus anticoagulant: negative	ACL Ig G: 15 GPL U/L

A discussion was held regarding future pregnancy. It was emphasized that pregnancy is not contraindicated and would be encouraged as the patient was approaching the age when fertility declines naturally.

★ **Learning point** Maternal and fetal outcomes in SLE

Maternal

The risk of developing pre-eclampsia is about 25%. This may result in hospital admission, antihypertensives, and early delivery. The renal function may show a transient improvement in early pregnancy, when plasma volume and glomerular filtration are increased, but will show deterioration in later pregnancy. This may lead to the need for early delivery. The renal function usually recovers to the pre-pregnancy baseline; however, persistent loss of function will occur in a proportion of patients (Table 14.4). Maternal death is rare, but may still occur.

Fetal

The chance of a live birth is high, over 70–90%. An explanation should be given regarding the presence of APL, but it should be emphasized that the clinical syndrome of APS is not present. The risk of early miscarriage is increased above the background risk, but quantification of this risk is difficult. The risk of FGR is 25%, similar to the risk of pre-eclampsia [15]. The risk of preterm delivery is also in the same order—30% [15]. This is usually iatrogenic preterm delivery due to pre-eclampsia or worsening renal impairment. The risk of extreme prematurity (delivery before 28 weeks) is low. With the presence of anti-Ro antibodies, there is a 2% risk of congenital heart block to the baby. In about 5% of babies, a transient lupus-like rash may occur especially on sun exposure. This may be associated with thrombocytopenia. Both are benign and resolve spontaneously.

✓ **Evidence base** Risk of flare in SLE

There have been many conflicting studies on the risk of flare in pregnancy in patients with SLE. Renal disease activity is more common post partum [16], while extra renal flare is more common in second and third trimesters [17]. In recent studies [5] as well as in a recent meta-analysis [18], the risk of flare was 15% in SLE without renal involvement, and 40% with lupus nephritis.

Permanent deterioration of renal function in/after pregnancy is rare; only 2–3% of women suffer this, and only 1% will need dialysis [19]. The reported maternal death rate in older studies was 3.4% [20].

The risk of complications in pregnancy with chronic kidney disease (CKD) from any cause is generally dependent on the pre-pregnancy creatinine [15] and stage of the disease. This is also true for SLE [21]. The risks of complications in CKD from SLE, however seems higher than in CKD from other conditions [22–24]. This applies especially to perinatal death [5, 18].

Table 14.4 Pregnancy outcome (%) in relation to creatinine, adapted from [15]

Creatinine (micromol/L)	Obstetric	Outcomes	(%)		> 25% loss of	kidney function
	FGR	PTD	Pre-eclampsia	PND	In Pregnancy	Persistent
> 125	25	30	22	1	2	0
125–180	40	60	40	5	40	20
> 180	65	> 90	60	10	70	50
On dialysis	> 90	> 90	75	10	N/A	N/A

> ✪ **Learning point** Anti-Ro and anti-La antibodies
>
> - Anti-Ro and anti-La antibodies cross the placenta and are associated with congenital heart block (CHB) in the fetus (Figure 14.2a and 14.2b).
> - The risk for the first pregnancy is 2%, increasing to 18–25% and 50% respectively, if one or two previous fetuses have been affected.
> - Complete atrio-ventricular block is irreversible and develops during weeks 16–24.
> - There is a significant fetal mortality rate (15–30%) resulting from cardiac failure. Two-thirds of the surviving neonates will require permanent pacing [25].
> - Babies with CHB need to be delivered by caesarean section as fetal heart monitoring in labour is not helpful to fetal well-being.
> - The presence of anti-Ro and anti-La autoantibodies confers a 5% risk of neonatal cutaneous lupus, a photosensitive rash (annular erythema) affecting the neonate, which is transient and resolves without sequelae once the maternal antibodies are cleared from the neonatal circulation.

A written plan was made for the patient, and a copy sent to her rheumatologist, her GP, and the patient herself. Prednisolone 5 mg/d was continued, azathioprine 100 mg/d was started, and lisinopril was switched to amlodipine 10 mg/d. She was advised to use paracetamol for simple pain relief. Aspirin 75 mg OD was added to reduce the risk of pre-eclampsia and pre-conception folic acid 400 micrograms/d was commenced. She was advised to book early with a multidisciplinary team.

Four months later, the patient presented to the antenatal clinic. She had already been booked with a high-risk midwifery team and had her 12-week ultrasound scan which confirmed the menstrual dates and a viable pregnancy with a

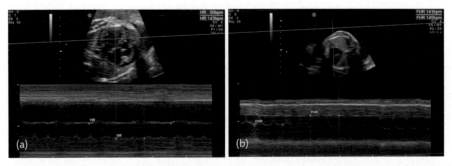

Figure 14.2 Congenital heart block: (a) shows atrio-ventricular block with an atrial rate of 143 bpm and ventricular rate of 50 bpm. (b) shows a normal heart with concordant, normal atrial and ventricular rate.

Images courtesy of Dr S Sankaran, Consultant in Fetal Medicine, Fetal Medicine Department, St Thomas' Hospital, London)

low-risk screening result for chromosomal abnormalities. Her current medications included azathioprine, prednisolone, aspirin, and amlodipine. She was well and on examination, there were no signs of active disease. Her BP was 128/86, there was proteinuria 2 + on urinary dipstick.

A multidisciplinary team consisting of an obstetric physician, high-risk obstetrician, and a fetal medicine consultant reviewed the history and full investigations and after a full explanation a plan was made for her antenatal care:

- Continue medication
- Fetal cardiology ultrasound at 16, 23, and 28/40
- Full fetal anatomy ultrasound and uterine artery Doppler at 20/40
- Fetal ultrasound for growth at 28, 32, and 36/40
- Fetal heart rate assessment at each antenatal visit (auscultation)
- Antenatal checks with BP and urinalysis monthly until 28/40, bi-weekly after or more often if necessary
- Not for LMWH unless admitted to hospital (e.g. hyperemesis) or immobile
- For LMWH thromboprophylaxis for one week following delivery
- Next antenatal visit at 20/40.

22 weeks

The patient was reviewed again at 22 weeks. Fetal anatomy including the heart was normal, with a normal heart rate. The uterine artery Doppler indicated bilateral notching. A further scan was booked for 24/40 to re-assess the uterine Dopplers and at 28, 32, and 36 weeks for fetal growth. The 24-week scan confirmed bilateral uterine artery notching, but the fetal growth and heart rate remained normal.

27 weeks

At 27 weeks, the patient reported increasing fatigue, shortness of breath, and joint pain. The BP was raised at 145/90 and there was 3 + proteinuria noted on dipstick. The physical examination detected bilateral wrist arthralgia. Investigations were repeated (Table 14.5).

The clinical picture and investigations were interpreted as a mild lupus flare. Prednisolone was increased to 20 mg OD and methyldopa was added at 250 mg TDS for blood pressure control. Azathioprine and aspirin were continued. The patient's

Table 14.5 Investigations at 27 weeks (abnormal in bold)

WBC: 6 × 10⁹/L	Albumin: 30 g/L
Hb: **9.8 g/L**	ALP: 230 IU/L
Plt: **96 × 10⁹/L**	ALT: 20 IU/L
Na:139 mmol/L	PCR: **150 mg/mmol**
K:4.6 mmol/L	C3: **0.63 g/L**
Creatinine: **122 micromol/L**	C4: **0.11 g/L**
	anti-ds-DNA titre: **100**

clinical condition improved. She remained as an outpatient, with weekly reviews. The 28-week scan confirmed growth along the fortieth centile and a normal fetal heart rate. The prednisolone dose was reduced to 15 mg OD.

29 weeks

One week later, the patient reported feeling generally unwell, with a mild headache. She appeared oedematous, her BP was elevated at 160/100, and the dipstick showed 4 + proteinuria. Reflexes were normal with no clonus.

She was admitted to the ward for increased surveillance and blood pressure control and investigations were repeated (Table 14.6), including the 24-hour urine collection. Methyldopa dose was increased to 500 mg TDS, prednisolone was increased to 20 mg OD and LMWH (enoxaparin) at 40 mg OD was added. The differential diagnosis at this stage was lupus flare and pre-eclampsia.

Table 14.6 Investigations at 29 weeks (abnormal in bold)

WBC: 6 × 10⁹/L	Albumin: 22 g/L
Hb: 10.2 g/L	ALP: 240 IU/L
Plt: 89 × 10⁹/L	ALT: 22 IU/L
Na:139 mmol/L	PCR: 400 mg/mmol
K:4.3 mmol/L	24h protein: 1.9 g/save
Creatinine: 145 micromol/L	Urine microscopy: RBC present
Urate: 35 mmol/L	no casts
C3: 0.6 g/L	anti-ds-DNA: 110
C4: 0.1 g/L	

> **❝ Expert comment**
>
> The differentiation between pre-eclampsia and any renal disease, but especially lupus nephritis, is difficult. The symptoms are very similar and the objective assessment is confused by the overlap (e.g. pre-existing SLE or flare associated with thrombocytopenia, proteinuria, hypertension). At times the differentiation is impossible and the two are not mutually exclusive but may well coexist. The features that may help distinguish between the two are highlighted in Table 14.7. Complement levels may not be as useful in pregnancy as outside pregnancy.
>
> Between 24 and 28 weeks' the differentiation is crucial as every effort should be made to prolong pregnancy safely. At earlier gestation a renal biopsy may be indicated as the result will influence management. This should be undertaken only by an experienced operator as there is an increased risk of bleeding due to increased renal blood flow. The BP and the clotting should be normal and platelets > 100 ×·10⁹/L and LMWH omitted for at least 12 hours prior to the biopsy. The treatment of a flare is usually with high dose, in severe cases, IV, steroids (methylprednisolone).
>
> After 28 weeks', delivery may be considered and the risk of continuing with the pregnancy should be weighed against the risk of prematurity.

During admission, there was a steady rise in the blood pressure and the patient required maximum doses of Methyldopa, and additional Labetalol, which was increased to 200 mg TDS. The rise in BP was accompanied by a further decline in the renal function. Blood results are shown in Table 14.8.

Table 14.7 Differential diagnosis of pre-eclampsia and lupus flare [6]

	Pre-eclampsia	Flare of lupus
Proteinuria	++ OR > 0.3g/day OR PCR > 30	++(in lupus nephritis)
Red cell casts in urine	Absent	Present (if lupus nephritis)
RBC on urine microscopy	Absent	Present if nephritic
Hypertension	Present	May be present
Involvement of skin and joints	No	Malar rash, photosensitive rash, or evidence of arthritis
Seizures	Present in eclampsia	Present if there is neurological involvement
Urate	Elevated	Not elevated unless CKD
Albumin	Low	Very low if nephrotic syndrome
LFT	May be deranged	Rarely deranged in a flare of SLE
C3 and C4	Unchanged from baseline in early pregnancy	Low
Anti-dsDNA	Unchanged	Elevated

Table 14.8 Investigations at 31 + 4 weeks (abnormal in bold)

WBC: 6 × 10⁹/L	**Albumin: 18 g/L**
Hb: 11 g/L	ALP: 240 IU/L
Plt: 90 × 10⁹/L	ALT: 22 IU/L
Na:139 mmol/L	**PCR: 800 mg/mmol**
K:4.6 mmol/L	
Creatinine: 159 micromol/L	

The fetal ultrasound performed at 31 +3/40 showed a reduction in the growth velocity, with the fetus now growing on the twenty-fifth centile. The liquor volume and umbilical artery Doppler were both normal. The decision for delivery was made for maternal indications (likely pre-eclampsia with creatinine and albumin levels as shown in Table 14.8). Two doses of IM Betamethasone were given for fetal lung maturation.

Labour was induced with prostaglandin and a baby girl was delivered in good condition, weighing 1800 grams. She was admitted to special care and made good progress.

The immediate postpartum period remained uncomplicated. The antihypertensives were changed back to enalapril on day 1. Nifedipine was required on days 2 and 3, when the BP spiked, but was discontinued prior to discharge. LMWH was prescribed for one week at the usual dose of 40 mg OD. Blood tests were repeated initially on a daily basis. There was a steady decline in the creatinine levels. The patient was discharged one week post delivery and warned regarding the risk of postpartum flare. The baby was discharged home at three weeks of age.

✪ Learning point Mode of delivery

About half of women with SLE are delivered by caesarean section. Neither SLE nor renal involvement is an indication for caesarean section, which should be performed for the usual obstetric indications, or the rarely occurring fetal CHB. In our case, there was no fetal compromise (normal liquor and Doppler) or CHB, and the patient had had a previous vaginal delivery. Therefore, although the baby is preterm, induction of labour is reasonable. Continuous CTG monitoring is mandatory.

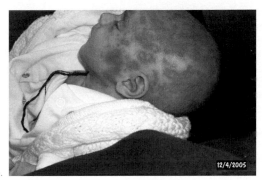

Figure 14.3 Neonatal lupus rash.

The patient was reviewed four weeks later in the postnatal clinic. She appeared well, her BP was controlled at 130/82, but with persistent proteinuria (2+ on dipstick). Her creatinine was almost back to baseline at 122 micromol/L. Interestingly, the baby had a discoid rash (Figure 14.3) that appeared after exposure to ultraviolet light therapy given in SCBU for jaundice. She was seen by the neonatologist, and additional investigations showed mild thrombocytopenia. As the baby was otherwise well, this was interpreted as neonatal lupus and managed conservatively and resolved spontaneously by six weeks.

Discussion

SLE with renal involvement (lupus nephritis) is a severe autoimmune disease. It predominantly affects women of childbearing age. Fertility is maintained, however the potential risk of pregnancy complications, both maternal and fetal, is significant. With good multidisciplinary care the risks can be minimized and outcomes improved.

Ideally, the patient should undergo pre-pregnancy counselling in order to ensure that conception occurs in remission and during treatment with non-teratogenic drugs. It is important that the patient has information and understanding regarding the potential risks to herself (PIH, pre-eclampsia, flare, transient or permanent decline in renal function), and to her baby (intra-uterine demise, growth restriction, prematurity).

During the antenatal period, it is imperative that the patient has regular multidisciplinary review, and fetal well-being is assessed regularly with ultrasound and fetal heart rate auscultation. Complications should be dealt with by an expert team and may require prompt intervention either in the form of drug treatment or delivery.

Following delivery, there is a risk of postpartum flare and neonatal lupus. Postnatal review of the mother and baby should be conducted by a team with experience in the disease.

A Final Word from the Expert

The case discussed has been deliberately chosen to illustrate the challenges and complications, but also a good outcome. While in retrospect one can deduce that the complication was that of early pre-eclampsia, pregnancy could progress to a gestation where delivery was safe and the birthweight was satisfactory. Although the patient has anti-Ro and antiphospholipid antibodies, none of the most worrying complications of these (neonatal CHB, maternal thromboembolism, very early onset pre-eclampsia) occurred. This is not always the case and serious complications may occur; the fetus may have to be born very preterm, and there still is an increased risk of *in utero* and neonatal death or sequelae from prematurity. Mothers can become very sick and have prolonged hospital admissions either because of active SLE, severe infection, or obstetric complications.

Therefore, pregnancy in lupus nephritis is never a clear 'yes or no', but a continuum, which requires individualized informed counselling, close surveillance, and a modern therapeutic arsenal.

References

1. Tan EM, Cohen AS, Fries JF, Masi AT, McShane DJ, Rothfield NF, *et al*. The 1982 revised criteria for the classification of systemic lupus erythematosus. *Arthritis Rheum* 1982 Nov; 25(11):1271–7.
2. Weening JJ, D'Agati VD, Schwartz MM, Seshan SV, Alpers CE, Appel GB, Balow JE, *et al*. The classification of glomerulonephritis in systemic lupus erythematosus revisited. *Kidney Int*. 2004 Feb; 65(2):521–30.
3. Fraga A, Mintz G, Orozco JOrozco JH. Sterilty and fertility rates, fetal wastage and maternal morbidity in systemic lupus erythematosus. *J Rheumatol* 1974;70:99–100.
4. Ramsey-Goldman R, Mientus JM, Kutzer JE, Mulvihill JJ, Medsger TA Jr. Pregnancy outcome in women with systemic lupus erythematosus treated with immunosuppressive drugs. *J Rheumatol* 1993 Jul; 20(7):1152–7.
5. Gladman DD, Tandon A, Ibanez D, Urowitz MB. The effect of lupus nephritis on pregnancy outcome and fetal and maternal complications. *J Rheumatol* 2010 Apr; 37(4):754–8.
6. Bramham KS, MC; Nelson-Piercy, C. Pregnancy and Renal outcomes in Lupus Nephritis: An update and guideline to management. *Lupus* 2011.
7. Stone S, Langford K, Nelson-Piercy C, Khamashta MA, Bewley S, Hunt BJ, *et al*. Antiphospholipid antibodies do not a syndrome make. *Lupus* 2002;11(2):130–3.
8. Miyakis S, Lockshin MD, Atsumi T, Branch DW, Brey RL, Cervera R, *et al*. International consensus statement on an update of the classification criteria for definite antiphospholipid syndrome (APS). *J Thromb Haemost* 2006 Feb; 4(2):295–306.
9. Khare M, Nelson-Piercy C. Acquired thrombophilias and pregnancy. *Best Pract Res Clin Obstet Gynaecol* 2003 Jun; 17(3):491–507.
10. Cervera R, Font J, Gomez-Puerta JA, Espinosa G, Cucho M, Bucciarelli S, *et al*. Validation of the preliminary criteria for the classification of catastrophic antiphospholipid syndrome. *Ann Rheum Dis* 2005 Aug; 64(8):1205–9.
11. Sifontis NM, Coscia LA, Constantinescu S, Lavelanet AF, Moritz MJ, Armenti VT. Pregnancy outcomes in solid organ transplant recipients with exposure to mycophenolate mofetil or sirolimus. *Transplantation* 2006 Dec 27;82(12):1698–702.
12. Cooper WO, Hernandez-Diaz S, Arbogast PG, Dudley JA, Dyer S, Gideon PS, *et al*. Major congenital malformations after first-trimester exposure to ACE inhibitors. *N Engl J Med* 2006 Jun 8;354(23):2443–51.

13. Kyle PM. Drugs and the fetus. *Curr Opin Obstet Gynecol* 2006 Apr; 18(2):93–9.

14. Carmichael SL, Shaw GM, Ma C, *et al*. Maternal corticosteroid use and orofacial clefts. *Am J Obstet Gynecol*. 2007 Dec; 197(6):585 e1–7; discussion 683-4, e1-7.

15. Williams D, Davison J. Chronic kidney disease in pregnancy. *BMJ* 2008 Jan 26; 336(7637):211–5.

16. Tandon A, Ibanez D, Gladman DD, Urowitz MB. The effect of pregnancy on lupus nephritis. *Arthritis Rheum* 2004 Dec; 50(12):3941–6.

17. Ruiz-Irastorza G, Lima F, Alves J, Khamashta MA, Simpson J, Hughes GR, *et al*. Increased rate of lupus flare during pregnancy and the puerperium: a prospective study of 78 pregnancies. *Br J Rheumatol* 1996 Feb; 35(2):133–8.

18. Smyth A, Oliveira GH, Lahr BD, Bailey KR, Norby SM, Garovic VD. A systematic review and meta-analysis of pregnancy outcomes in patients with systemic lupus erythematosus and lupus nephritis. *Clin J Am Soc Nephrol* 2010 Nov; 5(11):2060–8.

19. Imbasciati E, Tincani A, Gregorini G, Doria A, Moroni G, Cabiddu G, *et al*. Pregnancy in women with pre-existing lupus nephritis: predictors of fetal and maternal outcome. *Nephrol Dial Transplant* 2009 Feb; 24(2):519–25.

20. Oviasu E, Hicks J, Cameron JS. The outcome of pregnancy in women with lupus nephritis. *Lupus* 1991 Nov; 1(1):19–25.

21. Imbasciati E, Gregorini G, Cabiddu G, Gammaro L, Ambroso G, Del Giudice A, *et al*. Pregnancy in CKD stages 3 to 5: fetal and maternal outcomes. *Am J Kidney Dis* 2007 Jun; 49(6):753–62.

22. Julkunen H, Kaaja R, Palosuo T, Gronhagen-Riska C, Teramo K. Pregnancy in lupus nephropathy. *Acta Obstet Gynecol Scand* 1993 May; 72(4):258–63.

23. Carmona F, Font J, Moga I, Làzaro I, Cervera R, Pac V, *et al*. Class III-IV proliferative lupus nephritis and pregnancy: a study of 42 cases. *Am J Reprod Immunol* 2005 Apr; 53(4):182–8.

24. Moroni G, Ponticelli C. Pregnancy after lupus nephritis. *Lupus* 2005;14(1):89–94.

25. Julkunen H, Kaaja R, Wallgren E, Teramo K. Isolated congenital heart block: fetal and infant outcome and familial incidence of heart block. *Obstet Gynecol* 1993 Jul; 82(1):11–16.

26. RCOG. Reducing the Risk of Thrombosis and Embolism During Pregnancy and Puerperium. Green-top Guideline No. 37a. 2009.

27. Bower S, Bewley S, Campbell S. Improved prediction of preeclampsia by two-stage screening of uterine arteries using the early diastolic notch and color Doppler imaging. *Obstet Gynecol* 1993 Jul; 82(1):78–83.

28. Sau A, Clarke S, Bass J, Kaiser A, Marinaki A, Nelson-Piercy C. Azathioprine and breast-feeding: is it safe? *BJOG* 2007 Apr; 114(4):498–501.

29. Gisbert JP. Safety of immunomodulators and biologics for the treatment of inflammatory bowel disease during pregnancy and breast-feeding. *Inflamm Bowel Dis* 2010 May; 16(5):881–95.

30. Angelberger S, Reinisch W, Messerschmidt A, Miehsler W, Novacek G, Vogelsang H, *et al*. Long-term follow-up of babies exposed to azathioprine in utero and via breastfeeding. *J Crohns Colitis* 2011 Apr; 5(2):95–100.

31. Ostensen M, Motta M. Therapy insight: the use of antirheumatic drugs during nursing. *Nat Clin Pract Rheumatol* 2007 Jul; 3(7):400–6.

15 Management of a pregnant woman with morbid obesity

Carolyn Chiswick

ⓒ Expert Commentary Fiona Denison
ⓒ Guest Expert Ben Fitzwilliams

Case history

A 40-year-old primigravida booked with her community midwife at 12 weeks' gestation. Her weight was 136 kg and her body mass index (BMI) was 49 kg/m^2. In view of her obesity, she was referred for consultant led antenatal care. Her booking blood pressure (BP) was 120/78 and her urine was clear. She had a past medical history of asthma, which was well controlled with inhaled salbutamol. She was otherwise well. She was on no regular medication. She had taken 400 mcg folic acid per day during the first trimester. She had a normal dating scan and low-risk first trimester combined ultrasound and biochemical serum screening for Down syndrome.

> **✪ Learning point** Folic acid and risk of neural tube defects in obese women
>
> Obese women are at greater risk of having a fetus affected with a neural tube defect (NTD). A meta-analysis of 12 observational cohort studies reported an unadjusted odds ratio for a neural tube defect-affected pregnancy rising from 1.22 (95% CI, 0.99–1.49) in overweight women to 1.70 (95% CI, 1.34–2.15), and 3.11 (95% CI, 1.75–5.46) in obese and severely obese women compared with normal weight controls [1]. The mechanism for this is unclear but proposed theories include undiagnosed type 2 diabetes [2], lower serum folate levels in obese women [3], and decreased ultrasound detection of anomalies in obese women [4] leading to continuation of pregnancies that would otherwise have been terminated. The benefits of peri-conception folic acid in reducing risk of NTD are well established [5], and for those at increased risk (for example women with a previously affected pregnancy) a higher dose is beneficial [6]. However, this protective effect does not seem to benefit obese women. A Canadian study demonstrated no benefit in terms of reduction in incidence of neural tube defects, following introduction of flour fortification with folic acid in women with increased BMI [7]. Despite this lack of evidence, the Royal College of Obstetricians and Gynaecologists (RCOG) recommend that obese women should receive high dose supplementation [8].

Initially her pregnancy progressed normally. She had a fetal anomaly scan at 20 weeks' gestation but inadequate views of the face and thorax were obtained so this was repeated at 22 weeks' gestation with normal findings.

In accordance with the National Institute for Health and Clinical Excellence (NICE) guidance [11], she had a 75 g oral glucose tolerance test (OGTT) at 28 weeks' gestation. The results of this were within normal limits with reference to the World Health Organisation (WHO) standards currently adopted by NICE.

✪ **Learning point** Ultrasound and serum screening for fetal anomaly

Ultrasound is an invaluable tool in the care of the obese pregnancy woman. However, adipose tissue can significantly attenuate the ultrasound signal by absorbing the associated energy. The high-frequency, high-resolution signal used for detection of fetal anomaly is significantly absorbed at a lesser depth, sacrificing image quality. Obese women must be informed of the reduced sensitivity of ultrasound, and told that repeat visits are more likely to be required to obtain all the necessary images [9].

Placentally and fetally derived serum markers used for aneuploidy screening are subject to dilution in larger women [10]. Maternal weight is incorporated into risk calculations and must therefore be recorded accurately on the sample request card. If women are extremely heavy, then using serum markers is not possible and risk calculations must be based on ultrasound scan measurement and weight alone.

✪ **Learning point** Diagnosing diabetes

It is worth noting that diagnostic criteria for gestational diabetes vary around the world. The International Association of Diabetes and Pregnancy Study Group (IADPSG) [12] recommends that a lower fasting plasma glucose threshold be used, with a slightly higher two-hour level, compared to the current WHO guidance. These recommendations are based on the findings from the Hyperglycaemia and Adverse Pregnancy Outcomes (HAPO) study [13]. The Scottish Intercollegiate Guideline Network (SIGN) [14] has adopted the IADPSG recommendations. The NICE guideline is currently under review, and it is likely to lower its diagnostic fasting glucose threshold in line with the IADPSG recommendations. A summary of the different criteria is given in Table 15.1.

Table 15.1

Time	NICE venous plasma glucose	IADPSG venous plasma glucose
Fasting	≥ 7.0 mmol/l	≥ 5.1 mmol/l
2 hours after 75 g oral glucose load	≥ 7.8 mmol/l	≥ 8.5 mmol/l

✪ **Learning point** Treatment of gestational diabetes

Obesity is a well-recognized risk factor for gestational diabetes, and pre-gestational diabetes is more prevalent in obese women. There is no doubt that appropriate treatment of diabetes in pregnancy significantly reduces the risk of serious adverse perinatal outcome [14]. This patient's OGTT was normal but had it not been, treatment would have been initiated. Diet control should be used first line. If this is insufficient, pharmacotherapy with metformin is now widely used and endorsed by NICE [11]. Insulin may be required if glycaemic control is still not adequate.

🛈 **Expert comment**

There is no international consensus on when, how, and whom to screen for gestational diabetes. Both NICE [11] in the UK and ACOG [16] in the USA recommend screening at 24–28 weeks in women with a BMI > 30 kg/m². Consideration may be given to screening earlier if a woman has had gestational diabetes in a previous pregnancy.

◉ **Landmark trial** Metformin versus insulin for the treatment of gestational diabetes (MiG trial) [15]

751 women with gestational diabetes mellitus were randomized to treatment with metformin (plus supplemental insulin if required) or insulin alone. The primary outcome was a composite measure of perinatal morbidity. Secondary outcomes included neonatal anthropometry, maternal glycemic control, maternal hypertensive complications, postpartum glucose tolerance, and acceptability of treatment. There was no increase in perinatal complications in women on metformin (with or without supplemental insulin) compared to women on insulin (32.9% versus 32.2%, RR 0.99, 95% CI 0.8–1.23). Moreover, more women preferred metformin treatment to insulin.

This remains an issue of ongoing debate. In the UK, although it is routine for women to be weighed at the first antenatal appointment, NICE does not advocate repeated weighing of women throughout pregnancy, citing insufficient evidence of benefit, and indeed possible harm in terms of psychological distress [17,18]. Heavier women should be re-weighed at around 36 weeks to help stratify intrapartum and postnatal care, for example, to ensure weight-appropriate equipment is available. However, in the USA, repeated weighing is standard practice with reference to guidance set out by the Institute of Medicine [19]. There has not been universal acceptance of this guidance. Research from a large Swedish cohort recommended a smaller weight gain for all BMI categories. Furthermore, no guidance is provided for the increasing numbers of women who fall into BMI category > 40 kg/m^2.

A consultant anaesthetist reviewed the patient at 32 weeks' gestation. She was noted to have relatively straightforward venous access, Mallampati score of 3 (suggesting difficult intubation), and impalpable spinous processes. She was breathless on mild exertion. She had a normal ECG. The potential complications associated with anaesthesia were discussed and epidural analgesia for labour was discussed.

⭐ **Learning point** The anaesthetist and the obese patient

The anaesthetist plays an important role in the care of the obese parturient. A meeting between the patient and the anaesthetist in the antenatal period is important to discuss possible complications and mechanisms for reducing harm [20]. Good communication between obstetric and anaesthetic staff is essential to safe care.

Common challenges for the anaesthetist include difficulty with peripheral venous access, delay or failure of regional (epidural or spinal) anaesthesia, difficulty with tracheal intubation and ventilation, and increased risk of aspiration [21]. Failed intubation is as common as 1:300 in the obstetric population and is more frequent in the obese parturient. The anaesthetist should be informed when an obese patient is admitted in labour. Where venous access is difficult, the anaesthetist should have 'first go' rather than repeated failed attempts by less skilled staff [22].

In cases of suspected fetal compromise the safety of the mother is paramount and consideration should be given to intra-uterine resuscitation; e.g. discontinuing oxytocin and use of terbutaline, to 'buy time' and allow safe delivery of anaesthesia.

❝❝ **Guest expert comment** The anaesthetic clinic (anaesthetist)

An anaesthetic history is taken, asking about previous general or regional anaesthesia, in particular for previous deliveries, and any complications of these. The patient's previous experiences and concerns are noted. Pre-existing medical problems and complications of pregnancy are recorded.

Attention is paid to current medicines (especially anticoagulants), allergies, plans, and patient preferences for the forthcoming delivery.

The patient is examined with particular attention to the airway (to establish how challenging intubation of the trachea may be) and the spine (for scoliosis, degree of flexibility, palpability of spinous processes, and the presence of surgical scars or other lesions).

The patient is informed of the options for analgesia in labour, or anaesthesia for operative delivery, and the most likely scenarios for the individual patient are discussed. The patient is reassured regarding her anaesthetic care and any questions answered. This helps to build a rapport with the patient. Plans are documented for anaesthetic care should the pregnancy proceed as planned, and also in case the patient presents in an emergency. This will include plans should regional anaesthesia be unsuccessful.

(continued)

The obese patient is informed that regional anaesthesia may be more challenging, take longer, and have a higher failure rate than patients with a lower BMI. It may be suggested that if she would like an epidural for labour analgesia she should request it relatively early in labour. Epidural analgeisa is strongly advocated when the airway is potentially difficult and so general anaesthesia is best avoided when there is extreme obesity, and when operative delivery is considered likely. A working epidural in labour reduces the risks associated with performing a regional or general anaesthetic in an emergency.

As pregnancy progressed, the patient was increasingly troubled with reflux oesophagitis, which did not respond to alginate reflux suppressants. She was commenced on ranitidine with some benefit. She was also reviewed by the obstetric physiotherapist for advice regarding the management of pelvic girdle pain (PGP).

At 34 + 4 weeks' gestation she was referred to the day assessment unit (DAU) by her community midwife, with hypertension. Her blood pressure in the community was 155/97. However, a series of BP measurements in the DAU were in the region of 138/92. Urinalysis was clear. Clinical examination was unremarkable, including assessment of fetal size by abdominal palpation. Blood was taken to check renal and liver function and a full blood count. These were all within normal limits.

➕ Clinical tip Minor complications of pregnancy

Obesity is associated with an increased incidence of common minor morbidities of pregnancy [23]. Overweight women are more likely to suffer heartburn, carpel tunnel syndrome, pelvic girdle pain, and chest infection. They are also more likely to require medications to treat these conditions than women of normal weight (e.g. alginate reflux suppressants for heartburn).

❝ Expert comment

In the absence of proteinuria, or other symptoms or signs of pre-eclampsia, NICE guidance advises that it is not necessary to carry out blood tests as was done in this patient [26]. However, many women, particularly those at high risk of developing pre-eclampsia, have blood tests taken to serve as a useful baseline should she go on to develop proteinuria.

➕ Clinical tip Measurement of blood pressure

This can be difficult and is subject to error in obese women. An appropriate size of cuff must be used to achieve an accurate measurement. Too small a cuff will overestimate blood pressure, too large a cuff is associated with less error [24]. The Pre-eclampsia Community Guidelines advise using a different size of cuff depending on arm circumference, as shown in the Table 15.2 [25].

Table 15.2

Arm circumference	Appropriate cuff	Cuff size
Up to 33 cm	Standard	13 × 23 cm
33–41 cm	Large	15 × 33 cm
≥ 41 cm	Thigh cuff	18 × 36 cm

➕ Clinical tip Abdominal palpation

Estimation of fetal size by abdominal palpation is clearly more difficult in the obese patient; indeed it is sometimes impossible. The alternative is to perform serial ultrasound scans to measure growth but these too may be inaccurate [27], particularly as BMI increases.

Determining presentation by palpation can also be challenging. Where there is any doubt, it is wise to confirm presentation by ultrasound scan when the woman presents in labour or prior to arranging induction of labour.

She was allowed home with a plan to review again as an outpatient in 4 days. Her BP remained persistently elevated, in the region of 150/95, without proteinuria on dipstick testing. There was no excessive oedema. She felt well and was appreciating normal fetal movements. Given her history of asthma, β-blockers were relatively contraindicated and she was commenced on oral nifedipine modified release 10 mg bd, with thrice-weekly BP review. Her BP proved difficult to control and the dose of nifedipine was gradually increased to 20 mg bd. At 36 + 4 weeks' gestation the decision was made to induce labour as it was felt her BP was inadequately controlled. The recordings were all in the region of 140–150/90–100. Her urine remained clear and her blood results were within normal limits. Fetal monitoring by cardiotocography and liquor volume was normal.

⊗ **Learning point** Induction of labour

The decision to induce labour pre-term should be made by a senior obstetrician, preferably the patient's own consultant. In this case, the decision was made by a registrar who had not been involved in the patient's care previously. In the absence of proteinuria, or any other concerning features, it may have been appropriate to continue monitoring this woman's blood pressure as an outpatient, at least until she achieved 37–38 weeks' gestation [28]. Her antihypertensive treatment could also have been optimized further, e.g. by increasing her dose of nifedipine. This would be in line with NICE guidance [26]. A recent meta-analysis concludes that obese women do have an increased risk of preterm birth before 32 weeks and induced preterm birth before 37 weeks [29]. Clearly in many cases there will be a definite need for preterm induction. However, clinicians must be mindful to resist the temptation to induce labour for softer reasons.

She was admitted to the antenatal ward for induction of labour. The initial vaginal examination revealed an unfavourable cervix with a Bishop score of 3. Cervical ripening was achieved with a total of 5 mg of vaginal prostaglandin gel given over 24 hours. Amniotomy was performed at 15.00 hours. A consultant anaesthetist sited an epidural with some difficulty. Oxytocin infusion was eventually commenced. However, after 12 hours of oxytocin infusion, labour failed to be established. The cervix remained only 2 cm dilated. The patient had developed pyrexia (37.9°C). The CTG remained normal and the liquor was clear. The decision was made to deliver her by caesarean section.

The epidural was topped up adequately for caesarean section. The large abdominal pannus was retracted with the help of a second assistant. A low transverse suprapubic incision was used below the pannus. Delivery of a live female infant in good condition was relatively straightforward. Routine antibiotic prophylaxis of 1.5 g IV cefuroxime was given. A 5 IU bolus of oxytocin was given and an oxytocin infusion was commenced at a rate of 10 IU per hour. Despite this, the uterus failed to contract adequately. Intramuscular Carboprost was given, ergometrine being relatively contraindicated in view of her hypertension. Ultimately a uterine compression suture was inserted and adequate control of haemorrhage was achieved. The rectus sheath was closed with a polydiaxanone (PDS, Ethicon®) suture. The fat layer was sutured and the skin was closed with staples and interrupted polyester/Dacron (Ethibond, Ethicon®) mattress sutures. A drain was left in both the pelvis and the fat layer. The estimated blood loss was 3000 ml.

❻ **Expert comment**

Whenever possible it is sensible to try and organize induction of labour of high-risk patients so that delivery is likely to occur during daytime hours. In this case delivery occurred at around 06.30.

⊗ **Learning point** Surgical technique in the obese patient

There is a paucity of evidence to guide the surgeon as to the best approach to caesarean section in the obese individual. Most obstetricians are more familiar with a low transverse incision beneath the panniculus. This has a cosmetic advantage for the patient. Moreover, a transverse incision has a superior closed strength and is less prone to wound breakdown. It is also associated with less post-operative pain and therefore allows easier respiratory effort and earlier mobilization of the patient, with obvious advantages. However, the transverse incision may not provide sufficient surgical exposure. Also, the necessary cephalad displacement of the pannus can contribute further to cardiorespiratory compromise. The necessary division of the fascial and muscle layers may increase the risk of haematoma formation. Furthermore, the wound will invariably lie in the folds beneath the panniculus and be prone to infection. Care must also be taken when making the incision to incise perpendicular to the skin and avoid the risk of undermining the pannus.

(continued)

Expert comment

Obesity increases risk of postpartum haemorrhage. A retrospective study of > 30 000 women revealed that compared with women of normal weight, overweight and obese women were at greater risk of PPH (OR 1.4, 99% CI 1.3–1.5; OR 1.8, 1.6–2.0) with the risks increasing as BMI increased [33]. The obstetrician must anticipate risk prior to delivery (particularly if other risk factors are present).

A vertical midline incision provides the optimal exposure to the abdominal cavity. It does not necessitate division of the rectus muscles from the fascia, generally allowing quicker access and less blood loss. However, there is greater post-operative pain, contributing to a higher likelihood of respiratory complications and longer period of immobility. It is also cosmetically less acceptable.

With either approach, closure of the sheath should be with a delayed absorbable suture (e.g. polydiaxanone; PDS, Johnson&Johnson Medical Ltd, UK or polyglycolide-trimethylene carbonate; Maxon, Mansfiled, MA). These sutures invoke little tissue reaction and maintain tensile strength at four weeks.

There is some evidence that closure of the fat layer reduces the risk of subsequent wound dehiscence [30]. However, it is not clear whether the use of a fat drain provides any benefit. A Cochrane review concluded that, from the limited evidence available (seven small trials), there was no evidence of benefit from routine use of wound drain at caesarean section [31]. They recommend larger trials, a finding supported by a more recent meta-analysis which reached a similar conclusion [32].

The patient was transferred to the obstetric high-dependency unit for post-operative care. She had received one unit of packed red cells in theatre and required a further unit post-operatively to achieve a haemoglobin concentration of 9 g/l.

Low molecular weight heparin was prescribed at a weight-appropriate dose. There were no graduated elastic compression stockings of an appropriate fit available but calf compression was maintained during the immediate postnatal period with intermittent pneumatic compression boots. The initial post-operative period was uncomplicated. Assistance was provided with wound care and breastfeeding while she was in hospital. She was discharged home on the fourth post-operative day.

Learning point Thromboprophylaxis

Obesity is an important risk factor for thromboembolism. In the UK, 18 women died from thrombosis in the triennium 2006–2008 [22]. Fourteen of those women were overweight (BMI > 25 kg/m^2), of whom 11 had a BMI > 30 kg/m^2. The postpartum period is the time of greatest risk, attenuated by a period of immobility following surgical delivery. It should be routine practice to give thromboprophylaxis with low molecular weight heparin (LMWH) to all women following caesarean delivery. However, consideration should be given to treatment with LMWH even after vaginal birth for women with a BMI > 30 kg/m^2 and should be initiated in all women with a BMI > 40 kg/m^2 for seven days, regardless of mode of delivery [34].

The appropriate dose is weight-dependent and a suggested regime is illustrated in Table 15.3.

Table 15.3

Weight (kg)	Dose
91–130	60 mg Enoxaparin; 7500 units Dalteparin; 7000 units Tinzaparin daily
131–170	80 mg Enoxaparin; 10 000 units Dalteparin; 9000 units Tinzaparin daily
>170	0.6 mg/kg/day Enoxaparin; 75 units/kg/day Dalteparin; 75 units/kg/day Tinzaparin

Expert comment

The particular needs of the obese new mother must not be forgotten once the baby is delivered. Care should be taken to ensure the patient is nursed in a weight-appropriate bed with a suitable mattress to prevent the development of pressure sores. Staff should familiarize themselves with the safe operating weight limits of the standard furniture in the department. Help and advice regarding the availability of specialist equipment for morbidly obese patients is usually available from the bariatric or manual handling department of the hospital.

> **☉ Learning point** Breastfeeding
>
> Obese women are less likely than lean women to breastfeed [35]. This may be due to mechanical difficulties associated with larger breasts or self-consciousness about breastfeeding 'modestly'. There may even be a physiological contribution with obese women having a poorer prolactin response to suckling [36]. Regardless of the reason, cessation of breastfeeding clearly leads to higher rates of formula feeding, which in turn may be associated with childhood obesity, thus potentially perpetuating the cycle of disadvantage to the next generation [37]. Women must be supported in their decision to breastfeed and support maintained until breastfeeding is well established.

Unfortunately, she re-presented on the seventh post-operative day. She felt unwell and had a temperature of 37.9°C. Her wound was offensive-smelling and moist with surrounding erythema and tenderness, and a diagnosis of wound infection was made. Wound swabs and blood cultures were taken. She was admitted for a 24-hour period of intravenous antibiotics and then discharged home again to complete a course of oral antibiotics. The blood cultures were subsequently reported as negative but the wound swab grew a heavy growth of coliforms and anaerobes. The staples and sutures were removed and there was some gaping of the wound at one end. She was referred to the tissue-viability service for ongoing wound care for the duration of wound healing by secondary intention.

> **☉ Learning point** Post-operative infection
>
> Abdominal adiposity is a risk factor for post-operative infection. One study of 969 women demonstrated that for every 5 unit increase in BMI, the risk of post-operative infection doubles [38]. The fatty tissue has a poor vascular supply and this increases the susceptibility to infection. The wound is also often buried below the pannus and the patient may find it difficult, if not impossible, to clean and dry the area without assistance. There is strong evidence that antibiotic prophylaxis for caesarean delivery given before skin incision, rather than after cord clamping, decreases the incidence of postpartum endometritis and total infectious morbidities, without affecting neonatal outcomes [39]. Standard dosing is usually appropriate but in the morbidly obese a higher dose may be required [40], and repeat dosing may be necessary where there has been a prolonged operation or excessive blood loss.
>
> Where time allows, consideration should also be given to attempting to reduce skin colonization, and subsequent wound infection, by cleansing the skin prior to anaesthetic administration and then again immediately prior to commencing the procedure. The effectiveness of this regime has been demonstrated in other specialties [41]. Particular attention should be paid to the skin folds beneath the panniculus and in the groins.

Discussion

The global obesity epidemic presents a major challenge for healthcare providers in obstetrics. As demonstrated by the case illustrated in this chapter, obesity confers an increased risk of almost all pregnancy complications. It is important to recognise obese women as a high-risk group and as such they should be offered individualized, specialist multidisciplinary care before, during, and after their pregnancy. They should be made aware of the risks pregnancy poses to them and their baby, and advised about the strategies available to manage those risks to enable them to make informed decisions regarding their management. Primary care services have a responsibility to ensure that all women of childbearing age are aware of the excess risks associated with obesity. Any visit to a healthcare provider by a young woman who is overweight should be viewed as an opportunity to advise about the benefits of weight loss and the strategies to achieve this. For very obese women seeking a pregnancy, referral for pre-pregnancy counselling should be encouraged in order to emphasize this message and optimize treatment of common obesity comorbidities such as hypertension and diabetes. Specialist antenatal clinics for obese women are ideally placed to provide this care, but within a resource-poor health service this may not be a funding priority. It is therefore the responsibility of all obstetric practitioners to be aware of the implications of obesity on pregnancy and familiarise themselves with current best practice. Input from other specialties including endocrinology, anaesthetics, dietetics, physiotherapy, and psychological medicine can be extremely valuable.

A Final Word from the Expert

As illustrated by the case presented, maternal obesity is associated with significant morbidity and challenges for healthcare providers. Furthermore, increasing evidence suggests that the environment that the fetus is exposed to *in utero* can have lifelong implications for its health. Babies born to obese mothers are therefore at increased risk of developing obesity and the metabolic syndrome in childhood and adolescence compared to those born to women of normal weight. Maternal obesity has the potential to perpetuate the cycle of health disadvantage to the next generation. Unfortunately the evidence base underpinning many recent guidelines for managing maternal obesity remains poor. There is an urgent need for further research to optimize perinatal outcome. Until current management becomes evidence-based, women who are obese and their offspring will remain at increased risk of adverse perinatal outcome and long-term health disadvantage.

References

1. Rasmussen SA, Chu SY, Kim SY, Schmid CH, Lau J. Maternal obesity and risk of neural tube defects: a metaanalysis. *Am J Obstet Gynecol* 2008 Jun;198(6):611–9.
2. Jovanovic L. Definition, size of the problem, screening and diagnostic criteria: who should be screened, cost-effectiveness, and feasibility of screening. *Int J Gynaecol Obstet* 2009 Mar;104 Suppl 1:S17–9.
3. Mojtabai R. Body mass index and serum folate in childbearing age women. *Eur J Epidemiol* 2004;19(11):1029–36.
4. Dashe JS, McIntire DD, Twickler DM. Effect of maternal obesity on the ultrasound detection of anomalous fetuses. *Obstet Gynecol* 2009 May;113(5):1001–7.
5. Scholl TO, Johnson WG. Folic acid: influence on the outcome of pregnancy. *Am J Clin Nutr* 2000 May;71(5 Suppl):1295S–303S.
6. Group MVSR. Prevention of neural tube defects: results of the Medical Research Council Vitamin Study. MRC Vitamin Study Research Group. *Lancet* 1991 Jul 20;338(8760):131–7.
7. Ray JG, Wyatt PR, Vermeulen MJ, Meier C, Cole DE. Greater maternal weight and the ongoing risk of neural tube defects after folic acid flour fortification. *Obstet Gynecol* 2005 Feb;105(2):261–5.
8. Modder J, Fitzsimons KJ. CMACE/RCOG Joint Guideline: Management of women with obesity in pregnancy. London: Centre for Maternal and Child Enquiries and the Royal College of Obstetricians and Gynaecologists. 2010.

9. Phatak M, Ramsay J. Impact of maternal obesity on procedure of mid-trimester anomaly scan. *J Obstet Gynaecol* 2010;30(5):447–50.

10. Wald N, Cuckle H, Boreham J, Terzian E, Redman C. The effect of maternal weight on maternal serum alpha-fetoprotein levels. *Br J Obstet Gynaecol* 1981 Nov;88(11):1094–6.

11. Diabetes in pregnancy. NICE Guideline CG63. 2008 July.

12. Metzger BE, Lowe LP, Dyer AR, Trimble ER, Chaovarindr U, Coustan DR, *et al*. Hyperglycemia and adverse pregnancy outcomes. *N Engl J Med* 2008 May 8;358(19):1991–2002.

13. Network SIG. Management of Diabetes. A national clinical guideline. Report No. 116. 2010. http://www.sign.ac.uk/guidelines/fulltext/116/index.html.

14. Crowther CA, Hiller JE, Moss JR, McPhee AJ, Jeffries WS, Robinson JS. Effect of treatment of gestational diabetes mellitus on pregnancy outcomes. *N Engl J Med* 2005 Jun 16;352(24):2477–86.

15. Rowan JA, Hague WM, Gao W, Battin MR, Moore MP. Metformin versus insulin for the treatment of gestational diabetes. *N Engl J Med* 2008 May 8;358(19):2003–15.

16. ACOG Practice Bulletin. Clinical management guidelines for obstetrician-gynaecologists. Number 30, September 2001. Gestational Diabetes. *Obstet Gynecol* 2001;98: 525–38.

17. Dawes MG, Grudzinskas JG. Repeated measurement of maternal weight during pregnancy. Is this a useful practice? *Br J Obstet Gynaecol* 1991 Feb;98(2):189–94.

18. Dawes MG, Grudzinskas JG. Patterns of maternal weight gain in pregnancy. *Br J Obstet Gynaecol* 1991 Feb;98(2):195–201.

19. Institute of Medicine: Weight gain during pregnancy: Re-examining the guidelines. 2009. http://www.iom.edu/reports/2009/weight-gain-during-pregnancy-reexamining-the-guidelines.aspx

20. The Royal College of Anaesthetists. Guidance on the provision of obstetric anaesthesia services. 2009. http://www.rcoa.ac.uk/docs/GPAS-Obs.pdf

21. Saravanakumar K, Rao SG, Cooper GM. The challenges of obesity and obstetric anaesthesia. *Curr Opin Obstet Gynecol* 2006 Dec;18(6):631–5.

22. Cantwell R, Clutton-Brock T, Cooper G, Dawson A, Drife J, Garrod D, *et al*. Saving Mothers' Lives: Reviewing maternal deaths to make motherhood safer: 2006-2008. The Eighth Report of the Confidential Enquiries into Maternal Deaths in the United Kingdom. *BJOG* 2011 Mar;118 Suppl 1:1–203.

23. Denison F, Norrie G, Graham B, Lynch J, Harper N, Reynolds R. Increased maternal BMI is associated with an increased risk of minor complications during pregnancy with consequent cost implications. *BJOG* 2009 Oct;116(11):1467–72. Epub 2009 Jun 4.

24. Maxwell M, Waks A, Schroth P, Karam M, Dornfeld L. Error in blood-pressure measurement due to incorrect cuff size in obese patients. *Lancet* [Clinical Trial Randomized Controlled Trial]. 1982 Jul 3;2(8288):33–6.

25. Milne F, Redman C, Walker J, Baker P, Bradley J, Cooper C, *et al*. The pre-eclampsia community guideline (PRECOG): how to screen for and detect onset of pre-eclampsia in the community. *BMJ* 2005 Mar 12;330(7491):576–80.

26. NICE Clinical Guideline 107: Hypertension in pregnancy. 2010. http://www.nice.org.uk/CG107

27. Colman A, Maharaj D, Hutton J, Tuohy J. Reliability of ultrasound estimation of fetal weight in term singleton pregnancies. *N Z Med J* 2006;119(1241):U2146.

28. Koopmans CM, Bijlenga D, Groen H, Vijgen SM, Aarnoudse JG, Bekedam DJ, *et al*. Induction of labour versus expectant monitoring for gestational hypertension or mild pre-eclampsia after 36 weeks' gestation (HYPITAT): a multicentre, open-label randomised controlled trial. *Lancet* 2009 Sep 19;374(9694):979–88.

29. McDonald SD, Han Z, Mulla S, Beyene J. Overweight and obesity in mothers and risk of preterm birth and low birth weight infants: systematic review and meta-analyses. *BMJ* 2010;341:c3428.

30. Naumann RW, Hauth JC, Owen J, Hodgkins PM, Lincoln T. Subcutaneous tissue approximation in relation to wound disruption after caesarean delivery in obese women. *Obstet Gynecol* 1995 Mar;85(3):412–6.

31. Gates S, Anderson ER. Wound drainage for caesarean section. *Cochrane Database Syst Rev* 2005(1):D004549.

32. Hellums EK, Lin MG, Ramsey PS. Prophylactic subcutaneous drainage for prevention of wound complications after caesarean delivery—a metaanalysis. *Am J Obstet Gynecol* 2007 Sep;197(3):229–35.

33. Scott-Pillai R, Spence D, Cardwell CR, Hunter A, Holmes VA. The impact of body mass index on maternal and neonatal outcomes: a retrospective study in a UK obstetric population, 2004-2011. *BJOG* 2013;120:932–9.

34. RCOG. Reducing the risk of thrombosis and embolism during pregnancy and the puerperium. RCOG Green-top Guideline No. 37a: RCOG 2009. http://www.rcog.org.uk/womens-health/clinical-guidance/reducing-risk-of-thrombosis-greentop37a

35. Amir LH, Donath S. A systematic review of maternal obesity and breastfeeding intention, initiation and duration. *BMC Pregnancy Childbirth* 2007;7: 9.

36. Rasmussen KM, Kjolhede CL. Prepregnant overweight and obesity diminish the prolactin response to suckling in the first week postpartum. *Pediatrics* 2004 May;113(5):e465–71.

37. Armitage JA, Poston L, Taylor PD. Developmental origins of obesity and the metabolic syndrome: the role of maternal obesity. *Front Horm Res* 2008;36:73–84.

38. Tran TS, Jamulitrat S, Chongsuvivatwong V, Geater A. Risk factors for post caesarean surgical site infection. *Obstet Gynecol* 2000 Mar;95(3):367–71.

39. Costantine MM, Rahman M, Ghulmiyah L, Byers BD, Longo M, Wen T, *et al.* Timing of perioperative antibiotics for caesarean delivery: a metaanalysis. *Am J Obstet Gynecol* 2008 Sep;199(3):301 e1–6.

40. Cheymol G. Effects of obesity on pharmacokinetics implications for drug therapy. *Clin Pharmacokinet* 2000 Sep;39(3):215–31.

41. Zywiel MG, Daley JA, Delanois RE, Naziri Q, Johnson AJ, Mont MA. Advance pre-operative chlorhexidine reduces the incidence of surgical site infections in knee arthroplasty. *Int Orthop* 2011 Jul;35(7):1001–6.

16 Early-onset preeclampsia: balancing maternal and neonatal morbidity

Manju Chandiramani

ⓘ **Expert Commentary** Jason Waugh

ⓘ **Guest Expert** Ben Fizwilliams

Case history

A primiparous 30-year-old woman booked at 10 weeks' gestation, confirmed by ultrasound, at her local hospital, with level 2 neonatal care. She had a medical history of hypothyroidism, which was controlled with 50 μg thyroxine daily. She was Caucasian, a non-smoker, with no personal or family history of hypertension, diabetes, or cardiac disease. General examination was unremarkable apart from a BMI of 32 kg/m². Her booking blood pressure was 110/60 mmHg and her urine dipstick was negative for proteinuria. Her booking blood tests were normal and her first trimester ultrasound screening was unremarkable. Her anomaly scan at 21 weeks' gestation revealed no abnormalities with a placenta that was anterior and not low-lying.

At 27 + 4 weeks' gestation, she presented to the obstetric day assessment unit (DAU) with a one-day history of frontal headache, epigastric pain, and generalized oedema. She had also experienced a reduction in fetal movements in the preceding week. On admission, she was alert, her blood pressure was noted to be 173–189/100–121 mmHg, and she had 3 + of proteinuria on visual dipstick urinalysis. Abdominal examination confirmed epigastric and right upper quadrant tenderness, a symphyseal-fundal height of 24 cm, and a fetus with a longitudinal lie and breech presentation. Her reflexes were brisk but there was no clonus. Fundoscopy was normal. Fetal cardiotocography was normal.

> ✪ **Learning point** The epidemiology of pre-eclampsia
>
> - Multisystem disorder specific to pregnancy which usually occurs after 20 weeks' gestation.
> - Characterized by hypertension (diastolic blood pressure ≥ 100 mmHg on any one occasion or diastolic blood pressure 90 mmHg on two or more consecutive occasions ≥ four hours apart) and proteinuria (≥ 0.3 g in 24 hours), and can also affect other organ systems.
> - Thought to affect up to 4 % of all pregnancies, depending on the population [1, 2].
> - Risk factors for pre-eclampsia include antiphospholipid syndrome (relative risk [RR] 9.72), previous history of pre-eclampsia (RR 7.19), pre-existing diabetes (RR 3.56), multiple pregnancy (RR 2.93), nulliparity (RR 2.91), family history (RR 2.90), raised BMI before pregnancy (RR 2.47), raised body mass index at booking (RR 1.55), age over 40 years (RR 1.96), and raised diastolic blood pressure (> 80 mmHg) (RR 1.38) [3].
> - In women with at least 1 risk factor, the incidence can be as high as 15 % [4] however with multiple risk factors, the risk rarely exceeds 40 %.

➕ Clinical tip Accurate BP measurement

- Accurate blood pressure measurement is important.
- Automated blood pressure machines may significantly underestimate and occasionally overestimate blood pressures in women with pre-eclampsia.
- Validated devices must be used and be equivalent to standard sphygmomanometry [12].
- Women should be rested and sitting or reclining at a 45° angle when having their blood pressure checked.
- The blood pressure cuff should be appropriate in size and placed at the level of the heart
- Korotkoff phase 5 is used to measure diastolic blood pressure and multiple readings confirm the diagnosis [15].

➕ Clinical tip Accurate proteinuria assessment

Proteinuria estimation is also inherent to making an accurate diagnosis of pre-eclampsia, and routine dipstick urinalysis is fraught with limitations of false-positive and false-negative results. NICE recommends using an automated reagent-strip reading device or a spot urinary protein-to-creatinine ratio for estimating proteinuria in a secondary care setting. If an automated reagent-strip reading device is used to detect proteinuria and a result of 1+ or more is obtained, a spot urinary protein-to-creatinine ratio or 24-hour urine collection is recommended to quantify proteinuria. Significant proteinuria is diagnosed if the urinary protein-to-creatinine ratio is greater than 30 mg/mmol or a validated 24-hour urine protein excretion is greater than 300 mg protein. NICE also recommends that there is a recognized method for evaluating completeness of the sample of a 24-hour urine collection using a measure of total creatinine concentration or urinary volume [16]. As the use of spot urinary protein-to-creatinine ratio and spot urinary albumin-to-creatinine ratio to estimate proteinuria is well established in the management of chronic renal disease, research is currently aimed at establishing its use in the management of hypertensive disorders of pregnancy.

She was admitted to her local obstetric unit and her blood pressure was stabilized with oral labetalol (200 mg). The aim was to maintain a diastolic blood pressure between 80–100 mmHg and a systolic blood pressure less than 150 mmHg. Initial investigations revealed a protein-to-creatinine ratio (PCR) of 177 and a normal full blood count, renal function, electrolytes, and transaminases. Thromboprophylaxis in the form of thromboembolic stockings and low molecular weight heparin was commenced. Intramuscular bethamethsone was prescribed, 2 doses of 12 mg 24 hours apart, to accelerate fetal lung maturation. Further fetal assessment was undertaken; growth was confirmed with ultrasound and the estimated fetal weight was 847 g. The amniotic fluid volume was less than the fifth centile, umbilical artery end-diastolic flow was present. The local neonatalogists had a frank discussion with the woman and assured her that they would be present at delivery to assess and stabilize the baby but that an *in utero* transfer would be ideal for access to level 3 care, which would possibly include both cardiac and respiratory support, antibiotics, nasogastric feeding, and up to three months' admission to the neonatal unit. It was agreed that if she remained stable and her blood pressure adequately controlled then she would be transferred to the level 3 unit prior to delivery. She remained well overnight and was transferred to the nearest tertiary unit.

> ✪ **Learning point** Intra-uterine growth restriction (IUGR) and pre-eclampsia
>
> - Pre-eclampsia is associated with placental insufficiency which leads to IUGR.
> - IUGR occurs in more than one-third of pre-eclamptic pregnancies.
> - Growth is usually asymmetrical. The best method of assessment is the abdominal circumference.
> - In women who present with hypertension in pregnancy or pre-eclampsia, ultrasound assessment of the fetus is useful and serial scans may be necessary to monitor growth on a two-weekly basis.
> - Reduced liquor volume is also associated with placental insufficiency and serial assessment can detect compromise.

She remained well on labetalol 200 mg following transfer, but three days later, her blood pressure rose to 176–182/110–125 mmHg. She was started on the local pre-eclampsia protocol and had blood pressure measurements undertaken every 15 minutes. Her blood pressure was eventually controlled with an intravenous hydralazine infusion. She was fluid-restricted to 80 ml/h and had strict hourly input and output monitoring. Biochemical tests were repeated after arrival at the tertiary unit (see Table 16.1); her haemoglobin was 92 g/L, platelets 96×10^9/L, ALT 62 u/L, AST 78 u/L, creatinine 88 µmol/L, uric acid 0.46 mmol/L, and her clotting screen was normal. Her protein/creatinine ratio (PCR) was 700.

Table 16.1 Deterioration of biochemical profile in early-onset pre-eclampsia

Investigation	On admission	72 hours later
Haemoglobin (g/dL)	11.3	9.2
Platelets (10^9/L)	178	96
Alanine transaminase (u/L)	31	62
Aspartate transaminase (u/L)	28	78
Creatinine (µmol/L)	63	88
Uric acid (mmol/L)	0.27	0.46
Protein-to-creatinine ratio	177	700

> ➕ **Clinical tip** Pharmacological treatment of hypertension in pregnancy and pre-eclampsia
>
> Traditionally, the first-line treatment for hypertension in pregnancy has been methyldopa as a result of its safety profile and its history of no reports of serious adverse effects on the fetus followed by calcium antagonists (e.g. slow release nifedipine) and oral hydralazine, and finally by labetalol, a combined α- and β-adrenergic blocker. However, the recent NICE guideline [16] recommended the use of oral labetalol as first-line and suggested methyldopa and nifedipine as alternatives. Women with severe hypertension or who are in critical care during pregnancy or immediately postnatally should be treated with labetalol (oral or intravenous), intravenous hyralazine. or oral nifedipine.

> ✪ **Learning point** Magnesium sulphate for prophylaxis of eclampsia
>
> The use of magnesium sulphate in the UK for prophylaxis of eclampsia has become more commonplace in the last 20 years. An audit of UK practice undertaken in 2005 revealed that 99% of 295 women received magnesium sulphate with no associated deaths [19]. This study demonstrated improved outcome compared to a previous UK series undertaken in 1992, which described a death rate of 2% [20]. This improvement was possibly secondary to increased clinical vigilance and the introduction of management guidelines based on the evidence-based use of magnesium sulphate for eclampsia and pre-eclampsia, showing the practical benefits of translating research into practice. Nonetheless, five women still had strokes, reaffirming the recent CEMACE findings [12], which continue to suggest inadequate treatment of severe hypertension resulting in pre-eclampsia remaining the second leading cause of direct maternal deaths. Recent reports are reassuring as to the long-term effects of reduction in the risk of eclampsia following prophylaxis with magnesium sulphate in both mothers and children [21, 22].

> ➕ **Clinical tip** Fluid balance is important in reducing mortality from pulmonary oedema
>
> NICE recommends that volume expansion should not be used in women with severe pre-eclampsia unless hydralazine is the antenatal agent used. Women with severe pre-eclampsia should have maintenance fluids limited to 80 ml/hour unless there are other ongoing fluid losses, e.g. obstetric haemorrhage [15,16].

> ⊘ **Landmark trial** The Magpie Trial [21]—do women with pre-eclampsia, and their babies, benefit from magnesium sulphate? Immediate and long-term outcomes.
>
> - Compared magnesium sulphate with placebo for pre-eclampsia.
> - 99% of 295 women received magnesium sulphate; 24% reported side-effects compared with 5% of women who received placebo.
> - Women receiving magnesium sulphate had a 58% lower risk of eclampsia than those receiving placebo.
> - Maternal mortality was lower in women receiving magnesium sulphate and there was no clear difference in the risk of neonatal death.
> - Assessment of women at two to three years after delivery demonstrated that 3.5% of women allocated to magnesium sulphate died or had serious morbidity potentially related to pre-eclampsia, compared with 4.2% women allocated to placebo (RR 0.84, 95% CI 0.60–1.18) [22].
> - Assessment of children whose mothers had been recruited to the Magpie Trial at 18 months of age showed that there of those allocated magnesium sulphate, 15% were dead or had neurosensory disability compared with 14.1% allocated placebo (RR 1.06, 95% CI 0.90–1.25), and of the survivors, 1.3% had neurosensory disability at 18 months compared with 1.9% (RR 0.72, 95% CI 0.40–1.29) [23].

> ⊕ **Clinical tip** Magnesium sulphate
>
> **When should we consider magnesium sulphate?**
>
> - A woman with severe hypertension or pre-eclampsia who has or previously had an eclamptic fit.
> - A woman with severe pre-eclampsia in whom delivery is planned within 24 hours.
> - Consider in any women at risk of imminent delivery prior to 30 weeks' completed gestation (fetal neuroprotection, see Chapter 10).
>
> **What is the regime for magnesium sulphate?**
>
> - Loading dose of 4 g should be given intravenously over 5 minutes, followed by an infusion of 1 g/hour maintained for 24 hours.
> - Recurrent seizures should be treated with a further dose of 2–4 g given over 5 minutes.

> ⑥ **Expert comment**
>
> One of the top 10 recommendations of the recent CEMACE report [12] highlighted that all pregnant women with pre-eclampsia and a systolic blood pressure of ≥ 150 mmHg require urgent and effective anti-hypertensive treatment as per recent NICE Guidance [16]. The report also highlighted the need to consider treatment at lower levels of blood pressure if the clinical picture suggested rapid deterioration or blood pressure was thought to escalate rapidly. The aim of antihypertensive treatment is to reduce systolic blood pressure to less than 150 mmHg.

After a further 12 hours and with a deterioration in both her biochemical profile and right upper quadrant pain, the risk to the mother was thought to be significant and consideration was given to delivery. Her platelet count was repeated and was discovered to be 92×10^9/L. A blood film confirmed haemolysis. Her blood pressure remained somewhat difficult to control and required the addition of a labetalol infusion to maintain systolic pressures of below 150 mmHg. Vaginal assessment revealed a long, closed cervix, and as a result, the decision was made to deliver by emergency caesarean section.

❻ Expert comment

The delivery must be carefully planned and the mode of delivery determined depending on the favourability of the cervix and likelihood of success at induction, fetal presentation, and condition. Although vaginal delivery may be preferable overall, at gestations below 32 weeks, a caesarean section is often performed as the likelihood of successful induction is reduced [15]. Early dialogue between a referring unit and an accepting unit is paramount to a safe decision regarding *in-utero* or *ex-utero* transfer, and ensures consistent information is given to women regarding likely interventions as well as outcomes.

Once stabilized she had a combined spinal epidural for anaesthesia, and underwent a classical caesarean section, as her lower uterine segment was underdeveloped. The anaesthetists sited an arterial line prior to her anaesthesia but a joint decision was made with the obstetricians that central venous pressure monitoring was not required at this stage as urine output was adequate. Her caesarean section was uneventful and her estimated blood loss was 600 ml. She remained on magnesium sulphate for a further 24 hours following her delivery. Her blood pressure remained stable though she required her anti-hypertensive infusion for 48 hours after delivery. She was converted to a combination of oral labetalol and nifedipine, which safely allowed her to breastfeed and which were weaned off by the 12th week postnatally. She was debriefed in the antenatal clinic after 6 weeks and she was counselled regarding the management of future pregnancies. She was told that her recurrence risk in subsequent pregnancies could be as high as 40 %. She was advised that she would need low-dose aspirin prophylaxis and regular fetal growth surveillance. She was also informed that an obstetrician, in conjunction with her general practitioner and midwife, would manage her care.

❻ Guest expert comment (anaesthetics) Regional anaesthesia and thrombocytopaenia

Regional anesthesia is very safe, with a risk of permanent injury as low as 1:80,000 to 1:320,000 anaesthetics in the obstetric population [31]. One of the causes of morbidity is the rare but potentially devastating complication of epidural haematoma, which may lead to paralysis. In patients with impaired haemostasis this risk is increased, although it remains small. In some patients the risk is felt to outweigh the benefits. Different units will have different policies, but in general:

- In a patient with pre-eclampsia a platelet count from within the past 24 hours should be available. If this is above 100×10^9/L then regional anaesthesia can usually proceed. In severe pre-eclampsia and where there is a steep downward trend in the platelet count, a more recent result may be indicated. This may either encourage the anaesthetist to site an epidural before the platelets fall further, or to avoid regional anaesthesia.
- If the platelets are below 100×10^9/L and the clotting tests are normal, then consideration can be given to regional anaesthesia.
- It is highly unusual to perform regional anaesthesia when the platelets are below 50×10^9/L.

➕ Clinical tip Importance of pre-pregnancy assessment

Pre-pregnancy counselling is not universal for women who have had severe pre-eclampsia in the UK, and as a result, high-risk women may present at their booking visit with little knowledge of the pregnancy risk. Clinicians should continue to aim to identify women early in order to optimize health and initiate delivery of maternal care.

(continued)

Components of pre-conceptual care:

- Optimal hypertensive control in those with chronic hypertension.
- Weight loss in overweight and obese women.
- Adequate glycaemic control in women with type 1 and type 2 diabetes.

Prophylactic strategies may also be discussed in the pre-conception period and the use of low-dose aspirin is recommended once pregnancy is confirmed. Antiplatelet agents and possibly calcium supplementation have a limited role in the prevention of pre-eclampsia.

❝ Expert comment

If blood pressure is adequately controlled prior to conception, with appropriate agents for pregnancy the same agents may be used during pregnancy and in the postpartum period. Avoiding the use of angiotensin-converting enzyme (ACE) inhibitors or angiotensin II receptor blockers (ARBs) and reviewing the drug history for other prescription and non-prescription medication form an integral part of pre-pregnancy assessment and care. Interestingly, recent evidence demonstrates that the maternal use of ACE inhibitors in the first trimester has a risk profile similar to other anti-hypertensives regarding malformations and the apparent increased risk associated with the use of ACE inhibitors and other anti-hypertensives in the first trimester are likely secondary to the underlying hypertension [24].

✓ Evidence base Aspirin supplementation in women at risk of pre-eclampsia

Aspirin is thought to prevent vasoconstriction and pathological coagulative changes caused by inadequate perfusion and placental ischaemia. In a meta-analysis of individual patient data from 31 randomized trials ($n = 32\,217$ women), the use of antiplatelet agents, particularly low-dose aspirin, resulted in a significant 10% reduction in the relative risk of pre-eclampsia, delivery before 34 weeks, and a pregnancy with a serious adverse outcome [25]. In this population, the number needed to treat (NNT) to prevent pre-eclampsia was 114, making it important to consider in those women likely to develop pre-eclampsia. Earlier treatment can be even more useful, and the use of aspirin at less than 16 weeks has the ability to almost halve a woman's risk of pre-eclampsia (RR 0.47; 95% CI 0.34–0.65) with an NNT of 9 [26].

✓ Evidence base Calcium supplementation in women at risk of pre-eclampisa

Calcium, on the other hand, may be even more promising. In a review of 12 randomized controlled trials ($n = 15\,528$ women) [27], calcium supplementation resulted in a significant 52% reduction in the relative risk of pre-eclampsia with a higher effect in those at high risk (78%) and with low calcium intake (64%). Contrary to previous beliefs, even women with good dietary intake have a substantial benefit (38% reduction). However, in the largest study to-date in healthy nulliparous women ($n = 4589$) with no risk factors for the development of pre-eclampsia [28], there was no benefit from calcium supplementation. As a result, calcium supplementation is only used selectively for high-risk woman, but its use in the pre-conception period and in early pregnancy warrants further research.

✪ Learning point Postpartum hypertension

- Following an uncomplicated pregnancy, resolution of the pregnancy-related cardiovascular changes in pregnancy commonly results in a rise in BP.
- Most women will experience increased blood pressure over the first four days postpartum (an average of 6 mmHg systolic and 4 mmHg diastolic) [29].

(continued)

- A considerable number of previously normotensive women display elevations of BP in the puerperium; 12% will have documented diastolic BP > 100 mmHg [29].
- One-third of women with antenatal PIH or PET will experience sustained hypertension postnatally.
- Risk factors for development of postpartum hypertension include iatrogenic preterm delivery triggered by maternal BP; severe antenatal hypertension > 160/100; antenatal hypertension requiring antenatal pharmacotherapy; and antenatal pre-eclampsia[30], although it can develop in women with no previous history of hypertension.
- Up to 44% of eclampsia occurs post-partum [32].
- Symptoms of pre-eclampsia (such as headache, nausea. and visual disturbance) are more commonly reported in women with *de novo* postpartum pre-eclampsia/eclampsia than patients with antenatal or intrapartum pre-eclampsia/eclampsia [33].

⑥ Expert comment

Women with pre-eclampsia remain at high risk of complications postnatally and should be monitored closely as an inpatient post delivery. Following discharge, there should be clear plans in place for community monitoring of BP, and a hospital outpatient appointment should be arranged at six weeks postpartum to check BP and proteinuria and to discuss the implications both for future pregnancies, and future cardiovascular risk (see Figure 16.1).

⊕ Clinical tip Management of postpartum hypertension (adapted from NICE Guidelines) [33]

- A minimum of one blood pressure measurement should be carried out and documented within six hours of the birth.
- Women with severe or persistent headache should be evaluated and pre-eclampsia considered.
- Routine assessment of proteinuria is not recommended.
- A sustained blood pressure > 150/100 is an indication for antihypertensive treatment (see Table 16.2).
- Women with antenatal pre-eclampsia should be monitored as an inpatient for at least 72 hours post delivery, and on alternate days in the community until stable.
- Step-wise reduction of antihypertensive therapy can be considered when BP is persistently < 140/90.

Table 16.2 Treatment of postnatal hypertension.

Drug	Dose	Contraindications	Side effects
Chronic treatment			
Labetolol	100 bd–200 mg qds	Asthma, cardiac failure, bradycardia, 2nd or 3rd degree AV block	Postural hypotension, headache, urinary hesitancy, fatigue
Atenolol	25–100 mg daily		
Nifedipine (SR)	10–40 mg bd	Advanced aortic stenosis	Headache, tachycardia, palpitations, flushing
Amlodipine	5–10 mg od		
Enalapril	5–20 mg bd	Avoid in AKI	Hypotension, cough, renal impairment
Acute treatment			
Hydralazine	5–10 mg IV or IM repeated if necessary	Severe tachycardia, high-output cardiac failure	Headache, flushing, anxiety, arrhythmias
Labetolol	20 mg IV repeated if necessary at 20-min intervals	As chronic treatment	As chronic treatment
Nifedipine	10 mg sublingual repeated if necessary at 20-min intervals	Care to avoid profound hypotension when used alongside magnesium sulphate	As chronic treatment

AKI—acute kidney injury; AV—atrioventricular; bd—twice daily; IM—intramuscular; IV—intravenous; od—once daily; qds—four times daily; SR—sustained release

Smith M, Waugh J, Nelson-Piercy C. management of Postpartum hypertension. The obstetrician and gynaecologist. 2013; 15:45-50.

Relative risk (mean and 95% CI)

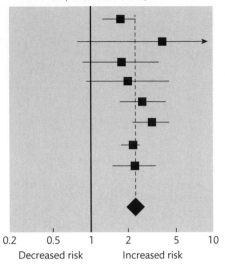

0.2   0.5   1   2   5   10
Decreased risk   Increased risk

Figure 16.1 Relative risk of developing non-fatal or fatal ischaemic heart disease after a pre-eclampsia affected pregnancy. Prospective and retrospective studies were included, providing a dataset of 3 488 160 women, with 198 252 affected by pre-eclampsia. Overall relative risk of ischaemic heart disease in pre-eclampsia was 2.16 (95% CI: 1.86–2.52)) [35].
Bellamy L, et al. (2007). Pre-eclampsia and risk of cardiovascular disease and cancer in later life: systematic review and meta-analysis. BMJ, 335, 974–77 with permission from BMJ Publishing Group Ltd.

Discussion

The case presented here is not unique: it is a scenario that confronts obstetricians working in all obstetric units on a regular basis. Hypertension itself complicates up to 15 % of all pregnancies and the structure of antenatal assessments in the UK has been designed to detect new-onset hypertension and proteinuria in a timely manner.

Widespread endothelial dysfunction, inadequate trophoblast invasion into the myometrium, and inhibition of physiological dilatation of maternal spiral arteries from narrow muscular vessels to wide non-muscular channels is thought to characterize pre-eclampsia [5,6]. As a result of the associated increase in utero-placental resistance, the 70 % reduction in resistance that usually occurs by the end of the first trimester is compromised. This leads to other insults including placental hypoperfusion and a harmful maternal inflammatory response with the production of reactive oxygen species and oxidative stress, possibly related to ischaemia in the placenta and reperfusion injury [7–9]. There is emerging evidence to suggest that early-onset severe pre-eclampsia has a unique pathophysiology, involving defective immunoregulatory pathways, potentially causing vascular and trophoblast damage at the implantation site [10]. Late-onset pre-eclampsia is thought to occur secondary to maternal microvascular diseases (chronic hypertension) or to reflect a maternal genetic disposition (11). Endothelial damage manifests as the two cardinal features of pre-eclampsia: hypertension and proteinuria. Pre-eclampsia remains difficult to diagnose because it commonly has an insidious onset and unpredictable course. It affects multiple organs including the liver, kidneys, brain, lungs, placenta, and haemotological systems, and when severe, may result in haemolysis, elevated liver enzymes and low platelets (HELLP) syndrome.

The clinical features may be variable in onset but left undetected can result in significant maternal and fetal complications, including placental abruption, fetal growth restriction, coagulopathy, haemolysis, liver and renal failure, eclampsia, and cerebral haemorrhage. The commonly used medications to control hypertension in the antenatal period include methyldopa, labetalol, and nifedipine, whilst the armamentarium used in peripartum management include oral or intravenous labetalol, oral nifedipine, intravenous hydralazine, and magnesium sulphate for eclampsia. Counselling in the postpartum and the periconceptual period is important as it allows individualized antenatal care to be planned, taking into account both NICE guidelines for antenatal care [36] and the Pre-eclampsia Community (PRECOG) guideline [37]. In this way, women are appropriately referred to specialists early when their input may be able to impact on prevention and early clinical detection of deterioration in maternal and fetal well-being. Careful history-taking, examination, and baseline investigations (renal and liver function) may result in initiation of prophylaxis (low-dose aspirin and possibly calcium), serial fetal growth surveillance (at 28, 32, and 36 weeks' gestation), and the formulation of shared antenatal surveillance by obstetricians, general practitioners, and midwives.

A Final Word from the Expert

The decision to deliver in early-onset severe pre-eclampsia remote from term is a difficult one and must be made by a senior obstetrician with discussion involving anaesthetists, neonatologists and haematologists. If both the mother and the fetus are stable, delivery may be deferred for 24–48 hours from the administration of corticosteroids to allow benefit. Although conservative management at early gestations may improve perinatal outcome, balancing maternal well-being is paramount. Two small randomized controlled trials have reported a reduction in neonatal complications with an expectant approach to the management of severe early-onset pre-eclampsia: pregnancy was prolonged for a mean of seven days and 15 days, respectively, at gestations of 28–34 weeks and 28–32 weeks, with no increase in maternal complications [17,18].

Pre-eclampsia continues to challenge obstetricians despite the immense progress being made in unravelling the complex molecular pathways that underpin this syndrome. There can be no doubt that management algorithms have improved the overall outlook for women with pre-eclampsia, but clinicians have to be constantly alert to its diverse presentations and the ability for multisystem disease to be rapidly progressive. Where next for pre-eclampsia? From the data we have on patterns of disease, maternal death, and severe morbidity, current emphasis is now focusing on management of the hypertensive component of the disease in the severely ill. The search for a better screening test or predictor of morbidity goes on and new points of care technologies for circulating angiogenic factors such as free placental growth factor (PLGF) are currently under evaluation.

Perhaps the greatest challenge to us all is to manage the longer-term risk that seems to be associated with hypertension in pregnancy (and more significantly pre-eclampsia). The association between these conditions and an excess of cardiovascular morbidity and mortality later in life may mean that we can use the occurrence of this condition to affect change for individuals and improve their long-term health (see Figure 16.1). As we wrestle with the ethics of informing women of increased levels of risk, we will have to look to large expensive clinical trials or the epidemiology of the future to see if a diagnosis of pre-eclampsia might not always be associated with just an increase in morbidity.

References

1. James PR, Nelson-Piercy C. Management of hypertension before, during, and after pregnancy. *Heart* 2004;90:1499–504.
2. WHO: Make Every Mother and Child Count. World Health Report, 2005. Geneva:WHO, 2005.
3. Shennan AH, Waugh JJS. *Pre-eclampsia*. London:RCOG Press, 2003.
4. Poston L, Briley AL, Seed PT Kelly FJ, Shennan AH; Vitamins in Pre-eclampsia (VIP) Trial Consortium. Vitamin C and vitamin E in pregnant women at risk for preeclampsia (VIP Trial): randomized placebo-controlled trial. *Lancet* 2006;367:1145–54.
5. Pijnenborg R, Anthony J, Davey DA, Rees A, Tiltman A, Vercruysse L, *et al.* Placental bed spiral arteries in the hypertensive disorders of pregnancy. *BJOG* 1991;98:648–55.
6. Moldenhauer JS, Stanek J, Warshak C, Khoury J, Sibai B. The frequency and severity of placental findings in women with pre-eclampsia are gestational age dependent. *Am J Obstet Gynecol* 2003;189:1173–7.
7. Visser N, van Rijn BB, Rijkers GT, Franx A, Bruinse HW. Inflammatory changes in preeclampsia: current understanding of the maternal innate and adaptive immune response. *Obstet Gynecol Surv* 2007;62:191–201.
8 Whiteley GS, Dash PR, Ayling LJ, Prefumo F, Thilaganathan B, Cartwright JE. Increased apoptosis in first trimester extravillous trophoblasts from pregnancies at high risk of developing pre-eclampsia. *Am J Pathol* 2007;170:1903–9.
9 Moll SJ, Jones CJ, Crocker IP, Baker PN, Heazell AE. Epidermal growth factor rescues trophoblast apoptosis induced by reactive oxygen species. *Apoptosis* 2007;12:1611–12.
10. Quinn KH, Lacoursiere DY, Cui L, Bui J, Parast MM. The unique pathophysiology of early-onset severe preeclampsia: role of decidual T regulatory cells. *J Reprod Immunol* 2011;91:76–82.
11. Raymond D, Peterson E. A Critical Review of Early-Onset and Late-Onset Preeclampsia. *Obstet Gynecol Surv* 2011;66:497–506.
12. Centre for Maternal and Child Enquiries (CMACE). Saving Mothers' Lives: reviewing maternal deaths to make motherhood safer: 2006-2008. The Eighth Report on the Confidential Enquiries into Maternal Deaths in the United Kingdom. *BJOG* 2011;118(Suppl. 1):1–203.
13. Wilton A, de Greeff A, Shennan A. Rapid assessment of blood pressure in the obstetric day unit using Microlife MaM Technology. *Hypertens Pregnancy* 2007;26:31–7.
14. De Greeff A, Reggiori F, Shennan AH. Clinical assessment of the DINAMAP ProCare monitor in an adult population according to the British Hypertension Society Protocol. *Blood Press Monit* 2007;12:51–5.
15. Tufnell DJ, Shennan AH, Waugh JJS, Lyons G, Mason GC, Russell IF, Walker JJ. The management of severe preeclampsia/eclampsia. Guideline No. 10(A). London: RCOG Press, 2006.
16. National Collaborating Centre for Women's and Children's Health. Hypertension in pregnancy: the management of hypertensive disorders during pregnancy. National Institute for Health and Clinical Excellence Guideline 107. London: RCOG, August 2010. http://guidance.nice.org.uk/CG107/
17.Murphy DJ, Stirrat GM. Mortality and morbidity associated with early onset pre-eclampsia. *Hypertens Pregnancy* 2000;19:221–31.
18. Haddad B, Deis S, Goffinet F, Paniel BJ, Cabrol D, Siba BM. Maternal and perinatal outcomes during expectant management of 239 severe preeclamptic women between 24 and 33 weeks' gestation. *Am J Obstet Gynecol* 2004;190:1590–7.
19. Knight M. Eclampsia in the United Kingdom2005. *BJOG* 2007;114:1072–8.
20. Douglas KA, Redman CW. Eclampsia in the United Kingdom. *BMJ* 1994;309:1395–400.
21. Magpie Trial Collaborative Group. Do women with pre-eclampsia, and their babies, benefit from magnesium sulphate? The Magpie trial: a randomised placebo-controlled trial. *Lancet* 2002;359:1877–90.

22. Magpie Trial Follow-up Study Collaborative Group. The Magpie Trial: a randomised trial comparing magnesium sulphate with placebo for preeclampsia. Outcome for women at 2 years. *BJOG* 2007;114:300–9.

23. Magpie Trial Follow-up Study Collaborative Group. The Magpie Trial: a randomised trial comparing magnesium sulphate with placebo for preeclampsia. Outcome for children at 18 months. *BJOG* 2007;114:289–99.

24. Li D-K., Yang C, Andrade S, Tavares V, Ferber JR. Maternal exposure to angiotensin converting enzyme inhibitors in the first trimester and risk of malformations in offspring: a retrospective cohort study. *BMJ* 2011; 343: d5931 doi: 10.1136/bmj.d5931.

25 Askie LM, Duley L, Henderson-Smart D, Stewart LA. Antiplatelet agents for prevention of preeclampsia: a meta-analysis of individual patient data. *Lancet* 2007;369:1791–8.

26. Bujold E, Roberge S, Lacasse Y, Bureau M, Audibert F, Marcoux S, *et al*. Prevention of preeclampsia and intrauterine growth restriction with aspirin started in early pregnancy: a meta-analysis. *Obstet Gynecol* 2010;116:402–14.

27. Hofmeyr GJ, Duley L, Atallah A. Dietary calcium supplementation for prevention of preeclampsia and related problems: a systematic review and commentary. *BJOG* 2007;114:933–43.

28. Levine RJ, Hauth JC, Curet LB, Sibai BM, Catalano PM, Morris CD, *et al*. Trial of calcium to prevent preeclampsia. *N Engl J Med* 1997;337:69–76.

29. Walters BN, Thompson ME, Lee A, de Swiet M. Blood pressure in the puerperium. *Clin Sci (Lond)* 1986;71:589–94.

30. Smith M, Waugh J, Nelson-Piercy C. Management of Postpartum Hypertension. *The Obstetrician and Gynaecologist* 2013;15:45–50

31. Cook TM, Counsell D, Wildsmith JAW. Major complications of central neuraxial block: report on the Third National Audit Project of the Royal College of Anaesthetists. *Br J Anaesth* 2009;102:179–190.

32. Douglas KA, Redman CWG. Eclampsia in the United Kingdom. *BMJ* 1994;309:1395–1400.

33. Atterbury JL, Groome LJ, Hoff C, Yarnell JA. Clinical presentation of women re-admitted with post partum severe pre-eclampsia or eclampsia. *J Obstet Gynecol Neonatal Nurs* 1998;27:134–41.

34. National Institute for Health and Clinical Excellence. Hypertension in pregnancy. NICE Clinical Guideline 107. London: NICE, 2010 (updated 2011).

35. Bellamy L, Casas JP, Hingorani AD, Williams DJ. (2007). Pre-eclampsia and risk of cardiovascular disease and cancer in later life: systematic review and meta-analysis *BMJ*;335:974–77.

36. National Institute for Health and Clinical Excellence. Antenatal care: routine care for healthy pregnant women. NICE Clinical Guideline 62. London: NICE, 2008.

37. Milne F, Redman C, Walker J, Baker P, Bradley J, Cooper C, *et al*. The preeclampsia community guideline (PRECOG): how to screen and detect onset of preeclampsia in the community *BMJ* 2005;330:576–80.

17 Vaginal birth after caesarean section

Natalie Atere-Roberts

⊕ Expert Commentary Lawrence W Impey
⊕ Guest Expert Geraint Lee

Case history

A 35-year-old multiparous woman attended the midwife led antenatal clinic at 20 weeks' gestation in her second pregnancy having been referred by her GP due to her previous obstetric history. In her first pregnancy with dichorionic diamniotic (DCDA) twins the previous year, she had had an elective caesarean section at 37 weeks' gestation, having developed pre-eclampsia with a breech presentation of the leading twin. This had been an uncomplicated procedure and she had made an uneventful post-operative recovery. Her blood pressure normalized and her GP was able to stop her anti-hypertensives at her 6-week postnatal check. She had no significant medical history of note and booked with a normal body mass index and blood pressure.

When seen in clinic she was counselled with regards to the good chance of achieving a vaginal delivery in this pregnancy, the small risk of uterine rupture, and the risks of repeat caesarean section. Having completed the discussion, she remained undecided regarding her preference, and was therefore seen in the vaginal birth after caesarean section (VBAC) clinic at 27 weeks' gestation, where she subsequently decided to aim for a vaginal delivery.

⊘ Evidence base Counselling for a VBAC

- The overall chances of successful vaginal delivery in women attempting VBAC are 72–76%[1].
- There is increased fetal and maternal morbidity associated with VBAC compared with repeat elective caesarean section (Tables 17.1 and 17.3).
  - The increased risk of maternal morbidity in women attempting VBAC is due to higher rates of complications in those who attempt VBAC but are unsuccessful (Table 17.2) [2].
  - Delivery related perinatal deaths are higher in the VBAC group. However, the absolute risk of this is low and comparable to that of women having their first birth [3]. The risk of transient tachypnoea of the newborn is increased in the babies of women having an elective repeat caesarean section versus VBAC (2–3% versus 3–4%)[1]; however, this additional risk can be minimized by delaying caesarean section until 39 weeks' gestation.
- Morbidity is reduced in women having a successful VBAC compared with elective repeat caesarean (2.4% versus 3.6%). They will benefit from a lower risk of blood transfusion and hysterectomy, as well as a shorter hospital stay [4].
- Minimizing repeat caesarean sections reduces risk of peri-partum hysterectomy and operative morbidity.
  - A retrospective Saudi Arabian study showed a linear increase in the risk of bladder injury (0.3%, 0.8%, 2.4%), hysterectomy (0.1%, 0.7%, 1.2%), and transfusion requirement (7.2%, 7.9%, 14.1%) with a second, third and fifth caesarean section, respectively [6].

(continued)

• The number of intended pregnancies must therefore inform any discussion regarding mode of delivery after caesarean section. One study has shown that in women planning just one further pregnancy, the risk of hysterectomy is higher in those attempting vaginal delivery versus those having a repeat section. However, for women intending on more than one subsequent pregnancy, the reverse is true [7].

Table 17.1 Maternal complications (Table adapted from [2])

Maternal outcome measure	VBAC (n = 17 898) %	Elective repeat caesarean section (15801) %	Odds ratio (95 % CI)
Uterine rupture	0.7	0	–
Uterine dehiscence	0.7	0.5	1.38 (1.04–1.85)*
Hysterectomy	0.2	0.3	0.77 (0.51–1.17)*
Thromboembolic disease	0.04	0.1	0.62 (0.24–1.62)
Transfusion	1.7	1.0	1.71 (1.41–2.08)*
Endometritis	2.9	1.8	1.62 (1.40–1.87)*
Maternal death	0.02	0.04	0.38 (0.10–1.46)

* p<0.05

Table 17.2 Maternal complications according to the outcome of VBAC [2]

Maternal Outcome measure	Failed vaginal delivery (n = 4759) %	Successful vaginal delivery (n = 13 139) %	Odds Ratio (95 % CI)
Uterine rupture	2.3	0.1	22.18 (12.7–38.72)*
Uterine dehiscence	2.1	0.1	14.82 (9.06–24.23)*
Hysterectomy	0.5	0.1	3.21 (1.73–5.93)*
Thromboembolic disease	0.1	0.02	3.69 (0.83–16.51)
Transfusion	3.2	1.2	2.82 (2.25–3.54)*
Endometritis	7.7	1.2	7.10 (5.86–8.60)*
Maternal death	0.04	0.01	5.52 (0.50–60.92)

* P<0.05

Table 17.3 Fetal complications of VBAC versus repeat elective caesarean section [2]

	VBAC (n = 15 338) %	Elective repeat caesarean (n = 15 014) (%)	Odds ratio (95 % CI)
Antepartum stillbirth:			
37–38 weeks	0.40	0.10	2.93 (1.27–6.75)
≥ 39 weeks	0.20	0.10	2.70 (0.99–7.38)
Intrapartum stillbirth:			
37–38 weeks	0.02	0	–
≥ 39 weeks	0.01	0	–
Hypoxic ischaemic encephalopthy	0.08	0	–*
Neonatal death	0.08	0.13	1.82 (0.73–4.57)

* P<0.05

❝ Expert comment

There are currently no randomized controlled trials to address the question of which birth option is associated with better maternal and fetal outcomes. The current evidence base is derived from observational studies which are associated with inherent bias and heterogeneity making their results difficult to interpret and compare. The design of any randomized trial would be hindered by the fact that some severe outcomes of interest are rare, and so most studies would be underpowered to detect them. In addition, a woman's decision to opt for either birth choice is dependent not only on her knowledge of the risks and benefits of each option but also her personal preferences, influenced by her past experiences, social factors, her doctor's opinion, and the local unit. The BAC (birth after caesarean) trial is a randomized controlled trial currently attempting to overcome these issues, the results of which are pending.

The two- to threefold difference in perinatal mortality between elective repeat caesarean section and VBAC is largely because labour tends to start at a later gestation than a caesarean section is usually performed. This cannot be ignored when counselling women, but of course elective delivery for all pregnancies at 39 weeks is not recommended.

Elective repeat caesarean section is, in many units, the commonest indication for elective caesarean section, and more widespread VBAC has the potential to reduce caesarean rates. The first pregnancy is, however, the best opportunity to avoid the need for subsequent VBAC in the first place.

✪ **Learning point** Determinants of VBAC success

Numerous factors are associated with a successful or unsuccessful VBAC outcome and these may allow some degree of individualisation in the counselling of women with regard to their own chance of success (Table 17.4). Previous vaginal birth, particularly previous VBAC, is the single best predictor and is associated with 87–90% success rate [1,8]. In addition, prior caesarean delivery for non-recurrent indications is associated with greater success; for example, placenta praevia or breech presentation has 77–89% success versus 60–65% for a history of dystocia. In women who are obese, have no previous vaginal birth, whose previous caesarean was for failure to progress, and have been induced, vaginal delivery will be achieved in only 40% [8]. Table 17.4 lists antenatal risk factors for an unsuccessful VBAC.

Table 17.4 Antenatal risk factors for unsuccessful VBAC [1]

Induced labour	Recurring indication
No previous vaginal birth	Short stature
Body mass index > 30	Cervical dilatation at admission < 4 cm
Previous caesarean for dystocia	Advanced maternal age ≥ 40 years
VBAC ≥ 41 weeks	Non-white ethnicity
Birthweight greater than 4000 g	Male infant

✔ **Evidence base** Risk scoring system for antenatal prediction of VBAC success

Given that successful VBAC is associated with the least risk of maternal morbidity and financial burden [4], a system that would allow risk stratification of those with a previous caesarean section would be invaluable to aid appropriate patient selection.

A validated assessment tool exists in order to categorize women into low, intermediate, and high risk of failed VBAC (Box 17.1) [9]. This method has the advantage of using only antenatal criteria and hence can be used to aid the counselling of women well prior to term. Factors included are maternal age, maternal height, method of induction if any, gestation at labour, sex of infant, and previous vaginal birth. For each variable they produced adjusted log likelihood ratios from which the probability of caesarean section can be derived (Table 17.5). In addition, they found that this risk of VBAC failure was also correlated with risk of uterine rupture.

Sample Calculation. Background risk of caesarean section = 26%. Convert into prior odds of caesarean section = 26/74 = 0.35.

Example. A 37-y-old woman, 160 cm tall, with no previous vaginal birth, and with a male infant wishes to know probability of caesarean section if she requires induction of labor at 41 wk gestation using prostaglandin.

Summary. ALLR = $1.40 \times 1.05 \times 1.51 \times 1.10 \times 1.13 \times 1.37 = 3.78$. Posterior odds = $0.35 \times 3.78 = 1.32$. Chance of caesarean delivery = $1.32/(1 + 1.32) = 0.57$ or 57%. (This is identical to the estimated risk using the logistic regression equation in the footnote of Table 4).

(continued)

Table 17.5 Adjusted log likelihood ratios (ALLR) for antenatal factors influencing VBAC outcome [9]

Category	Value	ALLR	Category	Value	ALLR
Height (cm)	143	2.68	Age (y)	18	0.62
	144	2.54		19	0.65
	145	2.40		20	0.68
	146	2.27		21	0.71
	147	2.15		22	0.74
	148	2.04		23	0.77
	149	1.93		24	0.81
	150	1.82		25	0.84
	151	1.72		26	0.88
	152	1.63		27	0.92
	153	1.54		28	0.96
	154	1.46		29	1.00
	155	1.38		30	1.04
	156	1.31		31	1.09
	157	1.24		32	1.13
	158	1.17		33	1.18
	159	1.11		34	1.23
	160	1.05		35	1.29
	161	0.99		36	1.34
	162	0.94		37	1.40
	163	0.89		38	1.46
	164	0.84		39	1.53
	165	0.80		40	1.59
	166	0.75		41	1.66
	167	0.71		42	1.74
	168	0.67		43	1.81
	169	0.64	Previous vaginal birth	Yes	0.30
	170	0.60		No	1.51
	171	0.57	Gestation (wk)	40	0.88
	172	0.54		41	1.13
	173	0.51		42	1.26
	174	0.48	Method of induction	None	0.93
	175	0.46		Non-prostaglandin	0.99
	176	0.43		Prostaglandin	1.37
	177	0.41	Sex of infant	Female	0.91
	178	0.39		Male	1.10
	179	0.37			
	180	0.35			
	181	0.33			
	182	0.31			

Derived from the following logistic regression model: log odds (caesarean) = 5.091 + 0.043 × age) + (−0.055 × height) + (0.193 × male) + (1.633 × no previous vaginal birth) + (0.067 × non-prostaglandin induction) + (0.393 × prostaglandin induction) + (0.248 × delivered at 41 wk) + (0.355 × delivered at 42 wk), where age is expressed in years and height is expressed in centimeters and all other variables are yes = 1 and no = 0. DOI: 10.1371/journal.pmed.0020252.t004

She was seen in the antenatal clinic at 36 weeks' gestation. She confirmed that she would like to aim for a vaginal birth. A plan was made for her to deliver on the consultant led unit and she agreed to have electronic fetal monitoring throughout labour. She was also counselled with regard to her options should she not go into spontaneous labour. She decided that she would be keen to be induced if amniotomy were feasible but she would prefer not to use prostaglandins. A plan was therefore made for her to be seen again in clinic at 41 weeks by the consultant obstetrician.

⊗ **Learning point** Can uterine rupture be predicted antenatally?

All women attempting VBAC should be assessed for risk factors for uterine rupture antenatally and have a plan for delivery documented in the notes, in an attempt to prevent its occurrence. Such risk factors include:

- Site of uterine scar
  - A classical uterine incision is associated with a risk of rupture of 2–9% and therefore planned VBAC is contraindicated in these women [10, 11]. The presence of a low vertical, inverted T- or J-shaped incision also carries an increased risk of rupture compared with a low transverse incision at 2% [2].
- Number of uterine scars
  - There is no apparent increase in the rates of uterine rupture in women with two or more previous caesarean births compared with women with a single section, and therefore the guidelines advise that women should not be prevented from attempting this. However, it may be that these findings are influenced by the small numbers of women with two or more uterine scars attempting VBAC compared with women with only previous section. Such women do need to be fully informed of the increased risk of hysterectomy however (0.6% versus 2%), and blood transfusion requirement (3.2% versus 1.6%), compared to women with a single uterine scar [12].
- Single or double uterine closure of uterus
  - The CESAR study is a randomized controlled trial to investigate the effect of surgical technique on adverse outcomes. The long-term data are yet to report on whether single or double closure at the time of primary caesarean section has a role to play in the subsequent risk of rupture. However, in the largest observational study to-date, including 2142 women, single layer closure was associated with a four fold increase in the risk of subsequent uterine rupture [13].
- Induction of labour
  - Induction of labour either with oxytocin or prostaglandins is an independent risk factor for uterine rupture although not an absolute contraindication (see later in this chapter)
- Black race
  - Despite increased rates of VBAC attempt and failure, black women are 40% less likely to suffer uterine rupture [14]. This may be secondary to racial differences in pelvic connective tissue, as highlighted by the variation in rates of pelvic floor prolapse observed amongst ethnic groups.
- Short inter-pregnancy interval
  - Inter-pregnancy interval of less than 6 months is associated with two- to threefold increase in rates of rupture [15].
- Scar thickness
  - A prospective observational study has shown that the risk of uterine rupture is related to thickness of the lower uterine segment in the late third trimester. A measurement of ≥ 3.5 mm carries a negative predictive value of 99.3%, however its positive predictive value is only 11.8%, and hence its clinical usefulness is limited [16].

⊕ **Clinical tip** Documentation of plans

It is important to have a clear plan for labour and delivery documented in the notes for all women opting for VBAC. This should include:

- Place of birth—ideally this should be on a consultant-led unit.
- Fetal monitoring during labour—continuous monitoring is advised, ideally using telemetry.
- Partographic documentation—this should be meticulous and senior medical review should be sought if there is a delay in either the first or second stage. It would be helpful to have time limits documented in the notes for the second stage, after which a medical review is needed.
- Augmentation—whether or not this is to be used should be clearly documented, and if it is to be used, the rate of increment and the target number of contractions per 10 minutes should be stated.
- Post dates— a discussion regarding whether or not induction should occur in the event of the woman going post dates should take place, and outcome documented. If the woman and her obstetrician opt for induction of labour, the method of induction and use of oxytocin augmentation should be clear in the notes.

For women opting for ERCS, a discussion must then take place regarding a plan of action should she go into labour prior to her elective section date, which occurs in 10% of cases [1].

At 37 weeks' gestation, the patient developed mild pregnancy-induced hypertension which did not require antihypertensive therapy and she was observed twice weekly in the antenatal day assessment unit. At 39 weeks' gestation her BP on presentation was 160/98 and she was admitted to the antenatal ward and treated with antihypertensives. There was no proteinuria on urine dipstick, and her urinary protein creatinine ratio was below the threshold for significant proteinuria at 16 mg/mmol. Elective delivery on the basis of deteriorating PIH was advised by her consultant obstetrician.

◑ Landmark trial Induction of labour versus expectant monitoring for gestational hypertension (PIH) or mild pre-eclampsia after 36 weeks' gestation (HYPITAT) [17]

- Multicentre, open-label randomized controlled trial ($n = 756$).
- Induction of labour ($n = 377$) versus expectant management ($n = 379$) for women with PIH or mild pre-eclampsia at term.
- Primary outcome: composite adverse maternal outcome—maternal mortality, maternal morbidity (eclampsia, HELLP, pulmonary oedema, thrombolytic disease, or placental abruption), progression to severe hypertension or proteinuria and major postpartum haemorrhage.
- Significant reduction in composite maternal morbidity (the contribution to this largely progression to severe hypertension) in the induction of labour group (117 (31%) versus 166 (44%); RR 0.71 95% CI 0.59–0.86).
- No significant difference in maternal clinical morbidity outcomes (HELLP [haemolytic anaemia, elevated liver enzymes, and low platelet count], thromboembolic disease, postpartum haemorrhage, eclampsia, placental abruption, length of hospital stay), caesarean section rate, or adverse neonatal outcome.

---

❻ Expert comment

HYPITAT did not discriminate between gestational hypertension and mild pre-eclampsia (conditions with potentially very different underlying pathologies). Subgroup analysis found that the reduction in progression to severe hypertension was significant only in the mild-pre-eclampsia group; for women with gestational hypertension, this was not the case. Furthermore, the findings from this trial are not directly applicable to a UK setting as in the Netherlands gestational hypertension is managed by offering immediate birth without antihypertensive treatment [18]. Thus, the current the recommendations from NICE [18] for management of women with gestational hypertension at term is that antihypertensive treatment should precede an offer of early birth. However, if the woman's blood pressure becomes severe (≥ 160/90 mmHg) the woman should be offered immediate birth after a course of corticosteroids if needed. After 37 weeks for women with a BP lower that 160/90 mmHg, the decision on timing of birth requires senior obstetric involvement.

On abdominal palpation, the head was 3/5 palpable and on vaginal examination her cervix was central, effaced, and 2 cm dilated. Her Bishops score was 8. Mode of delivery was discussed, and plans for a VBAC confirmed. She consented to induction of labour with artificial rupture of membranes and oxytocin augmentation, which was arranged for the following morning as the consultant felt it prudent to ensure her induction did not occur overnight.

⊕ **Clinical tip** Bishops score

The Bishops score is a scoring system (see Table 17.6) used to determine the favourability of the cervix for induction of labour and therefore which method of induction should be used. Scores of < 5 indicate the cervix is unfavourable and that if induction is required, cervical ripening with prostaglandins will be needed. Scores of > 7 indicate a favourable cervix and that induction is likely to be successful.

Table 17.6 Scoring system to assess cervical favourability

	Score			
	0	1	2	3
Dilatation	0 cm	1–2 cm	3–4 cm	5–6 cm
Effacement	0–30 %	40–60 %	60–70 %	> 80 %
Position	Posterior	Mid-position	Anterior	–
Station	–3 cm	–2 cm	–1/0 cm	1–2 cm
Consistency	Firm	Medium	Soft	–

✔ **Evidence base** Induction of labour in women having planned VBAC

Induction and augmentation of women with a previous caesarean delivery is an independent risk factor for uterine rupture and although not contraindicated, the decision to induce labour should be taken with caution after careful maternal assessment and counselling at a senior level. Women having a planned VBAC undergoing induced or augmented labours have 1.5 fold increased risk of caesarean section and two- to threefold risk of uterine rupture compared with spontaneous labours (Table 17.7) [2, 8, 19].

Method of induction is a determinant of risk of rupture. A recent prospective observational study showed that prostaglandin induction methods were associated with the highest risk of rupture (15.9/1000 births) [19]. Induction with oxytocin had the second highest risk of rupture (7.2/1000 births) whereas induction via mechanical means had similar risks of rupture as spontaneous labour (5.8/1000 versus 5.5/1000 births) [19].

Table 17.7 Association of induction of labour with uterine rupture and perinatal outcomes after previous caesarean section [19]

	Total no. (mothers)	Uterine rupture no. per 1000 (%)	OR (95 % CI)
Total	11 954	80 (6.6)	
Spontaneous labour onset	9239	51 (5.5)	1
Induction methods	2715	29 (10.7)	
Prostaglandins +/− amniotomy	1130	18 (15.9)	2.91 (1.7–5.0)
Prostaglandins, amniotomy, and oxytocin	168	2 (11.9)	1.30 (0.5–3.6)
Oxytocin +/− amniotomy	555	4 (7.2)	2.17 (0.5–8.9)
Mechanical methods	862	5 (5.8)	1.05 (0.4–2.6)

⑥ **Expert comment**

When VBAC is attempted, occasional uterine ruptures may be unavoidable. However, I virtually never use oxytocin or prostaglandins in women with a uterine scar because of the lower chance of success and higher chance of uterine rupture. Although often performed for minor indications, induction should generally only be performed if the risks of not inducing are greater: the presence of the scar adds another factor to consider. If labour has not started by 41+ weeks, I usually recommend caesarean section, although obstetric practice varies widely. Any decision must be discussed with the woman herself and risks and benefits of all options made clear. Use of oxytocin in a VBAC must be made by a senior obstetrician.

At 09.00 the next morning she was admitted to the delivery suite and the induction process was started with artificial rupture of membranes. Having been reviewed by the registrar on duty, cautious use of the syntocinon was recommended. The patient began contracting regularly at a rate of three in 10 minutes at 11.30 and the syntocinon infusion was therefore maintained at a rate of 12 mls/hour for the remainder of the labour. At 12.30 an epidural was sited and she continued to make good progress.

> ✚ **Clinical tip** The importance of the partogram in VBAC labour
>
> Women attempting VBAC who show signs of secondary arrest in labour are at high risk of uterine rupture, and hence all women require close observation and accurate documentation of progress using a partogram. This is evidenced by the results from a retrospective cohort study of 236 patients with seven uterine ruptures, in which a 1 cm/hour line was used after onset of active labour as an 'alert' line. They found that the partographic zone 2–3 hours after crossing the alert line in women undergoing VBAC represents a time of high risk of scar rupture [20].

At 16.00, the duty registrar was asked to review the patient as the midwife was concerned with regard to the presence of a small vaginal bleed. The patient was found to be comfortable, with no scar pain and a mild tachycardia. The head was 0/5 palpable per abdomen with no scar tenderness elicited, and the cervix was fully dilated with the head just below the spines on vaginal examination. Early decelerations were seen on the CTG with no non-reassuring features (Figure 17.1) and contractions maintained at a rate of 3 in 10. Active pushing was therefore commenced.

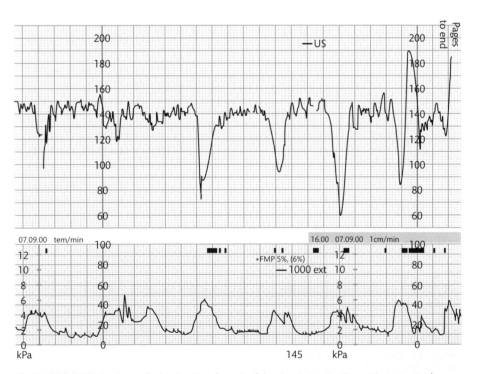

Figure 17.1 CTG showing early decelerations (trough of deceleration coinciding with contraction).

Reproduced from Sarris, Bewley, and Agnihotri, *Training in Obstetrics and Gynaecology*, 2009 with permission from Oxford University Press.

At 17.00, the midwife called for an urgent review of the CTG due to a bradycardia. Prior to the bradycardia, the CTG had become pathological with late decelerations and a fetal tachycardia (Figure 17.2). At vaginal examination the head was now –1 to the ischial spines and the decision was made to perform a category 1 caesarean section due to the possibility of uterine rupture.

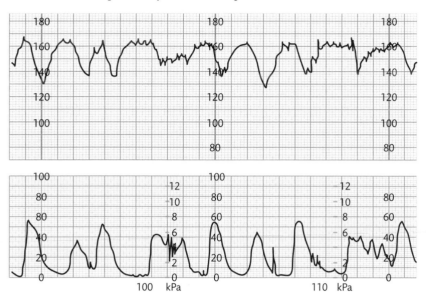

Figure 17.2 CTG showing late decelerations.

Adapted from Sarris, Bewley, and Agnihotri, *Training in Obstetrics and Gynaecology*, 2009 with permission from Oxford University Press.

> ⊗ **Learning point** Clinical and CTG features of uterine rupture
>
> Rapid diagnosis of uterine rupture is essential in order to reduce neonatal and maternal morbidity. Signs and symptoms of uterine rupture can be variable and hence a high index of suspicion is required, particularly in those presenting immediately prior to vaginal delivery and postpartum.
>
> **Clinical features:**
>
> - May be asymptomatic
> - Restlessness
> - Constant pain in lower abdomen
> - Sensation of something giving way or a 'pop'
> - Hypotension and tachycardia
> - Collapse
> - Difficulty palpating fetal parts or may be easy to palpate
> - Two swellings may be palpated; one being the fetus, and the other the contracted and retracted uterus
> - Loss of uterine contour
> - Vaginal bleeding
> - Haematuria
> - Loss of station of the presenting part on vaginal examination
> - There is no evidence that epidural anaesthesia masks these clinical features and is therefore not contraindicated for VBACs
>
> (continued)

Expert comment

Caesarean section scars are not uncommonly very thin or even dehisced at caesarean section. At elective procedures this is seldom important. Antenatal rupture of the scarred uterus is rare, but previous perforation, particularly with infection (e.g. bowel damage) or major myometrial scarring, are risk factors. Probably the most common cause of antenatal rupture is congenital abnormalities of the uterus and it often occurs at a pre-viable gestation.

Expert comment

Fetal mortality and morbidity from uterine rupture is largely because of extrusion of the fetus into the abdominal cavity, with consequent sustained contraction of the uterus. At this stage, *in utero* resuscitation is impossible. Maternal blood loss will be rapid and time is everything: this is one of the few real indications for a 'crash' caesarean section.

CTG features:

- The CTG will be abnormal in the majority of cases
- Bradycardia is most common occurrence
- Other characteristic CTG abnormalities that may be seen are:
  - Baseline tachycardia
  - Reduced baseline variability
  - 'Staircase' sign: gradual, stepwise decrease in contraction amplitude
  - Tachysystole

✚ Clinical tip Not all uterine rupture occurs in women with a scarred uterus

The vast majority of cases of uterine rupture occur in women with a scarred uterus. However, an increase in awareness and meticulous monitoring during labour has meant that despite the increase in caesarean section rate, the risk of catastrophic outcome remains low due to rapid diagnosis and expeditious management. In those women with rupture and an unscarred uterus, this may not be the case, resulting in increased maternal mortality as was highlighted in the 2003–2005 CEMACH report detailing a maternal death in a multiparous woman following the use of prostaglandins for induction [21].

Common risk factors for intrapartum rupture in an unscarred uterus are:

- Grand multiparity
- Fetal malpresentation, e.g. unrecognized brow, face, shoulder presentation
- Neglected dystocia
- Oxytocin augmentation in multiparous women
- Congenital uterine malformations

At caesarean section 20 minutes later, uterine rupture was confirmed with extrusion of the fetal head into the peritoneal cavity. At birth the baby was pale and floppy, with no respiratory effort and a heart rate of < 60 bpm. He was intubated, ventilated, received external cardiac compressions, and was given three boluses of epinephrine via an umbilical venous catheter, in addition to sodium bicarbonate, 0.9 % saline, and packed red cells. His heart rate increased > 60 bpm at 11 minutes of age. The first gasp was 14 minutes of age, and his heart rate remained above 100 bpm from 19 minutes of age. Once the baby was stabilized, he was shown to parents and transferred to the neonatal intensive care unit. Cord gases were: arterial pH 6.74 BE–21.3; venous pH 6.83 BE–20.2.

The uterine lacerations were extensive and despite repair, the ongoing haemorrhage was deemed to be life-threatening and hence a subtotal hysterectomy was performed. The total estimated blood loss was 4 litres, and the patient was resuscitated using 4 units of blood, 4 units of fresh frozen plasma (FFP), and one pool of platelets. She was subsequently transferred to the high dependency unit for her early post-operative care.

✚ Clinical tip Management of uterine rupture

Management of uterine rupture relies on prompt diagnosis, immediate resuscitation, and expeditious recourse to exploratory laparotomy in order to prevent maternal exsanguination and death, as well as severe neonatal morbidity and mortality. Anaesthetic and haematological involvement and early senior input is of paramount importance.

Once the baby is delivered, the surgical management will depend on the type and extent of uterine damage, the degree of haemorrhage, and the general condition of the mother. Repair of the uterus

(continued)

is possible in the majority of women, unless there is intractable uterine bleeding, broad ligament or cervical extensions, or the rupture sites are longitudinal and/or multiple. The requirement for future childbearing should be of low priority when deciding on the feasibility of conservative management in such circumstances. In parallel with the surgical management, the ongoing resuscitation and supportive care for the mother is of equal importance in achieving a favourable outcome, and as such, these women will require post-operative care in the intensive care unit.

⊘ Evidence base Maternal and fetal outcomes following uterine rupture

Fetal consequences

One study has reported the rate of perinatal asphyxia secondary to uterine rupture (defined as umbilical–artery pH < 7 with seizures and multi-organ dysfunction) to be 5% [22]. None of the neonates had clinically significant perinatal morbidity when delivery was accomplished within 18 minutes of an isolated and prolonged deceleration of fetal heart rate. However, if severe late decelerations preceded the prolonged deceleration, perinatal asphyxia was observed as soon as 10 minutes from the onset of the prolonged deceleration to delivery. Other studies have shown that even with rapid delivery of less than 18 minutes [23], hypoxic ischaemic encephalopathy can occur and that this may be related to the degree of fetal extrusion into the peritoneal cavity. A review of the literature found that 5% of uterine ruptures were associated with perinatal mortality and hence the additional risk of perinatal death from uterine rupture was 1.4 per 10 000 attempted VBACs. 7142 elective repeat caesarean sections would need to be performed to prevent one rupture-related perinatal death [24].

Maternal consequences

Hysterectomy occurs in 13% of women experiencing uterine rupture during trial of labour. This accounts for 3.4 hysterectomies per 10 000 attempted VBACs [24]. Uterine rupture is also associated with bladder injury which occurs relatively frequently (8–18% of cases) [22], massive transfusion [22], endometritis, and longer hospital stay. Maternal death is a rare occurrence quoted as 0.002% of women due to rupture following trial of labour [25].

The baby remained ventilated on intensive care and fulfilled the criteria for therapeutic cooling, with features of severe (grade 3) encephalopathy. Therapeutic hypothermia was commenced at 35 minutes of age.

✪ Learning point Hypoxic ischaemic encephalopathy

Hypoxic ischaemic encephalopathy (HIE) describes neonatal encephalopathy due to intrapartum asphyxia, and it represents a serious cause of mortality and long-term morbidity. In developed countries, perinatal asphyxia affects three to five infants per 1000 live births, with 0.5-1 infants per 1000 live births developing brain damage in the form of HIE [26]. It is characterized by the clinical evidence of acute or subacute brain injury such as the need for resuscitation at birth, neurological depression, seizures, and EEG abnormalities.

There are three grades of HIE based on clinical features and to which the degree of morbidity and mortality is correlated (see Table 17.8).

Table 17.8 Risk of death or severe handicap in remaining survivors associated with grade of HIE [27]

Grade HIE	Percentage	Likelihood ratio	95% CI
Mild	1.6	0.05	0.02–0.15
Moderate	24	0.94	0.71–1.23
Severe	78	10.71	6.71–17.1

❝ Guest expert comment (neonatology)

It is now a standard of care in the UK that all children with moderate or severe HIE should be offered therapeutic hypothermia, which may necessitate transfer to a cooling centre. Passive cooling can be safely commenced prior to transfer to a cooling centre, and continued by the neonatal transport team.

✪ Learning point Therapeutic hypothermia for HIE

Studies have shown that following hypoxic ischaemic injury, mild induced hypothermia (a reduction of body temperature by about 3 °C) preserves cerebral energy metabolism, reduces secondary cerebral tissue injury, and improves long-term neurological function. Randomized trials in full-term and near-full-term newborns demonstrate that treatment with mild–moderate hypothermia is safe and improves survival without disability up to 18 months of age (risk ratio 0.81, $p = 0.002$, number needed to treat–9); however, longer-term neurodevelopmental follow-up studies remain ongoing [26].

The aim of intervention with hypothermia is to maintain a cerebral temperature of approximately 33–34 °C for 72 hours, commencing as soon as possible after resuscitation, but before 6 hours of age. Two approaches have been used: head cooling combined with minimal to mild whole-body cooling or surface whole-body cooling to the target cerebral temperature. Therapeutic hypothermia is a relatively inexpensive, yet effective and safe treatment that should be offered to all infants that are ≥ 36 weeks' gestation, require resuscitation at birth, and develop seizures or moderate/severe encephalopathy after resuscitation. It should not be used in conditions that require immediate or imminent surgery, or in an infant that has a poor long-term outcome, or that is moribund.

The baby survived, however his long-term prognosis remains poor and he is likely to have four-limb cerebral palsy with associated sensory and cognitive difficulties. This obviously does not just have implications for the child, but also for the mother and wider family. The mother made a good post-operative recovery and was discharged on the 8th postnatal day. She was later seen in both the gynaecology and obstetric follow-up clinics for a full debrief of events.

❝ Guest expert comment (neonatology)

The national neonatal life support guidelines from the ALSG suggest that if a newborn term infant has no discernable cardiac activity by 10 minutes of age, then it is appropriate to consider discontinuing intensive care. The appropriate course of resuscitation is often less clear-cut in clinical practice, particularly when the heart rate is detectable but remains < 60 and further resuscitation measures are available, as in this case. The decision to stop resuscitation should always be made by the most senior paediatrician available.

It should be noted that despite the poor outcome for this baby, there are many babies who have suffered a perinatal asphyxial event who recover unaffected, particularly with moderate hypoxic ischaemic encephalopathy (HIE). 53% of children in the most recent meta-analysis [26] with moderate or severe HIE, who received therapeutic hypothermia, survived without severe disability. The assessment and grading of HIE takes time, and once the heart rate recovers following resuscitation, it is prudent to admit the baby to the neonatal unit for assessment and discussions with the parents, regardless of the perceived severity of the insult.

✪ Learning point Debriefing after an adverse event

Good communication with patients and their family after a poor outcome is of paramount importance. Whilst it is true that obstetrics remains one of the most litigious specialties in medicine, this does not mean that making a complaint or pursuing a medical negligence claim is at the forefront of every patient's mind. In the immediate aftermath, they should be counselled by the senior healthcare professional involved in the case, informed of what has happened, and what the consequences of this will be. In this case, this would have been done by the consultant obstetrician and neonatologist. At a later date, once the patient has had the opportunity to consider any questions she and her family may have and after a full investigation has been undertaken, a more detailed discussion of events should take place. It is usually at this stage, if this process has been mishandled

(continued)

and if questions remain unanswered that legal action may be under consideration [28]. It is therefore critical, in order to provide good patient care, which will in turn also limit litigation, that after a poor outcome communication with the patient and her family remains open, honest, and empathic.

A poor outcome is also highly distressing for those caring for the patient, and hence it is also important that those healthcare professionals involved have the opportunity to discuss the case in detail with a senior member of the team. This process should encompass both emotional and psychological support but should also provide a forum for the staff to learn from the incident [29].

✪ **Learning point** Risk management for maternity services

It should be the aim of all maternity units to identify and minimize risk in their department, and therefore an understanding of its process is important to all team members.

The definition of risk management is 'the culture, processes and structures that are directed towards realizing potential opportunities whilst managing adverse effects'. It forms one of the seven pillars of clinical governance (Figure 17.3) and is best approached in tandem with these other aspects.

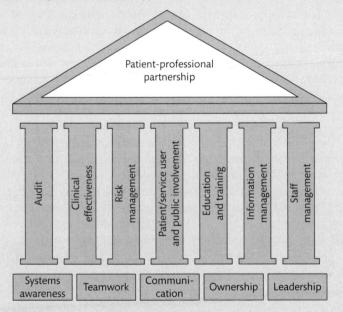

Figure 17.3 The seven pillars of clinical governance.

Adapted from NHS Clinical Governance Support Team, 1999.

It involves four basic steps [30]:

1. Risk identification: What could go wrong?
2. Risk analysis and evaluation: What are the chances of it going wrong and what would the impact be?
3. Risk treatment: What can we do to minimize the chance of this going wrong or to mitigate the damage if it does?
4. Risk control; sharing and learning: What can we learn from things that go wrong?

In addition to the local approach to risk management within an organization, it also exists on a national scale. The National Patient Safety Association (NPSA) was established in 2001 for this purpose. It acts to collect reports of patient safety incidents and near misses, analyses them to identify common risks, and it produces feedback and guidance to healthcare organisations to improve patient safety. This is known as the National Reporting and Learning System (NRLS).

The case underwent a detailed review by the risk management team and a root-cause analysis was performed in order to highlight areas in which the care might have been improved. The outcome of this was subsequently presented in a departmental meeting.

Discussion

Currently in the UK, 20–25% of births are undertaken by caesarean section [31]. In England, this number has increased significantly over the last 40 years: 4% in 1970, 9% in 1980, 13% in 1990, 21% in 2000, and 24.8% in 2009 [32]. There are also regional differences within the UK, with rates being highest in London 24.2% versus 19.3% in the north-east [32]. Similar increases have been seen in other developed countries although the absolute values differ; however, Nordic countries have still managed to maintain their rate below the WHO target of 15% despite similar rate of growth over this time period [31]. The National sentinel caesarean section report from 2001 has shown that the overall VBAC rate in the UK is 33%, however there was wide variation in this figure between geographical areas and between individual units [32].

Catastrophic consequences of unsuccessful VBAC are rare, and as clinicians we should not allow our fear of such events to cloud our ability to adequately counsel women according to the available evidence. Only half of women with one previous caesarean section will attempt VBAC despite the fact that the majority of women who do so will be successful with a favourable outcome achieved for both mother and baby. The key is to ensure careful patient selection which will not only encourage the majority of women who are likely to succeed but also identify the small number for which this birth option is inappropriate. This approach is vital to ensuring greater patient satisfaction, minimising maternal and perinatal morbidity and achieving significant financial savings. As this case demonstrates, even with seemingly appropriate management of the VBAC labour, uterine rupture may still occur, and the key to minimizing morbidity and mortality is in its early recognition and expeditious management at a senior level.

A Final Word from the Expert

There are four considerations surrounding elective caesarean section; of course their importance differs. First, is the safety of the mother. Second is that of the baby. Third, is the safety of them both in the next pregnancy. Finally, there is safety of other people.

For the baby, the risk of serious harm is lower with elective caesarean section. Indeed, this probably even applies for a first baby, providing the pregnancy is at 39 weeks. For the mother, the risk depends on the risk of an emergency caesarean section, and if this risk approaches 50%, then elective caesarean is probably safer for her. For the next pregnancy it is safer to deliver vaginally, unless of course the uterus ruptures, because of the accreta risk. There are also data suggesting an increased risk for the baby where a woman has had a caesarean section. Finally, the consideration 'other people' appears obtuse, and this issue applies perhaps more to the argument against elective caesarean section for all pregnancies.

There is the issue of finite funding, as well as operator skill. For instance, vaginal breech birth in the UK, which still occurs because of missed breeches and parent preference, has become more risky than at the time of the Term Breech Trial because of loss of operator skills.

The first pregnancy is the best opportunity to avoid the need for subsequent VBAC. Where a woman has had a previous caesarean section, informed choice is crucial, as is documentation of the risks and benefits. If VBAC is attempted, adequate monitoring of the baby, the mother and the progress are also crucial. Rupture will still happen occasionally, and the response must be decisive, coordinated, and fast.

References

1. Royal College of Obstetricians and Gynaecologists. Birth after previous caesarean birth. Green-top Guideline No. 45. 2007.
2. Landon M, Hauth JC, Leveno KJ, Spong CY, Leindecker S, Varner MW, *et al.* Maternal and perinatal outcomes associated with a trial of labor after prior caesarean delivery. *N Engl J Med* 2004;351:2581–9.
3. Smith GC, Pell JP, Cameron AD, Dobbie R. Risk of perinatal death associated with labor after previous caesarean delivery in uncomplicated term pregnancies. *JAMA* 2002;287:2684–90.
4. Hibbard JU, Ismail M, Wang Y, Te C, Karrison T, Ismail M. Failed vaginal birth after caesarean section: How risky is it? *Am J Obstet Gynecol* 2001;184:1365–73
5. Dunn EA, O'Herlihy C. Comparison of maternal satisfaction following vaginal delivery after caesarean section and caesarean section after previous vaginal delivery. *Eur J Obstet Gynecol Reprod Biol* 2005;121:56–60.
6. Makoha FW, Felimban HM, Fathuddien MA, Roomi F, Ghabra T. Multiple caesarean section morbidity. *Int J Gynaecol Obstet* 2004;87:227–32
7. Paré E, Quinones J, Macones G. Vaginal birth after caesarean section versus elective repeat caesarean section: assessment of maternal downstream health outcomes. *BJOG* 2006;113:75–85.
8. Landon MB, Leindecker S, Spong CY, Hauth JC, Bloom S, Varner MW, *et al.* The MFMU caesarean registry: factors affecting the success of trial of labor after previous caesarean delivery. *Am J Obstet Gynecol* 2005;193:1016–23
9. Smith GCS, White IR, Pell JP, Dobbie R. Predicting caesarean section and uterine rupture among women attempting vaginal birth after prior caesarean section. *PLoS Med* 2005;2:871–8
10. Guise JM, Hashima J. Evidence-based vaginal birth after caesarean section. *Best Prac Clin Obstet Gynaecol* 2005;19:117–30
11. Turner MJ. Uterine rupture. *Best Prac Res Clin Ostet Gynaecol* 2002;16:69–79
12. Landon MB, Song CY, Thom E, Hauth JC, Bloom SL, Varner MW, *et al.* Risk of uterine rupture with trial of labor in women with multiple and single caesarean delivery. *Obstet Gynecol* 2006;108:12–20
13. Bujold E, Bujold C, Hamilton EF, Harel F, Gauthier RJ. The impact of single layer or double layer closure on uterine rupture. *Am J Obstet Gynecol* 2002;186:1326–30
14. Cahill AG, Stamilo DM, Odibo AO, Peiper J, Stevens E, Macones GA. Racial disparity in the success and complications of vaginal birth after caesarean. *Obstet Gynecol* 2008;111:654–8
15. Stamilo DM, DeFranco E, Pare E, Odibo AO, Peiper JF, Allsworth JE, *et al.* Short interpregnancy interval: risk of uterine rupture and complications of vaginal birth after caesarean delivery. *Obstet Gynecol* 2007;110:1075–82

16. Rozenburg P, Goffinet F, Phillippe HJ, Nisand I. Echographic measurement of the inferior uterine segment for assessing the risk of uterine rupture. *J Gynecol Obstet Biol Reprod* 1997;26:513–9.

17. Koopmans CM, Bilenga D, Groen H, Vigen SM, Aarnoudse JG, Bekedam DJ, *et al.* Induction of labour versus expectant monitoring for gestational hypertension or mild pre-eclampsia after 36 weeks' gestation (HYPITAT): A multicentre, open-label randomised controlled trial. *Lancet* 2009;374;979–88

18. National Collaborating Centre for Women's and Children's Health. Hypertension in pregnancy; the management of hypertensive disorders during pregnancy. NICE clinical guideline 107, August 2010.

19. Al-Zirqui I, Stray-Pedersen B, Firsen L, Vangen S. Uterine rupture after previous caesarean section. *BJOG* 2010;117:809–20

20. Khan KS, Rivzi A. The partograph in the management of labour following caesarean section. *Int J Gynecol Obstet* 1995;50:151–7

21. Lewis G. (ed.). The Confidential Enquiry into Maternal and Child Health. Saving Mothers' Lives: Reviewing Maternal Deaths to Make Motherhood Safer 2003-5. The Seventh Report on Confidential Enquiries into Maternal Deaths in the United Kingdom. London: CEMACH, 2007.

22. Leung AS, Leung EK, Paul RH. Uterine rupture after previous caesarean delivery: maternal and fetal consequences. *Am J Obstet Gynecol* 1993;169:945–50

23. Bujold E, Gauthier RJ. Neonatal morbidity associated with uterine rupture: what are the risk factors? *Am J Obstet Gynecol* 2002;186:311–14.

24. Guise JM, Berlin M, McDonagh M, Osterweil P, Chan B, Helfand M. Safety of vaginal birth after caesarean: a systematic review. *Obstet Gynecol* 2004;103:420–9

25. Chauhan SP, Martin JN Jr, Henrichs CE, Morrison JC, Magann EF. Maternal and perinatal complications with uterine rupture in 142,075 patients who attempted vaginal birth after caesarean delivery: a review of the literature. *Am J Obstet Gynecol* 2003;189:408–17

26. Edwards AD, Brocklehurst P, Gunn AJ, Halliday H, Juszczak E, Levene M, Strohm B, Thoresen M, Whitelaw A, Azzopardi D. Neurological outcomes at 18 months of age after moderate hypothermia for perinatal hypoxic ischaemic encephalopathy: synthesis and meta-analysis of trial data. *BMJ* 2010;340:c363.

27. Evans DJ, Levene MI. Hypoxic-ischaemic injury. In Rennie JM, Roberton NRC (eds) *Textbook of neonatology.* 1231–51. Churchill Livingston, Edinburgh, 2000.

28. Woolfson J. What to do when things go wrong. *TOG* 2001;3(1):20–3

29. Vaithilingam N, Jain S, Davies D. Helping the helpers: debriefing following an adverse incident. *TOG* 2008;10:251–6

30. Royal College of Obstetricians and Gynaecologists. Improving Patient Safety: Risk Management for Obstetricians and Gynaecologists. Clinical Governance Advice, No. 2, 2009.

31. National Collaborative Centre for Women's and Children's Health. Caesarean Section. Clinical Guideline No. 132 London: NICE guidance; 2011.

32. Thomas J, Paranjothy S. College of Obstetricians and Gynaecologists Clinical Support Unit. *National Sentinel Caesarean Section Audit.* London: RCOG Press; 2001.

Maternal pyrexia: challenges in optimal perinatal management

Surabhi Nanda

Expert Commentary Kate Langford
Guest Expert Neil Marlow

Case history

A 33-year-old woman, Gravida 1 Para 0, presented to the antenatal day assessment unit (ADU) at 39 weeks and 6 days' gestation. The pregnancy was conceived spontaneously with an uneventful antenatal period. She had no significant past medical history and was not taking any regular medication. She had a history of penicillin allergy. Combined screening had indicated a low risk for trisomy 21 and the detailed scan at 20 weeks' gestation had not detected any concerns. All her

---

⊘ Landmark trial Birthplace study [1]

- A prospective UK nationwide cohort study carried out between April 2008–2010 comparing perinatal outcomes, maternal outcomes, and interventions in labour by planned place of birth at the start of care in labour for women with low-risk pregnancies.
- 64 538 singleton, booked, term (≥37 weeks' gestation) pregnancies from all NHS trusts providing intrapartum care at home, in free-standing and neighbouring midwifery units, together with a stratified random sample of obstetric units.
- Primary outcome: composite of perinatal mortality and specific neonatal morbidities: stillbirth after the start of care in labour, early neonatal death, neonatal encephalopathy, meconium aspiration syndrome, brachial plexus injury, fractured humerus, and fractured clavicle.
- Results—The study suggested that giving birth is generally very safe and that midwifery units appear to be safe for the baby and offer benefits for the mother.

  o For 'low-risk' women, the incidence of adverse perinatal outcome was low (4.3 events per 1000 births).
  o For nulliparous women, the odds of the primary outcome were higher for planned home births (adjusted OR 1.75, 95% CI 1.07–2.86) but not for either midwifery unit setting.
  o For multiparous women, there were no significant differences in the incidence of the primary outcome by planned place of birth.
  o For planned births in freestanding and alongside midwifery units there were no significant differences in adverse perinatal outcomes compared with planned birth in an obstetric unit.
  o Interventions during labour were substantially lower in all non-obstetric unit settings.
  o Transfers from non-obstetric unit settings were more frequent for nulliparous women (36–45%) than for multiparous women (9–13%).

- The key findings of this study suggest that:

  o **For women having a second or subsequent baby**, home births and midwifery unit births appear to be safe for the baby, and they offer benefits for the mother, reducing the odds of having an intrapartum caesarean section, instrumental delivery, or episiotomy.
  o **For women having a first baby**, a planned home birth increases the risk to the baby. There were significantly more adverse perinatal outcome events per 1000 planned home births (9.3 compared with 5.3 for births planned in obstetric units).

booking investigations had been normal. She was initially booked to deliver in the nearby midwifery-led birthing unit.

On presentation to the ADU, she gave a history of draining clear fluid per vaginum since 09.00 hours that morning. Pre-labour spontaneous rupture of membranes (PROM) was confirmed on speculum examination. After discussion she elected to wait 24 hours prior to stimulation of labour.

➕ Clinical tip Assessment of spontaneous pre-labour rupture of membranes (PROM)

Sterile speculum examination is the gold standard for confirmation or exclusion of ROM. It allows for assessment of liquor colour and gives the opportunity to rule out cord prolapse or presentation. Digital examination (VE) should be avoided where ROM is suspected until the woman is in labour, as it increases the risk of uterine infection.

Ultrasound measurement of the amniotic fluid volume can neither confirm nor exclude ROM; it can simply assess the current amniotic fluid volume.

Where there is a persuasive history of SROM but no liquor seen even on coughing, then a speculum examination can be repeated after 1 hour of the patient lying supine, which allows liquor to pool in the vagina.

Differential diagnoses:

I.   Urinary leakage—if secondary to urinary tract infection would present with nitrites in urine and no fluid in the vagina on speculum examination.
II. Transudate from bulging membranes—fluid is observed in the vagina with visibly intact membranes on speculum examination.
III. Vaginal discharge—vaginal discharge on speculum examination rather than a clear pool of liquor.

✷ Evidence base Management of PROM

The TERMPROM trial [4] showed no difference in neonatal infection rates or caesarean section rates with oxytocin versus prostaglandin for stimulation of labour; however, stimulation with oxytocin was associated with lower risk of maternal pyrexia. In the cohort of 5041 women with pre-labour rupture of membranes at term, clinical chorioamnionitis was less likely to develop in the women in the induction with oxytocin group than in those in the expectant management (oxytocin) group (4.0% versus 8.6%, P <0.001), as was postpartum fever (1.9% versus 3.6% P <0.008).

In the meta-analysis of studies included in the NICE guidance on intrapartum care [3], women in the planned early stimulation groups were less likely to develop chorioamnionitis or endometritis than women in the expectant management group RR 0.74 [95% CI 0.56–0.97] and RR 0.30 [95% CI 0.12–0.74] respectively, although there was no significant difference between groups regarding incidence of postpartum fever RR 0.69 [95% CI 0.41–1.17]. There was no difference between groups regarding mode of birth.

Babies born to women in the planned early birth groups were less likely to be admitted to neonatal intensive care unit or special care baby unit, RR 0.73 [95% CI 0.58–0.91]. No significant differences were found for any other investigated neonatal outcomes, including fetal/perinatal mortality, Apgar score less than 7 at 5 minutes, mechanical ventilation, or neonatal infection. Findings showed that longer periods of time from rupture of membranes to active labour were associated with a higher incidence of neonatal infection: 48 hours or longer versus 12 hours: OR 2.25 [95% CI 1.21–4.18]; 24 to 48 hours versus 12 hours: OR 1.97 [95% CI 1.11–3.48].

However, balancing the risks and benefits, the National Institute of Clinical Excellence (NICE) guidance on intrapartum care recommends that women with pre-labour rupture of the membranes at term (at or over 37 weeks) should be offered a choice of induction of labour or expectant management. If labour has not commenced approximately 24 hours after rupture of membranes, in those choosing expectant management, stimulation of labour is appropriate [3]. There was no consensus in the reviewed evidence on the method of stimulation, and the guideline development group suggested stimulation of labour with Prostin (prostaglandin E2) in the first instance, in view of it being less invasive than oxytocin.

Table 18.1 First blood results

Time	WCC	Hb	CRP
Normal values	4–11 10/S/9/L	11.5–15.5 gm/dl	<5 mg/L
Booking	7.1	12.3	–
Day 0 – 11.00hrs	9.2	11.5	13

The woman presented to the hospital birth centre the following morning at 11.00 for stimulation of labour. She was cannulated and baseline bloods FBC, G&S, CRP were sent (Table 18.1). She was apyrexial. Electronic fetal heart monitoring (CTG) was normal. She did not have any uterine contractions, and the fetus was cephalic in presentation, longitudinal lie, with around 3/5th palpable per abdomen. She was still draining clear liquor.

An internal examination suggested a closed cervix with a Bishop's score of 3 (Table 17.6). As she was a primigravida, with an unfavourable cervix, 2 mg of Prostin gel (prostaglandin E2) was administered vaginally at 11.30 with a plan to commence syntocinon six hours later.

Intravenous antibiotics (clindamycin 900 mg eight-hourly, due to previously known penicillin allergy) were commenced to reduce the risk of neonatal early-onset group B streptococcal infection (EOGBS), as per the departmental guidelines. Bloods were repeated three hours later (Table 18.2).

Table 18.2 Second blood results

Time	WCC	Hb	CRP
Booking	7.1	12.3	–
Day 0–11.00 hrs	9.2	11.5	13
14.00 hrs	13.1	11.2	32

She remained well and mobilized until her next examination six hours later at 17.30. The cervix was 1 cm dilated. There were no regular uterine contractions. Oxytocin infusion was commenced at 18.00hrs after epidural anaesthesia was sited at maternal request. CTG at the time of commencing oxytocin was normal (Figure 18.1). Oxytocin was increased as per the protocol in our unit and a partogram started for labour. She started contracting within an hour. The plan was to reassess her four hours after regular contractions on oxytocin.

By 22.00, she had dilated to 4 cm. The vaginal findings revealed the fetal head in LOT position, at station -1 with no caput or moulding. Clear liquor was seen draining. She was now pyrexial at 38.5 with a pulse of 110 bpm and respiratory rate of 18 per minute. The CTG remained normal (see Figure 18.1). One gram of PO paracetamol was given and IV Hartmann's was increased to run over four to six hours. Hourly observations were charted on a modified obstetric early warning score (MEOWS) chart (see Figure 18.3). Repeat bloods were sent for FBC, CRP, U&E blood cultures (Table 18.4). IV antibiotics were changed to a more broad-spectrum regime—cefuroxime 1.5 g and metronidazole 500 mg eight-hourly.

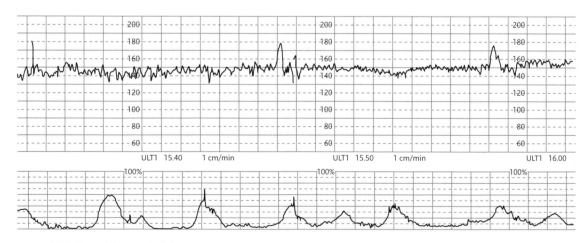

Figure 18.1 Normal CTG at admission.

❻ Expert comment

When a woman develops pyrexia in labour (38.0°C once or 37.5°C twice), it is often impossible to distinguish infective from non-infective causes acutely. Non-infective factors associated with pyrexia include nulliparity, long latent phase of labour and use of epidural analgesia. Measures in the management of pyrexia including administration of an anti-pyretic such as paracetamol, intravenous crystalloids, use of a fan, or tepid sponging.

Infective causes should always be considered, and intravenous antibiotics should be commenced after obtaining samples for investigation blood count (FBC), C-reactive protein (CRP), and blood cultures.

If severe sepsis is suspected, serum lactate should be measured. Many obstetric units would have an option of running venous lactate in their routine blood gas analyser. Serum lactate should be measured within six hours of the suspicion of severe sepsis in order to guide management and lactate ≥4 mmol/l is indicative of tissue hypoperfusion.

The CEMACH report from 2003–2005 suggested that respiratory rate is the most important for assessing the clinical state of a septic patient but it is not routinely recorded in labour. If sepsis is suspected consideration should be given to measuring respiratory rate in addition to pulse, BP, and temperature, and to plotting these on a MEOWS chart.

Table 18.3 Oxytocin regime in our unit (an example).

Oxytocin infusion regimen Time after starting (minutes)	Oxytocin dose (milliunits per minute)	Volume infused mL/hr (dilution 10 units in 49 mls N/saline)
0	2	0.6
30	4	1.2
60	8	2.4
90	12	3.6
120	16	4.8
150	20	6.0
Following discussion with senior obstetrician (ST6 or above)		
180	24	7.2
210	28	8.4
240	32	9.6

✪ Learning point What to do when you suspect severe sepsis?

If severe sepsis is suspected then a number of measures should be instituted in a care bundle. The Surviving Sepsis campaign care bundle is not pregnancy-specific, but adoption of its measures is endorsed by the RCOG Green-top Guideline on sepsis in pregnancy and includes the following tasks to be carried out within six hours of severe sepsis being suspected:

- Obtain blood cultures prior to antibiotic administration.
- Administer broad-spectrum antibiotic within one hour of recognition of severe sepsis.
- Measure serum lactate.
- In the event of hypotension and/or serum lactate >4 mmol/l, deliver an initial minimum 20 ml/Kg of crystalloid or an equivalent. Apply vasopressors for hypotension that is not responding to initial fluid resuscitation in order to maintain mean arterial pressure (MAP) >65 mmHg.
- In the event of persistent hypotension despite fluid resuscitation (septic shock) and/or lactate >4 mmol/l: a) achieve a central venous pressure (CVP) >8 mmHg, and b) achieve a central venous oxygen saturation >70% or a mixed venous oxygen saturation >65%.

✚ Clinical tip Venous Lactate analysis on the delivery suite

Venous lactate can be run in the blood gas analyser on the delivery suite. Some machines need the function to be 'activated' in the beginning of the analysis. A formal venous lactate sample in most units needs to be sent on ice to the lab.

✚ Clinical tip Causes of non-infective pyrexia

Non-infective causes of pyrexia include nulliparity, long latent phase of labour, and use of epidural anaesthesia. They should be considered in the overall risk assessment of a woman in labour.

✚ Clinical tip Clinical signs of fatal genital tract sepsis

CEMACH (2003–2005) [13] identified some women dying of genital tract sepsis before delivery where the sentinel sign of pyrexia was absent. The only outward clinical signs of overwhelming sepsis were tachycardia, fetal death, and the severity of abdominal pain. It is therefore important to assess the overall picture at presentation. Figure 18.5 depicts a CTG of a similar case where maternal pulse could easily be confused for the fetal heart rate.

⊘ Evidence base Confidential enquiries and MEOWS chart

The Seventh Report on Confidential Enquiries into Maternal Deaths in the United Kingdom (CEMACH 2003–2005) recommended the Modified Early Warning Scoring Systems (MEOWS) to improve the detection and subsequent management of life threatening illness. A recent validation study of the MEOWS score [7] on over 600 prospective admissions to a high-risk obstetric unit shows that the MEOWS was 89% sensitive (95% CI 81–95%), 79% specific (95% CI 76–82%), with a positive predictive value 39% (95% CI 32–46%), and a negative predictive value of 98% (95% CI 96–99%). The RCOG Green-top Guideline 'Sepsis in Pregnancy' also recommends use of a MEOWS chart when sepsis is suspected [14].

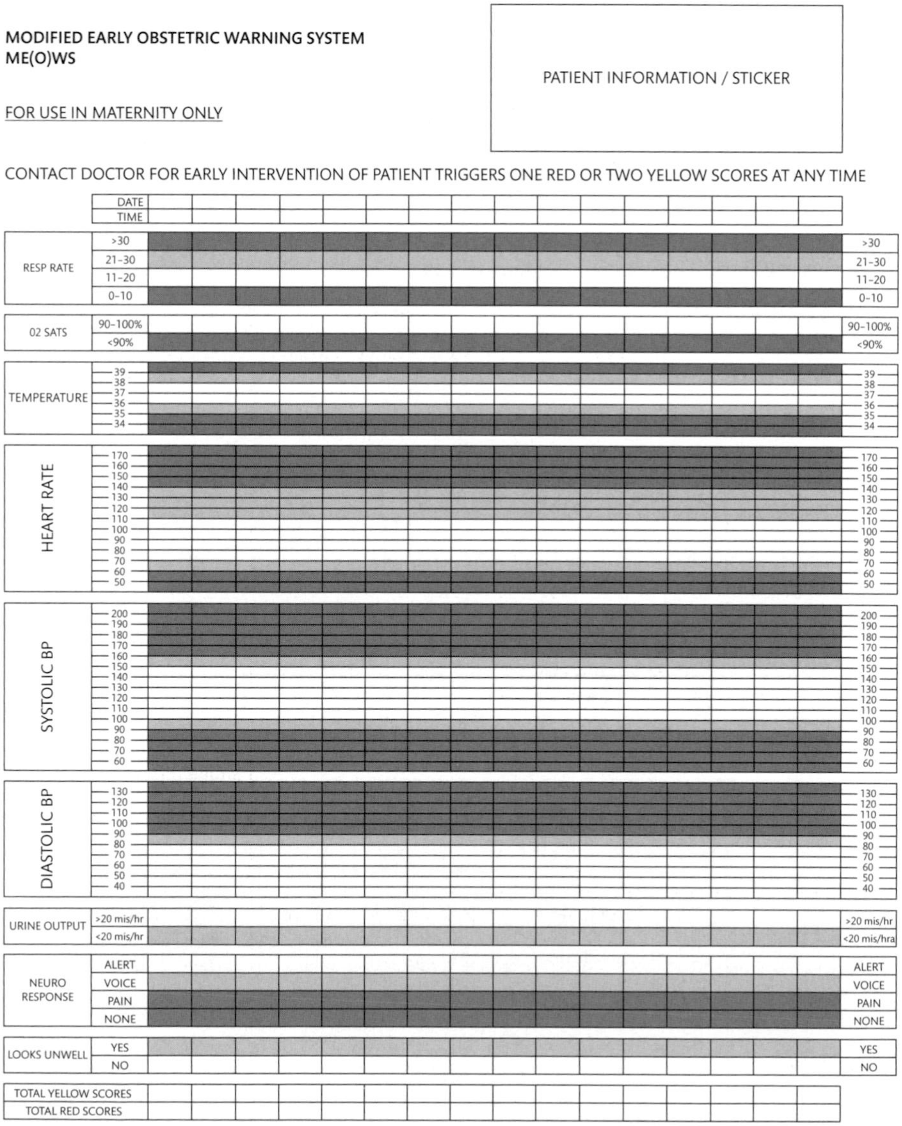

Figure 18.2 MEOWS chart.

Courtesy of St Thomas' Hospital.

Table 18.4 Further blood results

Time	WCC	Hb	CRP	Lactate
Day 0–11:00 hrs	9.2	11.5	13	–
14.00 hrs	13.1	11.2	32	–
01.00 hrs	19.6	11.1	54	3.1

> **❝ Expert comment**
>
> A 'fresh eyes' (Figure 18.3) approach to CTG review may minimize intrapartum complications and avert intrapartum fetal monitoring-related risk incidents. After being successfully piloted in Scotland and tried in Liverpool, the concept is now being adopted in other high-risk obstetric units. The system involves a 'buddy' reviewing the trace with the primary carer every 30 minutes. CTG assessment at each check is based on the standard criteria set by NICE. Our unit has developed a sticker to be inserted into the notes when the check is made.

GSTT RECORD OF CTG INTERPRETATION			
Determine **Risk factors**			Low High
Contractions	Rate _____ in 10 minutes Duration _____/seconds		Coordinate Incoordinate Hypertonic
Feature	**Reassuring** **0**	**Non-reassuring** **1**	**Abnormal** **2**
Baseline **Rate** = _____ bpm	110–150	100–109 OR 161–160	<100 OR >180
Variability	>5bpm	<5bpm for 40–90 min	<5bpm for >90 min Sinusoidal pattern >10 min
Accelerations	Present (a peak of >15bpm form baseline)	Absent (Absence of accelerations with otherwise normal trace is of uncertain significance)	
Decelerations	None OR Typical variables with <50% contractions for <90 min	Typical variables for >50% contractions >90 min OR Single prolonged up to 3 min	Atypical variables for >50% of contractions for >30 min OR Late >30 min OR Single prolonged >3 min
Overall score	0 = Normal	1 = Suspicious	≥2 Non-reassuring or 1 abnormal = Pathological
Plan	Continue/Observe	**Conservative measures** e.g. lateral position, IV fluids, treat pyrexia, consider reducing oxytocin	**Further measures:** e.g. FBS or expedite delivery if signs of fetal hypoxia or FBS not possible
Signature **Time** **Date**	1.	2.	

Figure 18.3 'Fresh eyes' review sticker.

Courtesy of St Thomas' Hospital.

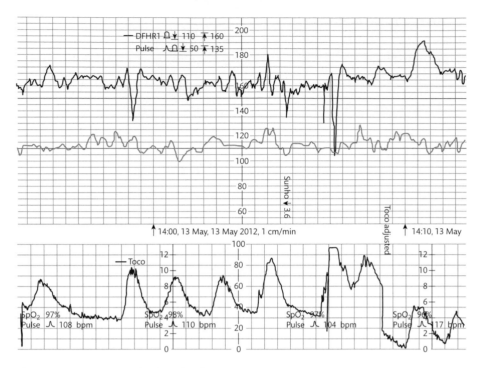

Figure 18.4 Uncomplicated tachycardia after commencing syntocinon.

By midnight, her temperature had slightly decreased to 37.5 °C and CTG findings were suggestive of uncomplicated tachycardia (Figure 18.4).

By 01.00 hours, the fetal tachycardia had settled, although the mother still remained pyrexial at 37.8 °C with a pulse of 100 bpm. She felt flushed, although did not have any rigors. The liquor was slightly blood-stained. The CTG became suspicious with variable decelerations. The CTG remained suspicious for more than 30 minutes despite physiological measures. A vaginal examination was performed to assess progress. She was 6 cm dilated with some head descent. As she was contracting 5–6 in 10, syntocinon was reduced from 6.0 ml/hr to 4.8 ml/hr.

By 02.00 hours, further CTG changes were noted making it pathological: tachycardia, reduced variability and with shallow variable decelerations (Figure 18.5). Oxytocin was therefore stopped and a decision was made not to perform fetal blood sampling in view of maternal sepsis. She continued to contract about 4 in 10. A vaginal examination was performed at 02.00 (eight hours from commencing oxytocin). She was 7 cm dilated, with an oedematous cervix and the fetal head was still LOT (left occipito transverse) at spines. The mother felt increasingly unwell and looked more flushed.

Her observations at 02.00 hours included BP 100/60 mmHg, pulse 125 bpm, and RR 20 per minute.

A decision was therefore made to deliver by caesarean section under a regional anaesthetic, based on failure to progress in the first stage of labour and a pathological CTG. Contractions spaced out after stopping oxytocin, but as the patient

⊕ Clinical tip Physiological measures in management of suspected intrapartum fetal acidemia

The majority of decelerations in active labour are due to cord compression. Physiological measures include: changing maternal position to either left or right lateral, ensuring mother is fluid replete, with IV crystalloids, and managing non-infective causes of pyrexia (if present) with paracetamol (oral or IV).

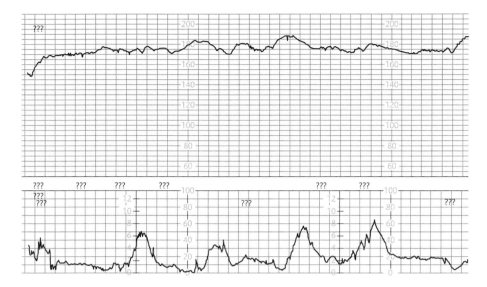

Figure 18.5 Complicated tachycardia with maternal pyrexia.

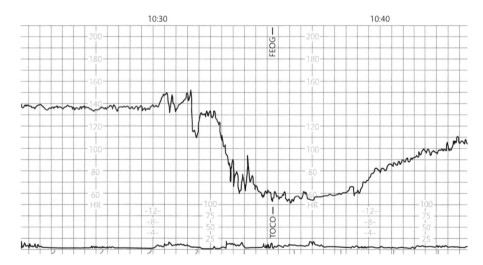

Figure 18.6 Fetal bradycardia.

was wheeled to theatre the fetal heart dropped to below 80 bpm with slow recovery (Figure 18.6). A category 1 CS under general anaesthesia was performed with delivery within 7 minutes of the onset of the fetal heart-rate drop. The baby was born at 02.25 hours with arterial pH of 7.013 (BE–8.3) and Apgar of $5_1 7_5 9_{10}$. The baby was taken to the neonatal unit for initial observations and intravenous antibiotics. The liquor was offensive at the time of CS. Placental swabs were sent for culture sensitivity and the placenta was sent for histology.

> ✚ **Clinical tip** The 3-6-9-12 min rule for fetal bradycardia [12].
>
> 3 min—call the doctor
> 6 min—prepare the woman
> 9 min—prepare for delivery
> 12 min—aim to deliver the baby

Expert comment

Uncomplicated CTG baseline tachycardia is common in women with intrapartum pyrexia, and the baseline may respond to measures to reduce maternal temperature. However, changes in baseline variability or new onset decelerations may be a warning of deterioration in maternal condition and should prompt reassessment of maternal mean arterial pressure, hypoxia, and acidaemia as well as consideration of fetal condition. Fetal scalp electrodes should be used with caution in women with pyrexia as they may provide a portal of entry for infection to the fetus. There is no evidence to support the use of ST Analysis (STAN) monitoring in women with intrapartum pyrexia.

Learning point Fetal bradycardia

The NICE guidance on intrapartum care [3] recommended that if a bradycardia occurs in the baby for more than three minutes, urgent medical aid should be sought and preparations should be made to expedite the birth of the baby urgently, classified as a category 1 birth. This could include moving the woman to theatre if the fetal heart has not recovered by nine minutes. If the fetal heart recovers within nine minutes, the decision to deliver should be reconsidered in conjunction with the woman if reasonable.

Table 18.5 Further blood results

Time	WCC	Hb	CRP	Lactate
Booking	7.1	12.3	–	–
Day 0–11.00 hrs	9.2	11.5	13	–
14.00 hrs	13.1	11.2	32	–
01.00 hrs	19.6	11.1	54	3.1
Day 1– 13.00 hrs	29.3	9.1	350	4.2

The patient was recovered in the delivery suite for six hours which coincided with the handover time for both obstetric and midwifery staff. During this time, her intravenous cannula fell out and as she was feeling much better and tolerating oral fluids, she was not re-cannulated. Her observations at 08.25 hours were BP 100/60 mmHg, P 105 bpm, RR 18 pm. On the ward round, she was deemed fit to go to postnatal ward, with a recommendation to change to oral antibiotics. These were, however, not charted on the drug chart.

By 12.30 hours on the postnatal ward, she started getting chills and rigors. She was pyrexial at 39.2, BP 90/50 mmHg and RR of 30 pm. As she was on 4-hourly observations, which were not on the MEOWS chart, it was difficult to assess the trend of observations since the transfer. The postnatal ward ST1 was asked to review her and promptly transferred the patient to the obstetric high-dependency unit (HDU) on the delivery suite.

At 13.00 hours, in the obstetric HDU, she was reviewed by the consultant obstetrician and anaesthetists. Intravenous fluids were commenced and clindamycin 900 mg IV eight-hourly with gentamicin 5 mg/kg daily for a maximum of two doses were commenced after seeking microbiology advice. Her observations at the time were: T 38.2, BP 100/50, P 120 bpm, RR 28 pm, urine output 30 ml/hr, GCS 15/15. Bloods are 13.00 hours are shown in Table 18.5.

The microbiology team contacted the obstetric registrar with findings of heavy growth of group A streptococcus in the blood cultures. He specifically asked about a contact with someone with sore throat and/or upper respiratory tract infection. The patient's husband confirmed that their 5-year-old nephew was suffering from sore throat and they had recently looked after him for a weekend.

The organism was sensitive to clindamycin and it was recommended that she completed a 7-day course. If becoming increasingly unwell, she would need the critical care team review and step up to critical care. There was some clinical improvement over the next 6 hours although she had some shortness of breath. However by 20.00 hours, she started feeling unwell with a very tender uterus, and became increasingly hypoxic. Her arterial blood gas showed evidence of metabolic acidosis with respiratory compensation. Her observations at the time were; T 39.4, BP 100/50, P 150 bpm, RR 40 pm, SpO2 95% on 5L 02, urine output 10 ml/hr. She was immediately seen by the outreach team (intensive care unit) and was stepped up to the intensive care unit. A CT-pulmonary angiogram ruled out a pulmonary embolus but was suggestive of acute respiratory distress syndrome. Her antibiotics were changed to imepenem and linezolid. Intravenous immunoglobulins were also added. She made a slow but steady recovery in intensive care and was discharged home after stepping down to obstetrics on day 17.

✪ Learning point History taking, communication, and follow-up

There should be a continuous evaluation of risk based on evolving clinical situation. In sepsis presenting in labour, although intrapartum causes of sepsis need to be assessed, a careful history may suggest the cause of sepsis to be pre-dating the onset of labour.

If a woman who is on prophylactic antibiotics to cover for EOGBS has sepsis in labour, it must be ensured that they are changed to broad-spectrum antibiotics, which would still cover EOGBS. Antibiotics should be continued intravenously for a period of apyrexia for at least 24 hours. A doctor would need to assess (with reference to microbiology) the duration of oral antibiotics depending on the culture results.

It is well established that effective patient handover is critical to patient safety. Patient handover is recognized as a vulnerable phase in patient care. There has to be a clear plan in the notes prior to patient transfer from one clinical setting (e.g. high-dependency unit) to another (e.g. postnatal ward). If there are pending results that would change clinical management, it is paramount that the team handing over should specify the urgency or the importance of follow-up of these results.

Discussion

Genital tract sepsis was identified as the leading cause of direct maternal death in the UK (2006–2008). The Confidential Enquiries into maternal deaths have identified substandard care in many of the cases, especially in recognition of signs of sepsis [13]. This prompted the development of RCOG Green-top Guideline on Sepsis in Pregnancy [14]. This guidance defines sepsis as infection plus systemic manifestations of infection and severe sepsis plus sepsis-induced organ dysfunction or tissue hypoperfusion.

The signs and symptoms of sepsis in pregnant women may be less distinctive compared to the non-pregnant population. Clinical signs suggestive of sepsis include one or more of the following: pyrexia, hypothermia, tachycardia, tachypnoea, hypoxia, hypotension, oliguria, impaired consciousness, and failure to respond to treatment. These signs, including pyrexia, may not always be present and are not necessarily related to the severity of sepsis. Severe sepsis has a mortality rate of 20–40%, which increases to 60% if septic shock develops. Early, goal-directed resuscitation, which has been shown to improve survival for non-pregnant patients presenting with septic shock, is therefore more important in the pregnant women. The appropriate management involves a multidisciplinary team framework including the obstetric and midwifery team, and an early liaison with the microbiology, infectious disease physicians, and obstetric anaesthetists. In severe or rapidly deteriorating cases, a discussion involving the consultant obstetrician and the critical care team, with a low threshold for transfer to intensive care unit, is important.

The Surviving Sepsis Campaign Resuscitation bundle [8] recommends broad-spectrum antibiotics in suspected cases of sepsis, with or without septic shock. The RCOG guidance therefore suggests that broad-spectrum antibiotics active against Gram-negative bacteria, and capable of preventing exotoxin production from Gram-positive bacteria, should be used according to local microbiology policy, and therapy narrowed once the causative organism(s) has been identified. Intravenous immuno-globulin has been tried successfully in pregnancy where other therapies have failed.

Group A streptococcus (GAS) has been recognized as a worrying cause of maternal death with severe genital tract sepsis in the recent Confidential Enquiries into Maternal Death in the UK [6]. GAS may present with common mild conditions, such as pharyngitis and impetigo, to less common but severe conditions, including septicaemia, pneumonia, and the potentially fatal streptococcal toxic shock syndrome. A recent literature review of 55 cases of GAS in pregnancy, including 20 from UK, 33 from Japan, and two from France has looked at the risk factors and potential prognostic indicators [22]. The review suggested that multiparous women (83%) in the third trimester (90%) were prone to the GAS infection from winter to spring (75%). Onset may be heralded by flu-like symptoms: high fever (94%), with upper respiratory (40%), and/or gastrointestinal symptoms (49%). Characteristic findings were early onset of shock (91%) and infection-induced strong uterine contraction (73%) suggestive of placental abruption. The clinical course was often too acute and severe to rescue the mother (58% mortality) and/or infant (66% mortality). However, early use of antibiotics (71% survival) and use of intravenous immunoglobulin (91% survival) were associated with favourable outcome.

Sepsis in labour is an indication for continuous electronic fetal monitoring (CEFM), although CEFM is not a sensitive predictor of early-onset neonatal sepsis [18–21]. A case control study from Baltimore found that CEFM parameters like baseline rate and variability had sensitivity of 29–65%, specificity of 46–93%, positive predictive value of 53–80%, and negative predictive value of 54–58% in identifying fetal systemic inflammation. If sepsis is suspected in labour, regional anaesthesia should be avoided. The effects of maternal sepsis on fetal well-being include the direct effect of infection in the fetus, the effect of maternal illness and the effect of maternal treatment. Table 18.6 shows the effect of infection with and without hypoxia on the neonatal outcome [15].

There is a dilemma regarding the safety of invasive fetal procedures like fetal scalp electrodes and fetal blood sampling (FBS) on a background of maternal sepsis. As the risk of neonatal encephalopathy and cerebral palsy is increased in the presence of intra-uterine infection, a normal FBS result therefore may not be as reassuring in a woman with pyrexia. It has been suggested that infection may lower the threshold at which fetal damage occurs and there is insufficient evidence to guide

Table 18.6 Synergistic effects of infection and hypoxia in brain injury [15]

	Cerebral palsy (RR)	95% CI
Clinical chorioamnionitis	4.7	1.3–16.2
Histological chorioamnionitis	13.2	1.2–144
Infection and intrapartum hypoxia-ischaemia*	78	4.8–406
Infection and intrapartum hypoxia-ischaemia**	367	19–1974

* spastic cerebral palsy;
** spastic quadriplegic cerebral palsy (term infants)

the use of FBS in this situation. In addition, significant maternal sepsis is itself an indication for delivery. Therefore, FBS in maternal pyrexia should always be discussed with a consultant before sampling.

Changes in CTG, however, must prompt reassessment of maternal mean arterial pressure, hypoxia and acidaemia. These changes may serve as an early warning sign for derangements in maternal end-organ systems, as recommended by the American College of Obstetricians and Gynaecologists.

The decision on mode and timing of delivery should be individualized by the consultant obstetrician with consideration of severity of maternal illness, duration of labour, gestational age, and viability. There is evidence that delivery in an unstable mother may increase the maternal and fetal mortality rates unless the source of infection is intra-uterine. Ideally, the source of sepsis should be sought if possible by delivery of the baby. The neonatologists should be informed at birth, so that prophylactic antibiotics can be promptly started for the baby. Asymptomatic term babies born to women with PROM (with or without sepsis) should be closely observed for the first 12 hours of life (at one hour, two hours, and then two hourly for 10 hours). The great majority of infants (89–94%) who develop infection exhibit signs within the first 24 hours after birth and the majority of such infants (65–67%) will have had one or more risk factors evident in or before labour.

A Final Word from the Expert

Sepsis is a significant cause of maternal death and women diagnosed with sepsis in labour should be managed using a surviving sepsis care bundle. As in this case, broad-spectrum antibiotics started promptly are key to effective therapy. Fetal heart-rate changes may indicate deterioration in maternal condition or developing fetal sepsis and should prompt urgent consideration of the need for delivery. Following delivery there is a continuing need for monitoring of both neonatal and maternal condition. Use of a MEOWS chart is recommended to facilitate early detection of the deteriorating septic woman.

Maternal pyrexia provides a major conundrum for the neonatologist after birth. Early-onset neonatal septicaemia has high mortality and morbidity. Maternal pyrexia, and illness as in this case, mandate an infection screen and antibiotics performed as quickly as possible after birth. Where antibiotics have been given to the mother it is not unusual to fail to identify an organism in the baby's infection screen. We try to minimize the effect on the family but frequently it is necessary to repeat blood tests and to maintain intravenous antibiotics for five to seven days if serological markers of infection are present (CRP, neutrophil, and platelet counts are most frequently used). In most centres, the presence of such a severe maternal illness may mitigate for a longer course of antibiotics assuming the baby is well, even if cultures are negative.

References

1. Brocklehurst P, Hardy P, Hollowell J, Linsell L, Macfarlane A. Perinatal and maternal outcomes by planned place of birth for healthy women with low risk pregnancies: The Birthplace in England national prospective cohort study. *BMJ* 2011;343:d7400.
2. NICE. Induction of labour (CG70). 2008. http://guidance.nice.org.uk/CG70

3. NICE (2007) Intrapartum care (CG55). http://guidance.nice.org.uk/CG55

4. Hannah ME, Ohlsson A, Farine D, Hewson SA, Hodnett ED, Myhr TL, *et al.* Induction of Labour compared with expectant management for prelabour rupture of membranes at term. *N Eng J Med* April 18; 334.16: 1005–10

5. RCOG (2012) Prevention of Early Onset Neonatal Group B Streptococcal Disease. Green-top Guideline 36. http://www.rcog.org.uk/files/rcog-corp/GTG36_GBS.pdf

6. Lewis, G (ed.). The Confidential Enquiry into Maternal and ChildHealth (CEMACH). Saving Mothers' Lives: reviewing maternal deaths to make motherhood safer- 2003–2005. The Seventh Report on Confidential Enquiries into Maternal Deaths in the United Kingdom. London: CEMACH, 2007.

7. Singh S, McGlennan A, England A, Simons R. A validation study of the CEMACH recommended modified early obstetric warning system (MEOWS). *Anaesthesia* 2012;67:12–18.

8. Surviving Sepsis Bundle. http://www.survivingsepsis.org/Bundles

9. RCOG electronic fetal monitoring eFM. https://e-learningforhealthcare.org.uk

10. Fitzpatrick T, Holt L. A 'buddy' approach to CTG. 2008. *Midwives* 11: 40–1.

11. Leighton BL, Halpern SH. The effects of epidural analgesia on labor, maternal, and neonatal outcomes: a systematic review. *Am J Obstet Gynecol* 2002;186:S69–S77.

12. Gibb D, Arulkumaran S. *Fetal Monitoring in Practice*, 3rd edn. Philadelphia: Elsevier, 2008.

13. Centre for Maternal and Child Enquiries (CMACE). Saving Mother's Lives: reviewing maternal deaths to make motherhood safer: 2006–2008. *BJOG* 2011;118(suppl. 1):1–203.

14. Royal College of Obstetricians and Gynaecologists. Bacterial Sepsis in Pregnancy. Green-top Guideline 64a. 2012. http://www.rcog.org.uk/womens-health/clinical-guidance/sepsis-pregnancy-bacterial-green-top-64a

15. Ugwumadu A. Infection and fetal neurologic injury. *Curr Opin Obstet Gynaecol* 2006;18:106–111.

16. Intrauterine Infection and Perinatal Brain Injury. Scientific Advisory Committee Opinion Paper 3. November 2002

17. Fein AM, DuVivier R. Sepsis in Pregnancy. *Clin Chest Med* 1992;13:709–22.

18. Yoon BH, Romero R, Park JS, Kim CJ, Kim SH, Choi JH, *et al.* Fetal exposure to an intra-amniotic inflammation and the development of cerebral palsy at the age of three years. *Am J Obstet Gynecol* 2000;182:675–81.

19. American College of Obstetricians and Gynaecologists Committee on Obstetric Practice. ACOG Practice Bulletin No. 100: Critical care in pregnancy. *Obstet Gynecol* 2009;113:443–50.

20. Buhimschi CS, Abdel-Razeq S, Cackovic M, Pettker CM, Dulay AT, Bahtiyar MO *et al.* Fetal heart rate monitoring patterns in women with amniotic fluid proteomic profiles indicative of inflammation. *Am J Perinatol* 2008;25;359–72.

21. Aina-Mumuney AJ, Althaus JE, Henderson JL, Blakemore MC, Johnson EA, Graham EM. Intrapartum electronic fetal monitoring and the identification of systemic fetal inflammation. *J Reprod Med* 2007;52:762–8.

22. Yamad T, Yamada T, Yamamura MK, Katabami K, Hayakawa M, Tomaru U, *et al.* Invasive group A streptococcal infection in pregnancy. *Journal of Infection* 2010;60:417–24.

Forewarned is forearmed in massive obstetric haemorrhage

Julia Kopeika

❻ Expert Commentary Susan Bewley
❻ Guest Experts Ben Fitzwilliams and Susan Robinson

Case history

A 33-year-old Jamaican multiparous woman with a BMI of 37 was booked for delivery in a large three-tier inner-city obstetric unit delivering 9 500 babies per year. Previously she had one normal delivery at term of a 3.0 kg baby, followed by a 2.4 kg term stillbirth secondary to growth restriction and undiagnosed gestational diabetes. In her current pregnancy, diabetes was confirmed by random blood sugar (RBS) at booking, and by 14 weeks' gestation she was commenced on insulin. Her BMI, stillbirth, and history of a growth restriction necessitated serial growth scans. The last, performed at 36 weeks, showed the baby's abdominal circumference and estimated fetal weight to be just below the 95th centile. Induction of labour was planned for 38 weeks' gestation.

> **❻ Expert comment** Induction of labour for gestational diabetes
>
> The role and timing of induction of labour in women with gestational diabetes have recently been questioned. The recommendation of induction of labour is mostly based on retrospective studies or a relatively small (n = 200) trial [1] that looked at the mode of delivery, birth weight, and neonatal morbidity and mortality as main outcomes. However, this trial has some methodological limitations [2], including the fact that the method of randomization was not reported, the sample population included both women with pre-gestational and insulin-requiring gestational diabetes, the size of the studied group was underpowered, and the unequal distribution of women with previous caesarean sections between arms was not taken into consideration. Even though retrospective studies suggest that elective induction in diabetic women may reduce the risk of stillbirth and shoulder dystocia, there are insufficient data to determine the precise gestation at which this should be offered [3].

Arriving early at 06.30 at the hospital on the day planned for induction of labour, she revealed a 34-hour history of leaking clear, non-offensive fluid vaginally, which was not associated with contractions. Speculum examination confirmed the diagnosis of ruptured membranes with a long closed cervix. Syntocinon was commenced for the stimulation of labour at 08.55. Labour progressed slowly. A sliding scale of insulin was started as her BMs remained above 6 mmol/l. An epidural was sited after 14 hours of labour to provide analgesia. After 18 hours of Syntocinon the cervix was fully dilated at 03.05. A temperature of 37.9 °C was noted on two occasions, unrelieved by paracetamol. The liquor remained clear and cardiotocograph was normal throughout.

❝ Guest expert comment (anaesthetist) Epidural analgesia and maternal pyrexia

Epidural analgesia for labour is associated with a significant incidence of maternal pyrexia [4]. The true mechanism for this is unclear. This effect unfortunately leads to some mothers being over-treated for pyrexia in labour, and to an increase in neonatal septic screens. However, epidural analgesia is not a reason to discount maternal pyrexia.

◔ Landmark trial The TERM PROM trial: Induction of labour in term pre-labour rupture of membranes (PROM) lowers risk of maternal infection

The TERM PROM study [5] (*n* = 5041, with approximately 1260 women in each of several arms) is regarded as the landmark trial for the management of pre-labour rupture of membranes without contractions at term. It demonstrated that induction of labour with intravenous oxytocin or with vaginal prostaglandin E2 gel, as well as an expectant management, are all reasonable options for women and their babies. There was no significant difference in neonatal infection rates or caesarean section. However, induction of labour with intravenous oxytocin resulted in a lower risk of maternal infection than expectant management.

✛ Clinical tip Second stage of labour

The NICE guideline [6] suggests:

'Upon confirmation of full cervical dilatation in women with regional analgesia, unless the woman has an urge to push or the baby's head is visible, pushing should be delayed for at least 1 hour and longer if the woman wishes, after which pushing during contractions should be actively encouraged.

Following the diagnosis of full dilatation in a woman with regional analgesia, a plan should be agreed with the woman in order to ensure that birth will have occurred within 4 hours regardless of parity.'

Since there was no concern about fetal well-being, two hours of passive second stage were allowed for descent after which time she commenced pushing at 05.10. After 1.5 hours of pushing, the midwife requested medical review as there were no signs of imminent delivery. The decision was made to perform a ventouse delivery in the room due to prolonged second stage (SHO supervised by senior registrar).[1] The head was delivered at 07.08 following three pulls with a ventouse and a mediolateral episiotomy. However, the rest of the delivery was complicated by a shoulder dystocia. Delivery of the shoulders was achieved three minutes after delivery of the head with McRoberts position and suprapubic pressure manoeuvres. Syntometrine (1 ml) was given intramuscularly. The baby had an Apgar score of 7 at one minute of life. Following delivery, there was a brisk blood loss of approximately 400 ml. At this point the senior registrar was called to attend a fetal bradycardia in another room. She told the junior to deliver the placenta and suture the perineum while she went to attend the other emergency. The patient had multiple vaginal wall and perineal tears in addition to the medio-lateral episiotomy.

✛ Clinical tip Anticipating postpartum haemorrhage

This patient had multiple risk factors for postpartum haemorrhage: obesity, stimulation with Syntocinon, prolonged first and second stages, pyrexia in labour, instrumental delivery, macrosomia, and shoulder dystocia. In anticipation of postpartum haemorrhage (blood loss of 500 ml or more), it would be appropriate that she has at least one established 16-gauge intravenous line, recent full blood count, and group-and-screen done. The third stage should be actively managed (oxytocin and controlled cord traction), and Syntocinon infusion be ready to aid contractions after the third stage of labour. If blood loss exceeds the normal threshold of 500 ml, a second intravenous line must be established promptly.

---

[1] SHO—senior house officer or ST1/ST2—usually trainee with at least 1-2 years of experience in obstetrics and gynaecology; Junior Registrar or St 3-5—usually specialty trainee with at least 3 to 5 years of experience in obstetrics and gynaecology; Senior Registrar or St 6/7—usually specialty trainee with at least 6 to 7 years of experience in obstetrics and gynaecology.

The placenta was delivered using controlled cord traction at 07.15. However, blood continued to soak the drapes heavily and drip onto the floor. The SHO assessed the perineal tear as second-degree and repairable in the room, and started at 07.24. A continuous 'trickle from above' made visibility and suturing difficult, particularly without the benefit of any assistant because the midwife was keen to clear up, write up her computerized notes, and hand over to the oncoming shift. Midwifery handover commenced at 07.30 and a new midwife replaced her colleague. At 07.45 she asked 'Do you want any help?' The junior doctor replied, 'No! I'm all right', and the midwife responded 'What about taking a blood sample?' The doctor agreed that the midwife should send a sample for FBC and coagulation and also asked her to commence an infusion of Syntocinon (10 IU/hour), since there was ongoing 'trickle'.

After suturing for over 45 minutes, and concerned about the extent of the tear, the junior doctor asked for help to call a senior. At 08.15, the junior registrar who had just arrived early for the day-shift responded to the call bell as he was passing by the room. He assessed the perineum and suggested that it might be a third-degree tear that needed to be repaired in theatre. The day registrar suggested that the night SHO place a pack in the vagina to stem the blood loss, give 800 mcg Misoprostol per rectum, consent the patient for theatre, and then join the formal labour-ward board handover, while the patient would be transferred to theatre by an anaesthetist and midwife. The extent of blood loss was 'guesstimated' by the SHO (who looked at the pads in the bucket) as '600 mls', unaware that the midwife (who had left the room to find a consent form) had already cleared away several swabs and pads and also placed a new inco-pad on the floor. None of the staff expressed their separate concerns about the blood loss.

Handover took some time that morning as it was a busy day with 17 patients to be discussed. The morning team included a newly appointed consultant, junior registrar, and SHO. They were told that the patient was 'stable', had been moved to theatre for repair of a third-degree tear, and her current **blood loss** was estimated at around 600 ml. Another patient needed immediate attention due to meconium and abnormal CTG.

> ✔ **Evidence base**   The role of Misoprostol as a prophylactic/treatment drug for PPH
>
> **Prophylactic:** Rectal Misoprostol is an unsuitable option for routine prophylaxis against PPH in high-income countries due to its slightly lower efficacy and higher side effects in comparison with oxytocin. It may be a reasonable alternative to oxytocin where storage and parental administration of the drugs are a problem [8].
>
> **Treatment:** The Cochrane review [9] demonstrates that there is insufficient evidence to show that the addition of Misoprostol is superior to the combination of oxytocin and Ergometrine alone for the treatment of primary PPH. Large multicentre, double-blind, randomized controlled trials are required to identify the best drug combinations, route, and dose of uterotonics for the treatment of primary PPH.

> ➕ **Clinical tip**   Assessment of PPH
>
> Always take a 'holistic approach' to a patient, no matter how time-restricted you are (indeed, it is more important to think carefully about the whole picture when under pressure or tired!)
>
> The registrar was asked to 'assess the tear', but he/she should also think of haemorrhage. Therefore, he/she should have performed a rapid assessment: what is the current and **running total** of blood loss? (The staff involved could be new, changing over, or the junior not familiar with the case).
>
> - Look around, on the bed, in the bins, and on the floor. Ask how many swabs and pads have been used?
> - Assess the patient clinically (is she pale, alert, feeling thirsty or dizzy?).
> - Check patient's vital signs: BP, pulse, urine output. They are **vital**. It is not acceptable to describe vital signs as 'stable', rather than 'normal' or 'abnormal' or, preferably, using the precise data.
> - Check if a recent haemoglobin is available. The patient might have been anaemic before the bleeding (anaemia will magnify the effect of haemorrhage).
> - Enquire about other underlying problems. This patient had pyrexia, long labour, and shoulder dystocia. Therefore, she was at increased risk of uterine atony that needed to be addressed as much as the perineal trauma to prevent further significant blood loss.

> ➕ **Clinical tip**   Management of atonic PPH
>
> According to the RCOG guideline [10], the following mechanical and pharmacological measures should be instituted, in turn, when uterine atony is perceived to be a cause of the bleeding until bleeding stops:
>
> - Bimanual uterine compression (rubbing up the fundus) to stimulate contractions.
> - Ensure bladder is empty (Foley catheter, leave in place).
> - Syntocinon 5 units by slow intravenous injection (may have repeat dose).
> - Ergometrine 0.5 mg by slow intravenous or intramuscular injection (contraindicated in women with hypertension).
> - Syntocinon infusion (40 units in 500 ml Hartmann's solution at 125 ml/hour) unless fluid restriction is necessary.
> - Carboprost 0.25 mg by intramuscular injection repeated at intervals of not less than 15 minutes to a maximum of eight doses (contraindicated in women with asthma).
> - Direct intramyometrial injection of Carboprost 0.5 mg (contraindicated in women with asthma), with responsibility of the administering clinician as it is not recommended for intramyometrial use.
> - Misoprostol 1000 micrograms rectally.

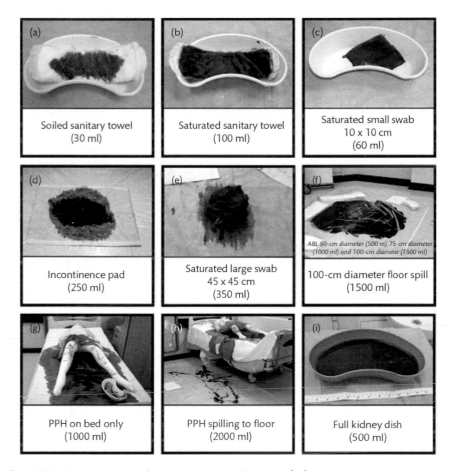

Figure 19.1 Pictorial guidelines for visual estimation of blood loss [11].

P Bose, F Regan, S Paterson-Brown. Improving the accuracy of estimated blood loss at obstetric haemorrhage using clinical reconstructions, *BJOG* John Wiley and Sons 2006.

> ➕ **Clinical tip** Guidelines for visual estimation of blood loss [11] (see Figure 19.1)
>
> | | |
> |---|---|
> | 60 ml | Small, 10 × 10 cm swab (maximum saturated capacity) |
> | 140 ml | Medium, 30 × 30 cm swab (maximum saturated capacity) |
> | 350 ml | Large, 45 × 45 cm swab (maximum saturated capacity) |
> | 500 ml | 50 cm-diameter floor spill |

> ✪ **Learning point** Communication and handover
>
> Early involvement of appropriate senior staff, including the anaesthetist, is of paramount importance in the management of postpartum haemorrhage [10]. It is well established that effective patient handover is critical to patient safety. Patient handover is recognized as a vulnerable phase in patient care. The RCOG [12] suggest applying the SBAR (situation— background—assessment—recommendation) tool for improving communication during handover.
>
> The steps involved in using SBAR are:
>
> - **Situation:** Describe the specific situation concerning a particular patient, including name, consultant, patient location, vital signs, resuscitation status, and any specific concerns.
> - **Background:** Communicate the patient's background, including age, ethnicity, parity, gestation, date of admission, diagnosis, current medications, allergies, laboratory results, progress during the admission, and other relevant information collected from the patient's charts.
> - **Assessment:** This involves critical assessment of the situation, clinical impression, and detailed expression of concerns.
> - **Recommendation:** This involves the management plan, making suggestions, and being specific about requests and time frame. 'Any order that is given, especially over the telephone or when discussed with a doctor who has been woken from sleep, needs to be repeated back to ensure accuracy' [12].

> ✪ **Landmark trial** Saline versus Albumin Fluid Evaluation (SAFE) study [13]
>
> The SAFE study ($n = 6997$) was a randomized controlled clinical trial that evaluated the outcomes of resuscitation in critically ill patients using albumin or crystalloid solutions. It found no evidence that albumin was associated with better or worse outcomes. The recent Cochrane review also showed no difference in mortality data whether resuscitation was done with colloids or crystalloids [14].

After handover was finished, the obstetric consultant went to theatre with the day SHO to repair the third-degree tear whilst the day registrar went to the room with the suspicious CTG to perform fetal blood sample (FBS). By this time, it was becoming clear that the blood loss had been considerably underestimated; the patient's pulse rate was 115 and BP 98/58, O_2 saturations 98%. Fluid resuscitation was commenced by the anaesthetic registrar and 4 units of blood were requested by urgent cross match.

Massage of a boggy uterus which remained above the umbilicus expelled a further 300 ml clot. Continued atony necessitated a further dose of Ergometrine injection 500 mcg IM, in addition to the Syntocinon infusion. Having read the notes and spoken to the case midwife, the consultant estimated that the running total blood loss now was at least of the order of **1.5 litres**. When the perineum was assessed, there was active bleeding from a 3b perineal tear in addition to uterine atony.

The consultant commenced repair of the tears at 09.25, while the midwife provided massage to the uterus abdominally. The patient continued bleeding and further uterotonics in the form of two doses of Carboprost (0.25 mg IM, 15 minutes apart) were given. At 09.35 the registrar on call informed the consultant that they needed to open a second theatre for urgent section for abnormal CTG as the fetal scalp pH had been found to be 7.19. The anaesthetic consultant was already with the second patient, and the SHO went to assist with that case, leaving the anaesthetic locum registrar and obstetric consultant with the current case.

The perineal suturing was performed promptly although the tissues were very friable. However, the bleeding did not settle as the uterus remained atonic. By 10.00, the measured blood loss in theatre was reaching **1.1 litres** (i.e. a total now of **2.6 litres**), and blood transfusion was commenced in addition to fluid resuscitation. Patient observations were also deteriorating (P 135, BP 86/52). Collapsed peripheral access made repeat blood sampling by the anaesthetic registrar difficult, although the result of the previous blood sample returned (sent nearly two hours earlier at 8.05), revealed the haemoglobin was 8.2 g/dl, but the coagulation sample was unprocessed. A more recent haemacue in theatre, following intravenous fluids, was 6.1 g/dl.

⓰ Guest expert comment (anaesthetist) Establishing invasive monitoring

Once adequate peripheral venous access is achieved in an unstable patient it is advisable to consider invasive monitoring using an arterial and or central venous pressure (CVP) line. This is easier to establish in a well-filled patient, and therefore should be considered early in an ongoing PPH. An arterial line allows:

- Beat-to-beat monitoring of the blood pressure.
- Avoidance of frequent inflation of the BP cuff, which many patients find irritating and anxiety provoking.
- Easy collection of blood samples, including for arterial blood gas analysis.

A CVP line allows:

- Measurement of the right atrial pressure. It is not always necessary to know this, and it is a poor estimate of the true left atrial pressure. Trends are of more value than absolute numbers.
- Taking of blood samples. A central venous gas sample can be informative in the absence of an arterial sample.
- Infusion of inotropes. This is rarely necessary even in massive obstetric haemorrhage.

However it takes time and the help of team members to insert a CVP line, which may be a distraction at a time when the information it offers is of limited use. Risks include pneumothorax and bleeding. Awake patients can find the procedure uncomfortable. Ideally the patient is placed head down during insertion which can cause further discomfort. In an awake patient, a peripherally inserted central line can sometimes be more easily inserted via the antecubital fossa. If a general anaesthetic is given, it is then easier to insert a CVP line.

> ❝ **Guest expert comment (anaesthetist) Moving to the operating theatre**
>
> It is seldom a mistake to move a patient you are concerned about to the operating theatre, before or after delivery, although it may frighten the patient to whom an explanation and reassurance should be given. The benefits are:
>
> - Easy monitoring of the patient and fetus.
> - Good access to equipment for insertion of lines, regional anaesthesia, general anaesthesia, and airway management.
> - The anaesthetist will be there, and working in a familiar environment.
> - Space and good lighting.
> - It focuses the attention of the entire team that this is a patient requiring close attention.
>
> Being in theatre does not mandate a surgical procedure, and the patient can return to her room when this is judged to be safe.

> ✪ **Learning point** Regional versus general anaesthesia (GA)
>
> Both regional anaesthesia (Table 19.1) (epidural and spinal) and GA (Table 19.2) have their advantages and disadvantages in the management of a PPH. The balance of these will change with the clinical situation.
>
> **Table 19.1 Regional Anaesthesia**
>
> | Advantages | Disadvantages |
> | --- | --- |
> | Awake patient's conscious level can be assessed | Patient may be traumatized by the experience |
> | Partner or other birth companion is allowed into theatre in some circumstances | Partner or other birth companion not normally in theatre |
> | Patient can be involved, give consent for additional procedures, and have an understanding of what took place and why | If conversion to general anaesthesia is required this may be at an unpredictable and challenging time |
> | No relaxation of the myometrium | Autonomic block may cause hypotension |
> | Airway protected whilst patient remains conscious | Block may take time to establish or be inadequate |
> | In antenatal cases, fetal condition typically better at delivery than with GA | Risk of epidural haematoma is increased if a new block is performed in a coagulopathic patient. This is a very rare complication but one that can lead to paralysis. |
>
> **Table 19.2 General anaesthesia**
>
> | Advantages | Disadvantages |
> | --- | --- |
> | Airway control is established | Risk of failed intubation approximately 1:300 in obstetric GA |
> | Anaesthetist can take control of ventilation | Risk of regurgitation and aspiration of gastric contents during induction of anaesthesia |
> | Anaesthetist can insert lines and perform interventions more readily | Myometrium is relaxed by inhaled general anaesthetic drugs, leading to increased blood loss |
> | | Myocardial depressant effects of anaesthetic drugs |
> | | Increased risk of DVT and allergic reactions |
> | | Small risk of awareness under anaesthesia |

**⑥ Guest expert
comment (anaesthetist)**

Just as obstetricians and midwives
vary in experience, seniority, and
familiarity with a given unit, so
do anaesthetists. Many obstetric
haemorrhages require a second
anaesthetist, and consultant help
should be called early. Support the
anaesthetist in decision making
here just as you would with any
other team member.

The obstetric consultant proceeded to perform a manual check of the uterine cavity. The uterine cavity contained clots only (400 ml) with no evidence of retained placental tissue (i.e. running total 3.2 litres) and the decision to insert a Rusch balloon was taken. Meanwhile the team continued to administer haemabate (250 mcg) every 15 minutes. By 10.30, the anaesthetic consultant and obstetric registrar returned to help since they had finished the caesarean section in the second theatre. The anaesthetic consultant was disappointed to learn that there was a haemodynamically unstable patient with suboptimally functioning intravenous access and no one had informed him about it. He established a central line and obtained a sample of blood that was immediately sent to the laboratory for FBC and coagulation.

The obstetric team requested 4 more units of packed red cells, 15 ml/kg of fresh frozen plasma (FFP) and 2 units of platelets. However, the biomedical scientist declined on the basis of having no recent FBC and clotting results as per the transfusion protocol. The obstetric consultant shouted at the SHO, *'Tell them to get the blood products now!'* The obstetric SHO went back to telephone the transfusion department and insisted that in view of the fact that bleeding was still uncontrolled and the blood loss was at least **3.2L** (possibly underestimated since the initial blood loss in the room was not clear), they could not afford to wait 30 minutes for the blood result to be processed and reviewed and then another 30 minutes for FFP/platelets to be prepared. Eventually, the scientist said he would ask the haematology registrar (who was new to this hospital) to ring back. The haematology registrar too was updated about ongoing major obstetric bleeding with a blood loss of **3.2L**. After involving his haematology consultant, agreement was reached that more packed red cells would be issued and blood components including platelets, FFP, and cryoprecipitate would be prepared urgently. The haematology consultant suggested administering 1 g of tranexamic acid intravenously.

> **✪ Learning point** Communication and handover
>
> Communication during an emergency must be clear and professional, and it is worth reflecting after the event 'how to do this better next time?' rather than 'blaming others'. The art of juggling competing priorities and recognizing changing risk is a key obstetric skill that needs honing continuously. For example, the SHO did not respond to the midwife's hint about the excessive blood loss. The handover was fragmented. A 'running blood loss total' wasn't kept initially. The obstetric consultant lost the respect of staff by shouting during the emergency. Even though they understood she was stressed, it frightened people that their leader appeared 'out of control' of the situation.
>
> - Bear in mind that there is a difference in the perceptions that midwifery and medical staff have of the harm to a patient, depending on their grade and position.
> - Assertive communication can also vary between individuals. Not everyone might 'speak up', in spite of perceiving a high potential for harm [15], and yet this is a vital 'check and balance' mechanism in team-working.
> - Cultivate approachability. Always ask for feedback about your clinical and communication skills in order to improve.
> - Catch your colleagues doing things well and tell them precisely what it is they do that works. Frame 'negatives' in a positive way, as areas for learning/ improving. Be prepared to give constructive comments to your peers and seniors—we all need it!

> **✔ Evidence base** Use of tranexamic acid in haemorrhage
>
> Presently, there is only one small (n = 144) randomized controlled trial [16] on the use of tranexamic acid for the treatment of PPH following vaginal delivery, although a large international trial is underway (the WOMAN Study). This showed that the use of high dose of tranexamic acid (loading
>
> (continued)

dose 4 g over one hour, then infusion of 1 g/hour over six hours) significantly (p < 0.041) reduces the blood loss. However, the trial was underpowered to assess the safety issues. Safety and efficacy are well addressed in a systematic review [17] of randomized controlled trials of antifibrinolytic agents in elective surgery. The review provides strong evidence that tranexamic acid reduces the risk of blood transfusion by 39%, whereas its efficacy does not appear to be offset by serious adverse effects.

❝ Guest expert comment (haematologist)

About 14 million mothers develop postpartum haemorrhage (PPH) each year, and about 2% of them will die, largely in resource poor countries. Systemic antifibrinolytic agents such as tranexamic acid are widely used in surgery to prevent clot breakdown (fibrinolysis) in order to reduce surgical blood loss. Trials in postpartum haemorrhage are too small to confirm or refute moderate effects. A simple, relatively cheap intervention such as tranexamic acid could prevent deaths and morbidity associated with postpartum haemorrhage. A large randomized placebo controlled trial (CRASH 2) [18] among trauma patients with or at risk of significant haemorrhage, of the effects of antifibrinolytic treatment on death and blood transfusion requirement, demonstrated a 10% reduction in deaths and no unexpected adverse events associated with tranexamic acid. The WOMAN Trial (tranexamic acid for the treatment of postpartum haemorrhage) is a currently open international, randomized, double blind, placebo controlled trial which aims to determine the effect of the early administration of tranexamic acid on mortality, hysterectomy, and other morbidities (surgical interventions, blood transfusion, risk of non-fatal vascular events) in women with clinically diagnosed postpartum haemorrhage. The use of health services and safety, especially thromboembolic effect, on breastfed babies will also be assessed. <http://www.womantrial.lshtm.ac.uk>.

The patient remained in theatre still under epidural. The Rusch balloon was inserted at 10.20 and filled with 400 mls of fluid, but the bleeding continued despite confirmation of position within the uterine cavity using transabdominal ultrasound, together with a Syntocinon infusion, five doses of Carboprost (1.25 mg) and Misoprostol (800 mcg). The uterus continued to relax and at 10.40, 20 minutes after insertion, the Rusch balloon fell out. The decision was made to try the Rusch balloon again, and if it failed to proceed with laparotomy. A scribe was appointed.

The second attempt at tamponade (using a larger infused volume) was also unsuccessful. The blood loss had reached **4.1L**.

❝ Expert comment

Massive PPH worsens rapidly. The UK blood transfusion handbook [19] suggests that in a patient *who is bleeding* and has evidence of a coagulopathy (or *is likely to develop* a coagulopathy), it is sensible to give blood components *before* coagulation deteriorates and worsens the bleeding.

The British Committee for Standards in Haematology guideline emphasizes that initial transfusion of blood components does not require to await results of coagulation tests. The RCOG guideline [10] also states: 'While acknowledging the general principle that results of coagulation studies and the advice of a haematologist should be used to 'guide transfusion of non cellular blood components in addition to appropriate use of red cells and platelets. 15ml/kg of fresh frozen plasma (FFP) and 2-3 pools of cryoprecipitate may be given empirically in the face of relentless bleeding, while awaiting the results of coagulation studies.

❝ Guest expert comment (haematology)

Ensure you are aware of the in-house communication cascade to manage massive obstetric haemorrhage. This should include detail of the primary haematology link to launch the cascade and should enable a rapid clear communication cascade, expedite blood component support via the

(continued)

laboratory, and sample receipt and turn-around times. Maintaining clear lines of communication, frequent blood sampling, and sample turn-around times is essential. Whilst recognizing that sample results will lag behind the evolving clinical scenario, these results, combined with detail of components transfused and current clinical situation, enable more individualized advice regarding ongoing component support.

✔ **Evidence base** Non-pharmacological treatment for PPH

Data on the effectiveness of second-line treatments for PPH is based mainly on observational studies. Reported success rates for second-line (non-medical) measures in the management of PPH are given in Table 19.3.

Table 19.3 Management of PPH

Second-line treatment	Success rate reported by UKOSS [20] % (95% CI)	Success rate reported by systematic review [21] % (95% CI)
Tamponade	–%	84% (77.5–88.8%)
Interventional radiology	86% (57–98%)	90.7% (85.7–94.0%)
Uterine compression sutures	75% (67–81%)	91.7% (84.9–95.5%)
Pelvic vessel ligation	36% (13–65%)	84.6% (81.2–87.5%)

There are no randomized control studies on the effectiveness of second-line treatments, and it would be very difficult to perform such studies. National population-based studies are the best evidence of efficiency that we have so far [20, 22, 23].

The patient's BP fell further to 84/42 in spite of aggressive resuscitation with fluid and blood products. By 11.00 she had received 5 units of blood, 8 litres of both crystalloid and colloid fluids, and had started the first unit of FFP. An inotrope in the form of adrenaline was given to maintain perfusion blood pressure. At 11.10 the help of a second consultant obstetrician/gynaecologist was requested, and the decision to proceed to laparotomy +/– hysterectomy was made. Radiological intervention was discussed (uterine artery embolization) but this would take some time to organize, and the patient was not thought stable enough to transfer across a large hospital site.

❝ **Guest expert comment (anaesthetist)**

Whilst vasopressors are frequently used in obstetric anaesthesia, and play a role in counteracting the autonomic block that goes hand-in-hand with effective regional anaesthesia, great care must be taken when using inotropes in haemorrhage. Maintenance of an adequate blood pressure for organ perfusion is clearly vital, but hypotension in the face of haemorrhage is almost invariably due to underfilling of the patient. The treatment for this is further fluid resuscitation, whose effect in the hypotensive patient can be judged by the response of the blood pressure and heart rate to further filling. Adrenaline, as used in this case, will raise the blood pressure by increasing cardiac contractility and systemic vascular resistance (SVR). At this stage there is no reason to suspect impaired myocardial function and a rise in the SVR will in fact decrease cardiac output, a key variable in oxygen delivery to the tissues, and which is by definition inadequate in shock. Inotropes can also give a misleading impression to team members glancing at the monitor, who may be falsely reassured by a 'normal' blood pressure. Where there is doubt about the filling status of the patient the urine output, acid/base status of the patient, and CVP can guide further fluid management. These add very little to the immediate care of a bleeding hypotensive patient for whom the correct treatment is fluid resuscitation.

After consenting the patient in the presence of her sister-in-law and establishment of general anaesthesia, subtotal hysterectomy was started at 12.00. The estimated total blood loss at completion of the hysterectomy was **5.4L**. Even after the hysterectomy, there was a continuous oozing of blood from all the pedicles, and again, interventional radiology was considered. As the problem appeared to be widespread, likely due to coagulopathy rather than being confined to one vessel, it was decided instead to leave three large rolled-up packs under pressure and correct the coagulopathy. The abdomen was closed. On removal of the theatre drapes a large pool of blood was found with continuing bleeding from the vagina noted. Re-examination of the vagina showed oozing from friable tissue and sutures, so a vaginal pack was also inserted. At completion of the procedure at 14.50, the EBL was revised to **6.1L**. The patient was transferred to ITU at 16.05 after cleaning up, further observation, and stabilization. In total, the patient received 10 units of blood, 2 pools of platelets, 4 units of FFP, and 3 units of cryoprecipitate. She was kept sedated in view of the plan to remove the abdominal packs the following morning (which was entirely uneventful). Two further 'top-up' units of blood were infused in ITU. Postnatal recovery afterwards was unremarkable apart from a swinging temperature that settled on day 4.

> ✪ **Learning point** Massive transfusion and DIC
>
> Massive blood loss is defined as loss of 1 blood volume within a 24h period, 50% blood volume loss within 3 hours or a rate of loss of 150 ml/min. In the presence of massive blood loss a specific massive haemorrhage protocol (specific to each hospital) should be launched.
>
> It is frequently associated with a reduction in clotting factor levels and thrombocytopenia. In addition, massive obstetric haemorrhage is associated with disseminated intravascular coagulopathy (DIC), especially if shock, hypothermia, or acidosis are also present, and these all necessitate rapid correction. DIC should be suspected where the fibrinogen is significantly reduced in conjunction with a ↑PT and ↑APTT and thrombocytopenia. Transfusion of FFP, cryoprecipitate and platelets should be given to maintain the PT/APTT < 1.5 × control value, fibrinogen > 1–1.5 g/dl, and the platelet count > 50–75 × 10^9/l, respectively. Whilst haemorrhage is ongoing, coagulation tests and blood counts should be checked at regular intervals proportional to rate and progression of blood loss [24].

An explanation of events was given to the patient and her family. Following discharge, she was given another appointment to be seen by her consultant in six weeks time for a check-up, a summary letter to her GP, and long-term advice about smears and ovarian function. An oral glucose tolerance test was arranged for six weeks postnatally. Uterine histology was as follows; '...at the deepest point of the cornu, just 2mm from the serosa, there is a large muscular vessel with cytotrophoblast within its wall, which has ruptured. Haemorrhage is seen spilling out both into endometrial cavity and into surrounding paratubal soft tissue from this vessel. On balance the large ruptured vessel deep in the cornu is considered the cause of this patient's post partum haemorrhage.' A three-month follow-up appointment was made in the perineal trauma clinic.

Seven months later a complaint letter was received focusing on the panic in the room at delivery; '*I thought I would die and never see my babies again*', together with '*unnecessary loss of fertility, continuing stress urinary incontinence, and postnatal depression*', all having had a negative impact on bonding and breastfeeding. The hospital gave a detailed explanation, but a year on, litigation continues.

⊗ **Learning point** Transfusion reactions

In spite of the importance of fluid and blood products resuscitation in patients with haemorrhage, clinicians should be also aware of the potential adverse effects of transfusion and the symptoms and signs of transfusion-related complications (Table 19.4 and Table 19.5) [19].

Table 19.4 Transfusion reactions

Adverse effect of transfusion/cause	Signs	Management
Acute haemolytic transfusion reaction (caused by transfusion incompatible blood products due to error)	Bleeding, tachycardia, hypotension, or Hypertension	Stop transfusion, check the unit of blood IV crystalloids, take blood cultures and sample for cultures from the pack May require an inotrope Urgent haematology and critical care involvement
Reaction to infusion of a bacterially contaminated Unit (more common for platelets stored at 22°C)	Rapid onset of hyper- or hypotension, rigors, and collapse. The signs and symptoms may be similar to acute haemolytic transfusion reactions or severe acute allergic reactions.	As above + antibiotics Microbiologist involvement
Transfusion-related acute lung injury / It is often found that plasma of the donor has antibodies that react strongly with recipient leucocytes	Shortness of breath, non productive cough within 6 hours of transfusion Hypotension, fever Chest X-Ray—bilateral nodular infiltrates in a batwing pattern	Urgent critical care and haematology advice Diuretics should be avoided Inform blood service, so implicated donor could be taken off donor service
Acute fluid overload/ when too much fluid transfused too rapidly	Dyspnoea, tachypnoea, non-productive cough, raised jugular venous pressure (JVP), basal lung crackles, frothy pink sputum, hypertension, and tachycardia	Stop transfusion Diuretics Oxygen
Severe allergic reaction or anaphylaxis	Hypotension, bronchospasm, periorbital and laryngeal oedema, vomiting, erythema, urticaria and conjunctivitis, dyspnoea, chest pain, abdominal pain, and nausea.	If mild reaction (e.g. urticaria): give chlorpheniramine 10 mg IV and restart transfusion at slower rate + more frequent observations If severe: stop transfusion, and give chlorpheniramine , O_2, salbutamol, adrenaline (0.5 ml of 1 in 1000 intramuscular)
Febrile non-haemolytic transfusion reactions	Fever (> 1.5 °C above the baseline), rigors towards the end of the transfusion or up to 2 hours after it	Reduce the transfusion rate, IV paracetamol, remember to watch for other signs of more severe reactions

> ⊕ **Clinical tip**
>
> **Table 19.5 Example of transfusion management [19]**
>
> | Objective | Action | Notes |
> |---|---|---|
> | Control the bleeding Restore circulating volume | Early intervention—surgical, radiological Insert wide-bore cannulae Give adequate volume of crystalloids/ blood Aim to maintain normal BP and urine output | Interventional radiology Blood loss is often underestimated Monitor arterial pressure and CVP if unstable |
> | Avoid exacerbating coagulation problems | Keep patient warm | |
> | Monitor laboratory data to guide/improve the management | Request laboratory investigations: FBC, INR, APTTr, fibrinogen, biochemical profile, blood gases Repeat FBC, PT, APTT, fibrinogen frequently | Colloid solutions can prolong clotting times Take samples early FFP, cryoprecipitate, and platelets may be required before results are available in addition to red cells |
> | Platelets | Anticipate platelet count $< 50 \times 10^9/l$ after 1.5–2 blood volume replaced | Target platelet count: $> 75 \times 10^9/l$ |
> | FFP | Anticipate coagulation factor deficiency after blood loss of $1–1.5 \times$ blood volume Aim for PT and APTT $< 1.5 \times$ mean control and fibrinogen $> 1.0–1.5$ g/l Allow for 30 minutes thawing time Dose: 12–15 ml/kg body weight | May need to use FFP before laboratory results are available Take sample for PT, APTT, fibrinogen before FFP transfused |

Discussion

Postpartum haemorrhage is one of the leading causes of maternal deaths worldwide. Up to 50 % of the estimated 530 000 maternal deaths that annually occur across the globe are attributed to haemorrhage (CMACE 2006–2008) [25]. The number of maternal deaths due to haemorrhage in the UK continues to decline and is the lowest since the UK-wide Confidential Enquiry Reports began in 1985. Although the number of deaths decreased, substandard care was a contributing factor into mortality in 66 % of cases (six out of nine). In four women who died, it was thought that different management may have altered the outcome [25]. It was disappointing that the leading cause of 'failure' in the last CMACE report was not a lack of expensive drugs, complex technologies, or highly skilled professionals, but the more elementary lack of routine observations in a high-risk patient or failure to appreciate the extent of bleeding.

This case illustrates several important points in the diagnosis and management of postpartum haemorrhage, and typical challenges on the frontline of care. The value of early recognition, senior involvement, efficient communication, and multidisciplinary teamwork is central to the successful management of a sick patient. The chain of events might have been different (or more promptly managed) if the senior registrar had not been distracted and had not delegated the case at an early stage to the most junior doctor at the end of a night shift. Blood loss was underestimated at the beginning, and communication was hampered by multiple handovers and interruptions. The diagnosis of the third-degree tear and move to theatre could have been achieved earlier. This would have involved the anaesthetic team in a joint approach, to monitor vital observations continuously, and to recognize the need for appropriate intravenous access and fluid resuscitation before the patient became haemodynamically unstable. Having more senior staff involved earlier might have helped the recognition that there was more than one cause of bleeding that needed to be addressed. Initially the causes were perineal trauma and atony, but these were followed by surgical site bleeding and coagulopathy. Having recognized the severity earlier would have allowed more accurate information at handover. The morning team might have distributed their staff differently and asked the most senior anaesthetist (consultant) to help deal with major haemorrhage, rather than the fetal compromise case in the second theatre. The involvement of senior haematology at an earlier stage might also have helped prevent multiple unnecessary phone calls and debates, potentially speeding up time regarding the blood product transfusion.

Postpartum haemorrhage is the commonest life-threatening obstetric emergency that justifies our professional existence. We treat it successfully most of the time, but cannot take any haemorrhage for granted, as the case shows. However, a combination of training, regular drills and skills, clinical experience, and reflection will help prepare doctors for future cases.

A Final Word from the Expert

Later that week, the two obstetric consultants were talking in the coffee room and the first wondered aloud whether she should have performed a Brace suture first. A third consultant colleague (a well-known plaintiff's medico-legal opinion-giver), intending to be helpful, butted in that 'I wouldn't have done a hysterectomy. Why didn't you use a tourniquet around the uterus? That would have controlled the bleeding and enabled you to re-establish clotting'. This was taken as criticism rather than educational by the consultant. it was also overheard by junior doctors, and 'gossip' rapidly circulated. The senior consultant with responsibility for risk and clinical governance heard about the disquiet in the unit and made it his business to talk quietly to a number of individuals on a one-to-one basis, both offering his support and pointing out that serious incident investigations should be performed calmly after the event. They should not be held in public and nor is it wise for people to give opinions without full information and access to the facts. He fixed a date for the incident to be discussed at the morbidity meeting (sometimes called the 'significant event analysis' meeting).

It is very difficult to make the decision that is also fertility-destroying, but hesitation can lead to maternal death. Retrospectively, the histology did lend some support to hysterectomy being the correct, life-saving, decision for the patient, and the consultants who had been present had thought the patient was in extremis. However, on looking back, they wondered if they could have done more to avoid hysterectomy, at the same time as wondering whether it might have been performed at an earlier stage.

It can be very hard to look back self-critically, and it is upsetting to be criticized (e.g. by colleagues, or in formal complaints or legal actions). We all need support when things go wrong, but have professional obligations to be able to defend our actions (under ethical, legal, and GMC requirements).

It is impossible to put the clock back. One can only 'try to be a better doctor tomorrow than yesterday'. A safe, learning, multidisciplinary culture of challenge when things go well, and support when they go badly, helps all of us cope with the stresses and strains of midwifery and medical practice. Remember to look after yourself and other people.

Action is the key to success in postpartum haemorrhage

- Measure blood loss accurately, and remember it is safer to overestimate than underestimate.

- Act quickly, and treat several causes at once.

- Watch the clock and keep planning ahead in case present action does not work.

- Examination under anaesthesia (EUA) at 1500 ml especially to look for retained products.

- Get senior help and bodies earlier rather than later.

- Early recourse to hysterectomy.

References

1. Kjos SL, Henry OA, Montoro M, Buchanan TA, Mestman JH. Insulin-requiring diabetes in pregnancy: a randomized trial of active induction of labor and expectant management. *Am J Obstet Gynecol* 1993;169(3):611–15.

2. Maso G, Alberico S, Wiesenfeld U, Ronfani L, Erenbourg A, Hadar E, Yogev Y, Hod M; GINEXMAL RCT: Induction of labour versus expectant management in gestational diabetes pregnancies. *BMC Pregnancy Childbirth* 2011;11(1):31.

3. National Collaboration Centre for Women's and Children's Health, National Institute for Health and Clinical Excellence. Diabetes in pregnancy management of diabetes and its complications from preconception to the postnatal period. Clinical guideline CG 63 2008:226. <http://www.nice.org.uk/nicemedia/live/11946/41320/41320.pdf>

4. Segal S. Labor epidural analgesia and maternal fever. *Anesth Analg* 2010;111(6):1467–75.

5. Hannah ME, Ohlsson A, Farine D, Hewson SA, Hodnett ED, Myhr TL, *et al*. Induction of labor compared with expectant management for prelabor rupture of the membranes at term. TERM PROM Study Group. *N Engl J Med* 1996;334(16):1005–10.

6. National Collaboration Centre for Women's and Children's Health, National Institute for Health and Clinical Excellence. Intrapartum care: care of healthy women in their babies during childbirth. Clinical guideline CG 55. 2007. <http://www.nice.org.uk/nicemedia/live/11837/36280/36280.pdf>

7. WHO guidelines for the management of postpartum haemorrhage and retained placenta. World Health Organisation 2009.

8. Belfort MA, Dildy GA. Postpartum haemorrhage and other problems of the third stage. In:James DK, Steer PJ, Weiner CP,vGonik B, Crowther CA, Robson SC (eds). *High Risk Pregnancy: Management Options*, 4th edn. Philadelphia, PA: Elsevier/Saunders; 2011. 1283–313. <http://whqlibdoc.who.int/publications/2009/9789241598514_eng.pdf>

9. Mousa HA, Alfirevic Z. Treatment for primary postpartum haemorrhage. *Cochrane Database Syst Rev* 2007;(1):CD003249.

10. Arulkumaran S, Mavrides E, Penney GC. Royal College of Obstetricians & Gynaecologists. Postpartum haemorrhage. Green-top Guideline No. 52 RCOG, 2009. <http://www.rcog.org.uk/files/rcog-corp/GT52PostpartumHaemorrhage0411.pdf>

11. Bose P, Regan F, Paterson-Brown S. Improving the accuracy of estimated blood loss at obstetric haemorrhage using clinical reconstructions. *BJOG* 2006;113(8):919–24.

12. Toeima E, Morris EP, Fogarty PP. "Improving patient handover." Good Practice No. 12 RCOG, 2010. <http://www.rcog.org.uk/files/rcog-corp/GoodPractice12PatientHandover.pdf>

13. Finfer S, Bellomo R, Boyce N, French J, Myburgh J, Norton R; SAFE Study Investigators. A comparison of albumin and saline for fluid resuscitation in the intensive care unit. *N Engl J Med.* 2004;350(22):2247–56.

14. Perel P, Roberts I Colloids versus crystalloids for fluid resuscitation in critically ill patients. *Cochrane Database Syst Rev* 2011;(3):CD000567.

15. Lyndon A, Sexton JB, Simpson KR, Rosenstein A, Lee KA, Wachter RM. Predictors of likelihood of speaking up about safety concerns in labour and delivery. *BMJ Qual Saf* 2012 Sep;21(9):791–9. doi: 10.1136/bmjqs- 2010-050211. <http://www.ncbi.nlm.nih.gov/pubmed/21725045>

16. Ducloy-Bouthors AS, Jude B, Duhamel A, Broisin F, Huissoud C, Keita-Meyer H, *et al.* The EXADELI Study Group, Susen S. High-dose tranexamic acid reduces blood loss in postpartum haemorrhage. *Crit Care* 2011;15(2):R117.

17. Henry DA, Carless PA, Moxey AJ, O'Connell D, Stokes BJ, McClelland B, *et al.* Anti-fibrinolytic use for minimising perioperative allogeneic blood transfusion. *Cochrane Database Syst Rev* 2007;(4):CD001886.

18. CRASH-2 trial collaborators, Shakur H, Roberts I, Bautista R, Caballero J, Coats T, Dewan Y, *et al.* Effects of tranexamic acid on death, vascular occlusive events, and blood transfusion in trauma patients with significant haemorrhage (CRASH-2): a randomised, placebo-controlled trial. *Lancet* 2010 Jul 3;376(9734):23–32. doi: 10.1016/S0140-6736(10)60835-5.

19. McClell DBL (ed.) *Handbook of Transfusion Medicine*, 4th edn. United Kingdom Blood Service, TSO: London, 2007.

20. Kayem G, Kurinczuk JJ, Alfirevic Z, Spark P, Brocklehurst P, Knight M. Specific second-line therapies for postpartum haemorrhage: a national cohort study. *BJOG* 2011;118(7):856–64.

21. Doumouchtsis SK, Papageorghiou AT, Arulkumaran S. Systematic review of conservative management of postpartum hemorrhage: what to do when medical treatment fails. *Obstet Gynecol Surv* 2007;62(8):540–7.

22. Knight M, UKOSS. Peripartum hysterectomy in the UK: management and outcomes of the associated haemorrhage. *BJOG* 2007;114(11):1380–7.

23. Zwart JJ, Dijk PD, van Roosmalen J. Peripartum hysterectomy and arterial embolization for major obstetric hemorrhage: a 2-year nationwide cohort study in the Netherlands. *Am J Obstet Gynecol* 2010;202(2):150.e1–7.

24. Macphail S, Fitzerald J. Massive post-partum haemorrhage. *Curr Obstetr Gynaecol* 2001;11:108–14.

25. CEMACE. Saving Mothers' Lives: Reviewing maternal deaths to make motherhood safer: 2006-2008. The Eighth Report of the Confidential Enquiries into Maternal Deaths in the United Kingdom. *BJOG* 2011;118Suppl 1:1–203.

Premature ovarian failure: not the same as the 'normal' menopause

Beth Cartwright

❻ Expert Commentary Janice Rymer

Case history

A 29-year-old woman was referred to a premature ovarian failure (POF) clinic by her GP. She had stopped the combined oral contraceptive pill (COCP) 6 months earlier and had only had one period since. The GP had measured two serum follicle-stimulating hormone (FSH) levels, taken four weeks apart, which were significantly elevated at 60 and 45 IU/l. The GP had expressed surprise at these levels and told her that she was 'too young to be going through the menopause'.

✪ Learning point Diagnosis of premature ovarian failure

- The average age of menopause in the UK is 51–52 years.
- POF is defined as a loss of ovarian function before the age of 45 [1].
- POF is diagnosed by two serum follicle-stimulating hormone (FSH) levels over 30 IU/l taken at least 4 weeks apart, combined with amenorrhoea or oligomenorrhoea of at least 4 months, and a low serum oestradiol.
- POF is not a rare condition—it affects approximately one in 1000 women before the age of 30, one in 100 by 40 years, and one in 20 by 45 years. Although it is not a common cause of oligomenorrhoea or secondary amenorrhoea, it should always be considered and promptly excluded or confirmed.

✚ Clinical tip Asking about symptoms of POF

Many young women will not volunteer symptoms, either because they are embarrassed, they have not realized that they may be associated with POF, or because they are preoccupied with their fertility. Therefore it is important to ask about symptoms directly. This will aid subsequent discussions about oestrogen replacement and will also help women to recognize potential symptoms. Possible symptoms are described in (Table 20.1).

Table 20.1 Menopausal symptoms

Vasomotor	Urogenital	Psychological	Other
Hot flushes	Vaginal dryness	Anxiety	Joint pains
Night sweats	Urinary frequency	Depression	Itching
Palpitations		Mood changes	Hair thinning
		Irritability	Skin changes
		Tiredness	Decreased libido
		Difficulty concentrating	

❻ Expert comment

POF should always be considered and promptly investigated in cases of oligomenorrhoea or secondary amenorrhoea. Many women with menstrual irregularity are not investigated promptly and this can lead to a delay in diagnosis of POF. One study reported that over half of the participants with menstrual irregularity visited their doctor three or more times before any tests were carried out. Diagnosis was delayed by over five years for a quarter of women in this study [3].

➕ **Clinical tip** Timing of gonadotrophin levels

It is important to obtain a correctly timed FSH level and to be aware of the limitations of interpretation if the sample is not correctly timed. Due to the intermittent nature of POF, FSH levels may fluctuate. One cross-sectional study revealed that 11% of women with previously confirmed POF had an FSH level which did not meet the criteria for diagnosis [2]. FSH is known to have a high cycle-to-cycle variability, and to rise only during the later stages of ovarian failure [3].

In the case of complete amenorrhoea, the level can be obtained at any time. However, if there is any cyclical activity, the FSH should be measured on day 2–5 when the oestradiol level is at its lowest. High oestradiol levels later on in the cycle may suppress FSH secretion, producing a falsely reassuring low FSH. FSH also rises to over 30 IU/l immediately prior to ovulation. An oestradiol level taken at the same time as the FSH aids interpretation.

❝ **Expert comment**

If a woman has been taking the combined oral contraceptive pill for some years, the symptoms and signs of POF (a change in menstrual pattern, menopausal symptoms) are masked and do not become apparent until she stops the pill. It is important that she understands that the pill did not cause her to develop POF as this can lead to a distrust of medications, particularly hormone replacement therapy (HRT).

❝ **Expert comment**

Although 30 IU/l is typically taken as the cut-off for diagnosing POF, a correctly timed FSH level in a young woman of above 8–10 IU/l indicates reduced ovarian reserve. Due to the problems of using FSH for diagnosis, interest has turned to new, more direct, markers of ovarian reserve, such as antral follicle count (measured on transvaginal ultrasound), and anti-Mullerian hormone (AMH), which is produced by developing antral follicles. However, their role in the diagnosis of POF is yet to be determined and their use is currently being evaluated.

⭐ **Learning Point** Communicating the diagnosis of POF

Premature ovarian failure is a very difficult diagnosis to communicate and sensitivity is vital. The woman is unlikely to anticipate the diagnosis and it is useful to warn her that it is not good news. The diagnosis should then be explained clearly and directly using simple language. She may wish to have her partner or a family member present. On the other hand, especially in some cultures, the woman may choose not to reveal the diagnosis to her partner for various reasons. The setting of a fertility clinic where a woman attends with her partner but has not told him about her lack of periods is especially difficult, and in some situations it may be appropriate to speak to the woman in the first instance on her own.

Distress, denial, and anger may be felt and expressed on receiving a diagnosis. For these reasons, it is advisable to have a senior colleague either present or easily accessible. Early follow-up is often helpful, and it is not unusual to need to explain the diagnosis on several occasions before it is accepted. The Daisy Network (<http://www.daisynetwork.org.uk>) is a UK-based charity run by women with POF. It provides information and support to women diagnosed with POF through internet resources, leaflets, and a networking system. Many women find this support invaluable, especially as they may not wish to tell family or friends about the diagnosis.

❝ **Expert comment**

POF is a devastating condition. Affected women may suffer menopausal symptoms, depression, and feelings of loss. They also have to cope with loss of fertility and the prospect of associated long-term health sequelae. They deserve specialist care, which is different from that required by a woman experiencing menopause at the normal age, to address all of these aspects. Realistically, this is unlikely to be available in a primary care setting.

Multidisciplinary POF clinics with the direct input of a fertility specialist enable women to access the best care. This also avoids the need for attendance at the general menopause and fertility clinics, where women with POF can feel very out of place.

Further history revealed that she underwent normal puberty and menarche was at the age of 12. She had a regular 28-day cycle with normal periods, starting the combined oral contraceptive pill at the age of 26. She stopped it because she was about to get married and wanted to start a family. She had never been pregnant. She had no previous medical problems. She experienced joint pains but no other menopausal symptoms. There were no stigmata of Turner's syndrome. Her mother went through menopause at the age of 48. She had one brother and no sisters. A cousin on her father's side had POF which developed at the age of 24. There was no other family history of POF and no history of learning difficulties. There was also no family history of breast/ovarian/bowel cancer, cardiovascular disease or venous thromboembolism.

⊘ **Learning point** Investigations in secondary amenorrhoea

- BHCG to rule out pregnancy.
- Serum FSH, LH, and oestradiol.
- Serum TSH and prolactin.
- Serum dehydroepiandosterone and testosterone if clinical signs of hyperandrogenism are present.
- Ultrasound of pelvis to assess ovaries for polycystic appearance.

Once diagnosis of POF is confirmed

- Karyotyping and FMR1 (fragile X) premutation
- Associated autoimmune disorder screening: POF can occasionally be associated with autoimmune disease. Anti-thyroid (antithyroid peroxidase, antithyroglobulin), and anti-adrenal antibodies are used to identify women who may have an autoimmune aetiology for the POF (Table 20.2). Testing for anti-adrenal antibodies will also identify the tiny subset of women at risk of developing Addison's disease, which is of particular importance to those considering egg donation because of the dangers of adrenal insufficiency in pregnancy.
- There is no value in measuring anti-ovarian antibodies as they are present in a large proportion of the general population [7].
- Blood glucose testing can rule out associated autoimmune diabetes.
- A DXA scan should be offered to all women to obtain a baseline bone density. This will inform current treatment decisions as well as allowing future comparisons to be made.

Table 20.2 Aetiology of POF and differential diagnosis

Causes of spontaneous POF	Causes of secondary POF	Differential diagnosis (secondary amenorrhoea)
No cause found (idiopathic) (the majority of cases)	Bilateral oophorectomy	Hypothalamic causes (low BMI, excessive exercise, hypothalamic lesions, systemic disease)
Autoimmune disease	Chemotherapy	Pituitary causes (adenomas, pituitary infarction secondary to hypotension [Sheehans syndrome])
Fragile X premutation (5% overall)	Radiotherapy	Ovarian causes (PCOS, POF)
Other genetic causes—e.g. Turner's syndrome, Down's syndrome, rare mutations such as FSH receptor polymorphism and inhibin B mutation	Interruption of ovarian blood supply due to pelvic surgery or uterine artery embolization	Genital tract causes (intrauterine adhesions [Ashermans syndrome], Cervical stenosis)
Enzyme deficiencies – e.g. galactosaemia	Infections—mumps, tuberculosis, HIV	Certain drugs (e.g. progestogens, dopamine antagonists)
		Systemic disease (e.g. Cushings disease, diabetes mellitus, renal failure, liver disease)

❝ **Expert comment**

It is worthwhile taking time to explain that in most cases no cause is found, and that even if a cause is found, this will not lead to a way to restore ovarian function; management options including the need for egg donation to achieve pregnancy are unchanged. This will avoid a difficult situation at the next clinic visit when, if this had not been explained previously, she may ask about the cause and cure for the POF.

> ✪ **Learning point** Family history in POF
>
> Premature ovarian failure often appears to be familial although estimates have varied widely from around 4–31% [4]. Whilst causative mutations in some genes have been identified [5], routine testing for most of these is unavailable and it is likely that there are many more which are as yet undiscovered. The two genetic causes of POF which can be readily tested for are the FMR1 (fragile X) premutation and chromosomal disorders, such as Turner's syndrome and translocations of the X chromosome, which can be assessed on karyotype. If there is a family history of POF, there is a 10% chance of finding a FMR1 premutation, compared with 2% if there is no family history [6].

There was no need to repeat the serum FSH level as she already had two levels above 30 taken over four weeks apart, confirming the diagnosis of POF. Blood was taken for thyroid-stimulating hormone, glucose, thyroid auto-antibodies, adrenal auto-antibodies, karyotype, and FMR1 (fragile X) premutation screening. A dual energy X-ray densitometry (DXA) scan of the lumbar spine and hip was performed which was normal.

> ✔ **Evidence base** Loss of bone density at the menopause and in POF
>
> An accelerated phase of bone loss due to oestrogen deficiency occurs in the early post-menopausal years, with subsequent slowing to a rate seen in older men. The clinical consequence of reduced bone density is fracture. For each standard deviation the bone density drops below the young adult mean, the risk of sustaining a fracture doubles [8].
>
> Several cross-sectional studies have shown that women with POF have a 2–3% lower bone density compared with matched controls [9-11], and one retrospective study has shown that women who have an earlier menopause have a life-long increased risk of bone fracture (odds ratio for fracture 1.5 CI 1.2–1.9 [12].
>
> Numerous studies have shown that HRT prevents bone loss [13]. The Women's Health Initiative trial found that HRT reduces hip and vertebral fractures by one-third; other fractures were also reduced [14]. Factors contributing to risk can be estimated in women over 40 using the FRAX™ model (see Clinical tip: The Frax™ model).

> **❝ Expert comment**
>
> There is little published research in the field of premature ovarian failure, and findings from trials conducted in older menopausal women cannot be extrapolated to this age group, particularly regarding cardiovascular outcomes. Unfortunately this is not always appreciated, and women may be given conflicting advice from different clinicians.

> ✔ **Evidence base** Cardiovascular disease after the normal menopause and in POF
>
> For many years, it was considered that the use of HRT after the menopause decreased the risk of developing CVD, based on data from observational studies, including the large Nurses' Health Study, in which a 33% reduction was seen in those starting HRT close to the menopause [16]. This association was not confirmed in the initial Women's Health Initiative (WHI) publications, which reported that combined HRT increases coronary heart disease by 29% [14]. A recent re-analysis of the WHI data showed that in women under 60 and those who commenced HRT within 10 years of the menopause, there was a trend towards cardiovascular benefit [17]. This correlates with knowledge about the direct effects of oestrogen on the cardiovascular system.
>
> Epidemiological studies have associated an earlier menopause with increased cardiovascular risk. A recent meta-analysis reported that early menopause increases the risk of developing CVD by 38% [18]. A previous study suggested that for each year the menopause is delayed, the risk of cardiovascular mortality decreases by 2% [19]. However, the amelioration of risk with oestrogen treatment in POF and the optimal form of oestrogen replacement to use is unknown. There are very few studies in this area.

➕ **Clinical tip** The FRAX™ model

The FRAX™ model is an online model to quantify risk of osteoporotic fracture which has been developed from meta-analysis of risk factors and calibrated to the UK population [15]. It is quick and easy to complete in clinic when seeing a patient over the age of 40, with or without a DXA result, and is a useful way to help a patient understand her risk of fracture. It is available online at <http://www.shef.ac.uk/FRAX>. It cannot be used to calculate risk on women under 40 due to a lack of available data to construct models.

✔️ **Evidence base** Ovulation and spontaneous pregnancy in POF

Ultrasound studies have demonstrated ovarian activity and ovulation in POF. One study followed 49 women with POF over 12 weeks and demonstrated ovulation in 49% and ovarian activity without ovulation in another 37% [20]. The ovaries were completely inactive in only 14%. This may account for the wide variation in symptoms observed in clinical practice. Sadly, the rates of ovulation observed do not translate to pregnancy rates.

Spontaneous pregnancy occurs in approximately 5–10% of women with POF [21]. No hormonal or ovulation induction regimes (including oestrogens, clomiphene citrate, corticosteroids, gonadotrophins, and gonadotrophin-releasing hormone agonists) have been shown to produce a higher pregnancy rate than the background observed rate. Studies to-date are limited by short follow-up periods, wide variations in inclusion criteria, and few randomized controlled trials. Many studies have used ovulation rather than pregnancy as an end-point.

It is impossible to predict accurately which women will conceive spontaneously, but weakly positive prognostic factors identified were: shorter duration of amenorrhoea, autoimmune aetiology of POF, and the presence of ovarian activity on ultrasound scan [21–22].

💬 **Expert comment**

The possibility of spontaneous conception means that if a woman does not want to get pregnant, it is vital that she is advised to use contraception. Pregnancy can occur even after many years of amenorrhoea, and an unplanned pregnancy in POF may be especially difficult for the patient to handle. The combined oral contraceptive pill may be a suitable option as it provides both oestrogen replacement and contraception.

She was counselled about the long-term complications of POF due to a low oestrogen level. She also saw the fertility specialist who explained that her only option for future fertility treatment would be egg donation.

⭐ **Learning point** Oestrogen replacement therapy (HRT)

Oestrogen replacement is recommended in POF to protect against bone loss and cardiovascular disease and to alleviate menopausal symptoms. Women with POF should be strongly advised to take some form of oestrogen replacement until the age of 51–52 (average age of menopause), at which point it should be reviewed.

There is a paucity of evidence to recommend a particular regime and route of oestrogen replacement over another. Currently, either HRT or the COCP is commonly prescribed.

- HRT is considered to be more 'physiological', but some young women dislike taking a preparation associated with older women. Women with POF may need significantly higher doses of oestrogen than women at the average age of menopause.
- The COCP contains synthetic oestrogen at a higher dose with a 'pill-free' week. It may be considered more 'peer friendly' than HRT (it is taken by 16% of women aged 16–49 [23]), and there is no prescription charge.

HRT

- Preparation

    For women with a uterus, progesterone must be included in the HRT regime to avoid the action of unopposed oestrogen on the endometrium and the risk of endometrial cancer. An option for women who do not wish to become pregnant is a Mirena intra-uterine system combined with oral

(continued)

or transdermal oestrogen. This may be particularly suitable for women who experience significant progestogenic side effects or who wish to be period-free, but who experience break-through bleeding on continuous combined HRT.

HRT can be sequential (simulating monthly menstrual cycles), or continuous (which avoids menstrual flow). Continuous combined HRT is suitable for women who have been amenorrhoeic for at least a year and who do not wish to have periods. If continuous combined HRT is started too early (whilst there are still periods), it is likely to be complicated by break-through bleeding. Sequential combined HRT produces cyclical bleeding, which some women prefer. It can be started before the complete cessation of periods. Women with previous hysterectomy can take oestrogen only HRT.

Some women continue to experience symptoms despite adequate oestrogen replacement. If the symptoms are suggestive of hypo-androgenism (tiredness, low libido), it may be worth considering testosterone replacement. This can be as an implant, patch, or gel.

- Route

HRT comes in various preparations and may be delivered orally, transdermally, subcutaneously, or vaginally. Many women with POF choose to take an oral form rather than a patch which can act as a continuous reminder of the diagnosis and may be visible. For women who suffer from migraine, or who have a personal or family history of venous thromboembolism (VTE), transdermal delivery methods have a lower risk of VTE.

- Dose

Women with POF may need a higher dose of HRT than older women, for whom HRT was originally designed. It is important to warn them of this and explain that the dose can be increased if necessary. Some women who take the COCP complain of symptoms during the pill-free week and they can be advised to take packets back-to-back.

She was counselled on her options for oestrogen replacement but decided that she would like to wait and see what happened, and hope for spontaneous ovarian activity leading to conception. She decided to enroll in the no-treatment arm of a two-year trial comparing the use of HRT and COCP in POF, and observing women who decide to take no treatment.

> ✪ **Learning point** Egg donation
>
> In vitro fertilization (IVF) using an egg donor carries high success rates of over 50%, dependent on the age of the donor. NHS funding may be available, subject to the usual criteria, but is not guaranteed and is usually considered on a case-by-case basis. Finding a suitable donor may be another challenge. There is a shortage of egg donors in the UK due to payment for the process being illegal, and the fact that the recipient is able to track the donor when he/she is 18. The ideal donor is under 35 and has already completed her own family. A related donor may not be ideal due to the familial nature of POF and therefore the increased risk of poor ovarian response to stimulation. For women who have not identified a donor, egg sharing, or advertising for a donor are other options. Egg-sharing schemes are offered by some IVF centres and involve a woman who is undergoing conventhional IVF sharing her eggs. The incentive for the donor is usually to reduce the cost of IVF or the waiting time. The disadvantage is that it may reduce the donor's chance of achieving a pregnancy herself. Altrui (<http://www.altrui.co.uk>) is a recently set up organization which helps women find anonymous altruistic donors.
>
> For ethnic minorities, finding a suitable donor can be very difficult and may prompt women to seek treatment overseas. Other reasons that women go abroad for treatment include cost and anonymity. Some things to consider in this situation are safety, ethical sourcing of donors, and limiting the number of embryos replaced in order to avoid multiple pregnancy.
>
> There are many ethical issues involved in egg donation and extensive counselling is required for both donor and recipient prior to embarking on the process.

There are a significant proportion of women who decline treatment, for various reasons. It is important to try to elucidate these reasons as some may be unfounded. For example, many women have heard about the media 'health scares' of HRT being associated with cardiovascular disease and breast cancer and do not realize that these risks do not apply to their age group. One way to alleviate anxiety is to explain that in POF oestrogen replacement is simply replacing the hormones that the ovaries should be producing at this age. However, some women feel that their best chance of achieving a spontaneous pregnancy is to delay starting oestrogen treatment for a while in order to reduce the chance of suppressing any ovarian activity. This is reasonable given that we do not have any evidence either way of how to optimize chances of conception.

Expert comment

It is important to recognize that some women do not wish to take oestrogen replacement. The diagnosis of POF is hard to accept and it is unreasonable to expect women to make decisions at their first clinic visit. These women need support and long-term follow-up, including bone scans, the results of which may influence treatment decisions. If a sympathetic approach is not adopted they will not re-attend the clinic and the chance of future uptake of oestrogen treatment is further reduced.

When she came for her first visit for the trial, she reported a positive pregnancy test four weeks previously followed by heavy bleeding. She had assumed that she had experienced a miscarriage and had not sought medical attention. A pregnancy test was positive and a transvaginal ultrasound scan revealed an empty irregular gestation sac measuring 15×17×10 mm. An ultrasound scan the following week confirmed a non-viable pregnancy, and she underwent evacuation of retained products of conception.

The initial blood results were reviewed at this time. The karyotype, TSH, glucose, and auto-antibodies were normal, but genetic testing revealed an FMR1 premutation with 162 repeats.

⭐ **Learning points** The FMR1 gene

The FMR1 gene is located on the long arm of the X chromosome and consists of CGG repeats. The normal number of repeats is less than 55. The full mutation of over 200 repeats causes fragile X syndrome in men. The phenotype is very variable. In women, over 200 repeats may cause mild symptoms, or may have no effect. These women are carriers for fragile X syndrome—a male baby has a 50% chance of being affected by fragile X syndrome. The premutation consists of 55–200 repeats. The chance of a woman with the premutation developing POF is approximately 15% [24]. The exact mechanism behind this is unknown and the full mutation does not cause POF. The premutation can also occasionally lead to a neurodegenerative disorder in later life [25]. The premutation is unstable and the number of CGG repeats may develop to become a full mutation in offspring. For this reason, women with the fragile X premutation are at risk of having a child with fragile X syndrome.

Expert Comment:

Overall, the FMR1 premutation is responsible for 4–5% of cases of POF [6,26].

IVF with pre-implantation genetic diagnosis (PGD) is an option for couples where one partner is affected by the mutation or premutation. However, PGD is not an option for this woman as her ovaries would not respond to stimulation.

She was referred to a geneticist to discuss what the FMR1 premutation meant for her and other members of her family. Family members identified as possible carriers of the gene were offered genetic counselling and testing.

A year later, she continued to take part in the POF trial in the no-treatment arm. Her bone density remained stable and she was relatively symptom-free. The potential benefits of oestrogen replacement were reiterated but she decided to opt for no treatment for the time being. However she was thinking about starting HRT in the long-term in order to decrease her cardiovascular risk and maintain bone density and uterine size. She and her husband had come to terms with the diagnosis and were considering the options of egg donation or adoption.

Discussion

This case illustrates that POF and its management are different from the 'normal' menopause. It is vital to bear these physiological and psychological differences in mind when managing these women. They deserve to be provided with accurate

Expert comment

It is always important to explain any investigations you are carrying out, and this is especially relevant with genetic testing, which may have implications both for the individual and for other family members. Some women decline genetic testing and this should be documented. There are reports of women with POF having children with fragile X syndrome [27], and this could potentially result in legal action if FMR1 premutation testing had not been offered.

and honest information regarding their diagnosis, fertility prospects, and long-term health during what is a very difficult time in their life.

Most women want to know what caused them to develop POF and in the majority of cases there is no clear answer. Genetic studies may shed some light on this area in the future.

There is currently a lot of interest in predicting the timing of menopause using AMH and other markers of ovarian reserve. This would enable women, especially those with a family history of POF, to assess their risk of POF. However, this is not possible at the moment, especially in young women.

It is vital that women with POF are advised to take oestrogen replacement until the average age of menopause [51,52]. This will treat vasomotor symptoms, prevent bone loss, and reduce their risk of cardiovascular disease. Education is extremely important as this is the factor which most strongly influences a woman's decision to take and to continue oestrogen replacement.

A Final Word from the Expert

One of the greatest difficulties in managing POF is making the initial diagnosis. It is often not considered when younger women present with irregular cycles or amenorrhoea. Taking a thorough history is important, as is conducting a hormone profile in order to establish the diagnosis. Management at a specialist clinic where there are menopause experts as well as fertility experts is ideal. These women require long-term management, and denial of the diagnosis is often a major hurdle to overcome in the beginning.

References

1. Pitkin J, Rees MCP, Gray S, Lumsden MA, Marsden J, Stevenson JC, *et al*. Management of premature menopause. *Menopause Int* 2007;13(1):44–5.
2. Knauff EAH, Eijkemans MJC, Lambalk CB, ten Kate-Booij MJ, Hoek A, Beerendonk CCM, *et al*. Anti-Mullerian hormone, inhibin B, and antral follicle count in young women with ovarian failure. *J Clin Endocr Metab* 2009;94(3):786–92.
3. Henrich JB, Hughes JP, Kaufman SC, Brody DJ, Curtin LR. Limitations of follicle-stimulating hormone in assessing menopause status: findings from the National Health and Nutrition Examination Survey (NHANES 1999–2000)*. *Menopause* 2006;13(2):171–7.
4. van Kasteren YM, Hundscheid RD, Smits AP, Cremers FP, van Zonneveld P, Braat DD. Familial idiopathic premature ovarian failure: an overrated and underestimated genetic disease? *Hum Reprod* 1999 Oct;14(10):2455–9.
5. Vujovic S. Aetiology of premature ovarian failure. *Menopause Int* 2009 Jun;15(2):72–5.
6. Sherman SL. Premature ovarian failure in the fragile X syndrome. *Am J Med Genet* 2000 Fall;97(3):189–94.
7. Luborsky J, Llanes B, Davies S, Binor Z, Radwanska E, Pong R. Ovarian autoimmunity: greater frequency of autoantibodies in premature menopause and unexplained infertility than in the general population. *Clinical Immunology*. 1999 Mar;90(3):368–74.
8. Johnell O, Kanis JA, Oden A, Johansson H, De Laet C, Delmas P, *et al*. Predictive value of BMD for hip and other fractures. *J Bone Miner Res* 2005;20(7):1185–94.
9. Jones KP, Ravnikar VA, Tulchinsky D, Schiff I. Comparison of bone density in amenorrheic women due to athletics, weight loss, and premature menopause. *Obstet Gynecol* 1985;66(1):5–8.

10. Miller KK, Klibanski A. Clinical review 106: Amenorrheic bone loss. *J Clin Endocr Metabol* 1999;84(6):1775–83.

11. Uygur D, Sengul O, Bayar D, Erdinc S, Batioglu S, Mollamahmutoglu L. Bone loss in young women with premature ovarian failure. *Arch Gynecol Obstet* 2005;273(1): 17–19.

12. van Der Voort DJM, van Der Weijer PHM, Barentsen R. Early menopause: increased fracture risk at older age. *Osteoporosis International* 2003;14(6):525–30.

13. Wells G, Tugwell P, Shea B, Guyatt G, Peterson J, Zytaruk N, *et al*. Meta-analyses of therapies for postmenopausal osteoporosis. V. Meta-analysis of the efficacy of hormone replacement therapy in treating and preventing osteoporosis in postmenopausal women. *Endocr Rev* 2002;23(4):529–39.

14. Rossouw JE, Anderson GL, Prentice RL, LaCroix AZ, Kooperberg C, Stefanick ML, *et al*. Risks and benefits of estrogen plus progestin in healthy postmenopausal women: principal results From the Women's Health Initiative randomized controlled trial. *JAMA* 2002;288(3):321–33.

15. Kanis JA, Johnell O, Oden A, Johansson H, McCloskey E. FRAX and the assessment of fracture probability in men and women from the UK. *Osteoporosis International* 2008;19(4):385–97.

16. Grodstein F, Manson JE, Stampfer MJ. Hormone therapy and coronary heart disease: the role of time since menopause and age at hormone initiation.[see comment]. *J Women's Health* 2006 Jan-Feb;15(1):35–44.

17. Rossouw JE, Prentice RL, Manson JE, Wu L, Barad D, Barnabei VM, *et al*. Postmenopausal hormone therapy and risk of cardiovascular disease by age and years since menopause. *JAMA* 2007;297(13):1465–77.

18. Atsma F, Bartelink M-LEL, Grobbee DE, van der Schouw YT. Postmenopausal status and early menopause as independent risk factors for cardiovascular disease: a meta-analysis. *Menopause* 2006;13(2):265–79.

19. van der Schouw YT, van der Graaf Y, Steyerberg EW, Eijkemans JC, Banga JD. Age at menopause as a risk factor for cardiovascular mortality. *Lancet* 1996 Mar 16;347(9003):714–18.

20. Welt CK, Hall JE, Adams JM, Taylor AE. Relationship of estradiol and inhibin to the follicle-stimulating hormone variability in hypergonadotropic hypogonadism or premature ovarian failure. *J Clin Endocr Metab* 2005;90(2):826–30.

21. van Kasteren YM, Schoemaker J. Premature ovarian failure: a systematic review on therapeutic interventions to restore ovarian function and achieve pregnancy. *Hum Reprod Update* 1999;5(5):483–92.

22. Bidet M, Bachelot A, Touraine P. Premature ovarian failure: predictability of intermittent ovarian function and response to ovulation induction agents. *Curr Opin Obstet Gynecol* 2008 Aug;20(4):416–20.

23. Opinions survey report No. 41. Contraception and Sexual Health Office for National Statistics 2008–2009.

24. Wittenberger MD, Hagerman RJ, Sherman SL, McConkie-Rosell A, Welt CK, Rebar RW, *et al*. The FMR1 premutation and reproduction. *Fertil Steril* 2007 Mar;87(3):456–65.

25. Hagerman RJ, Leavitt BR, Farzin F, Jacquemont S, Greco CM, Brunberg JA, *et al*. Fragile-X-associated tremor/ataxia syndrome (FXTAS) in females with the FMR1 premutation. *Am J Hum Genet* 2004 May;74(5):1051–6.

26. Murray A, Webb J, Grimley S, Conway G, Jacobs P. Studies of FRAXA and FRAXE in women with premature ovarian failure. *J Med Genet* [Research Support, Non-U.S. Gov't]. 1998 Aug;35(8):637–40.

27. Corrigan EC, Raygada MJ, Vanderhoof VH, Nelson LM. A woman with spontaneous premature ovarian failure gives birth to a child with fragile X syndrome. *Fertil Steril* 2005;84(5):1508.

21 Treating urinary incontinence: an evolving challenge for us all

Eduard Cortes and Louise Webster

ⓘ **Expert Commentary** Con Kelleher

Case history

A 61-year-old woman was referred to urogynaecology clinic by her general practitioner, complaining of a five-year history of worsening urinary frequency and a dragging sensation in her vagina. She described urgency to pass urine, associated with occasional urge urinary incontinence, increased daytime frequency of micturition, and nocturia three to five times/night. She also reported episodes of urinary leakage and dribbling after sneezing, coughing, and laughing. The social difficulties this condition presented were expressed, including becoming increasingly house-bound 'in case accidents happen', and the continual need to wear sanitary protection. She had also noticed that sexual intercourse had become more uncomfortable during penetration, and this, together with her urinary symptoms, had worsened considerably over the previous weeks. She did not complain of dysuria or haematuria. Her bowels functioned normally and she did not experience abdominal pain. Her urine cultures sent by the GP had always been negative.

She was Para 3 having had one forceps delivery during which she suffered a second-degree tear, and two spontaneous vaginal deliveries. Her BMI was 30 and she had no significant past medical history. Her past surgical history included a total abdominal hysterectomy for heavy periods together with a Burch colposuspension for urodynamic stress incontinence at the age of 45. She reached the menopause at age 48 and had never been on hormonal replacement therapy.

⭐ **Learning point** Burch colposuspension

Although first described by Dr JC Burch in 1961 [8], the Tanagho modification is now considered the standard method for this operation. Indicated for urodynamic stress incontinence in association with a cystourethrocoele, the goal of the retropubic procedure is to suspend and stabilize the urethra so that the urethrovesical junction (UVJ) and proximal urethra are replaced intra-abdominally. The theoretical mechanism of action of colposuspension is the anatomic restitution of the normal pressure transmission to the urethra during increased intra-abdominal pressure. The more modern urethral hammock hypothesis of Delancey [9] would also explain the mechanism of action of colposuspension whereby the sub-urethral hammock is shortened and therefore more supportive of the urethra.

The procedure is performed via a low transverse suprapubic incision or laparoscopically and sutures are placed alongside the bladder neck in the vagina and attached to the ipsilateral iliopectineal ligament (Figure 21.1).

(continued)

The subjective and objective cure rate of colposuspension is reported at around 90% [8]. Prior to the introduction and widespread use of the mid urethral tension-free tapes, there was a brief interest in the procedure of laparoscopic colposuspension although this did not appear to be as successful as the TVT procedure [10]. When looking at the cost-effectiveness of laparoscopic versus open colposuspension, there was no advantage of the laparoscopic procedure 6 months post-operatively [11]. The Burch colposuspension remains a valuable surgical alternative in younger patients and those patients with persistent USI following failure of less-invasive surgical options such as tension-free vaginal tapes.

✪ Learning point Post void residual volumes

Post void residual (PVR) volume is the volume left in the bladder at the completion of micturition. If the PVR is high, the bladder is emptying incompletely (which may represent outflow obstruction or disordered intrinsic bladder function).

High PVR (>50 mls[0]) can be associated with the following conditions [15]:

- Bladder outflow obstruction.
- Pelvic floor prolapse can lead to mechanical outlet obstruction of the bladder and is associated with a progressive decline of maximum and average urine flow rates. Elevated PVR is one of the hallmarks of such obstruction [16].
- Other causes of outflow obstruction include a bladder stone, urethral, or meatal blockage.
- Bladder hypocontractility.
- Bladder diverticulum.

Chronic urine retention has been defined as a non-painful bladder with a chronic, high PVR of 200 ml average [17]. In patients with significant vaginal prolapse, it is important to rule out chronic urinary retention presenting as stress incontinence or OAB.

A high PVR of urine (>50 mls) has clinical implications for the upper and lower urinary tracts; the incidence of recurrent UTI is increased in patients with high PVR (often presenting with symptoms mimicking those of OAB). Preventing high PVR (and subsequent recurrent UTI) can help prevent complications to the upper urinary tract level such as pyelonephritis and upper urinary tract dilatation which may have long-term implications for renal function, in particular for the elderly patient.

✚ Clinical tip The Modified Oxford scale [14]

Patients attending pelvic floor muscle training are instructed by their physiotherapist to contract their pelvic floor in an inward and upward lifting manoeuvre. With two fingers inserted in the vagina, the physiotherapist feels for the patient's ability to contract the levator ani. This can be recorded according to the Modified Oxford scale in four grades:

0 = no contraction
1 = flicker
2 = weak
3 = moderate contraction
4 = good contraction

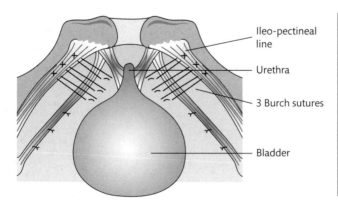
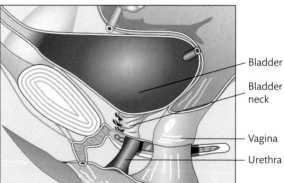

Ileo-pectineal line
Urethra
3 Burch sutures
Bladder

Bladder
Bladder neck
Vagina
Urethra

Figure 21.1 Burch colposuspension technique.
Two to four sutures are inserted bilaterally, lateral to the urethra and anchored onto the ileo-pectineal line (A). Elevation of the vagina with a gloved hand in the vagina helps with tying the sutures. When tying the sutures, no tension should be present. The goal is to approximate the vaginal wall to the lateral pelvic wall, where it will become adherent with healing (B).

> ★ **Learning point** Lower urinary tract symptoms
>
> Lower urinary tract symptoms (LUTS) are common, affecting millions of women throughout the world, with a reported prevalence in European countries estimated as high as 35% [2]. The joint International Urogynaecology & International Continence Society (ICS) standardized the terminology used to describe lower urinary tract function in 2010 [3].
>
> LUTS are a subjective indicator of a disease or change in condition as perceived by the patient, carer, or partner, and may lead him/her to seek help from healthcare professionals.
>
> - Urgency is the complaint of a sudden compelling desire to pass urine which is difficult to defer.
> - Urge urinary incontinence is the complaint of involuntary leakage accompanied by or immediately preceded by urgency.
> - Increased daytime frequency is the complaint by the patient who considers that he/she voids too often by day.
> - Nocturia is the complaint that the individual has to wake at night one or more times to void.
> - Stress urinary incontinence is the complaint of involuntary leakage on effort or exertion, or on sneezing or coughing.
> - Mixed urinary incontinence is the complaint of involuntary leakage associated with urgency, and also with exertion, effort, sneezing, or coughing. In the absence of underlying pathological or metabolic conditions (such as UTI, fistulae, polyuria, and neurological conditions), incontinence can be broadly divided into stress incontinence and urgency incontinence (characterized by the associated symptom of urinary urgency).
>
> Symptoms may correlate poorly with diagnosis and history alone is regarded as a poor predictor of underlying pathology particularly when the symptoms are complex. Risk factors for urinary incontinence are shown in Table 21.1.

> ★ **Learning point** Health-related quality of life (HRQoL) tools
>
> Quality of life questionnaires are almost always used in clinical trials of treatment for lower urinary tract dysfunction. These questionnaires are also of value in clinical practice; particularly those such as the Kings Health Questionnaire [1] which combines a symptom and quality of life questionnaire. They are usually multi-item questionnaires, covering various domains related to the patient's life, including sleeping pattern, emotions, social limitations, sexual, or work problems.
>
> Questionnaires available include:
>
> - Screening questionnaires
> - Symptom assessment questionnaires (female and male)
> - Condition specific assessment questionnaires (e.g. OAB, nocturia)
> - Symptom-bother questionnaires
> - Treatment satisfaction questionnaires
> - Sexual function questionnaires
> - Quality of life questionnaires

Table 21.1 Risk factors for urinary incontinence (UI, including stress, mixed, and urge), and stress urinary incontinence (SUI) in middle-age women [7]

	Relative Risk (95% CI)	
	UI	SUI
Age > 40	2.16 (1.86–2.57)	2.18 (1.66–2.87)
Pregnancy	2.22 (1.71–2.87)	2.36 (1.55–3.58)
Previous vaginal delivery	2.15 (1.72–2.69)	2.47 (1.7–3.59)
Vaginal delivery versus caesarean section	1.77 (1.19–2.62)	2.43 (1.17–5.05)
Postpartum UI	2.57 (2.22–2.96)	2.78 (2.14–3.61)
Hysterectomy	1.52 (1.11–2.08)	2.83 (1.93–4.15)

> **✚ Clinical tip** Urine dip testing
>
> - Due to overlapping of symptoms between urinary tract infection (UTI) and other causes of LUTS, clinicians should always exclude a diagnosis of UTI.
> - All patients with a history of LUTS should have a urine dipstick at their first appointment, and if positive for leucocytes or nitrites, a mid-stream urine (MSU) sample should be sent for culture and sensitivity.
> - If a diagnosis of UTI is established, the patient should be treated with an appropriate antibiotic.
> - A repeat MSU is advised following treatment to check for the clearance of any infection.
> - In the presence of haematuria or glycosuria, the presence of other systemic or urinary tract pathology should be excluded.

> **❝ Expert comment**
>
> By the time women with urinary incontinence (UI) seek treatment from health professionals, they have usually tried different strategies to mitigate the impact of urinary symptoms/incontinence on their day-to-day activities. These non-medical coping strategies include fluid restriction, regular toileting, toilet mapping, wearing a pad, or restricting outdoor activities [4]. In a survey of all women with UI, 42% used protective pads, 33% did regular toileting pre-emptively, and 30% toilet-mapped their outdoor activities. Of those who were incontinent, only 23% fluid restricted, and 20% regularly performed pelvic floor exercises [5,6].

> **❝ Expert comment**
>
> Many different questionnaires have been designed for the purpose of clinical trials and clinical practice to assess urinary symptoms and the bother they cause. In our clinic the patients are sent the questionnaire to complete at home and bring with them when they attend the hospital. A full review of the many different measures available can be found in the latest International Consultation on Incontinence (ICI) triennial review. A modular approach to questionnaire administration for the assessment of LUTS is available from the ICI via their website: <http://www.ICIQ.net>.

> **❝ Expert comment**
>
> Despite its widespread recognition in the international forums as a standard tool for the classification of prolapse, the POP-Q system only appeared in 30% of the literature regarding pelvic floor support and is used only by 40% of the members of the above international societies. This is, however, likely to change and for the purpose of any future presented or published studies of prolapse treatment, POPQ scoring is likely to be required [13].

In order to assess the severity of her symptoms and their impact on her quality of life, the patient was asked to fill in the King's Health questionnaire (KHQ) [1], a condition specific Quality of Life (QoL) questionnaire for lower urinary tract symptoms (LUTS).

Abdominal examination revealed a low transverse suprapubic scar with no other abnormal findings. Pelvic floor prolapse grading was assessed using the pelvic organ prolapse quantification (POP-Q) scoring system with the patient in lithotomy and left lateral position using a Sims speculum. Examination revealed atrophic vaginal changes, with a well-supported anterior vaginal wall (Ba -7; Aa -3), and a stage 2 rectoenterocele (D -2; Bp 0; Ap +2). Urinary leakage was demonstrated on coughing. Using the Modified Oxford scale, digital examination of pelvic-floor muscle strength was graded as level 2. Urine dipstick was negative. Post-micturition urine residual volume was assessed using a bladder scan showing volumes between 30 ml and 50 ml of urine.

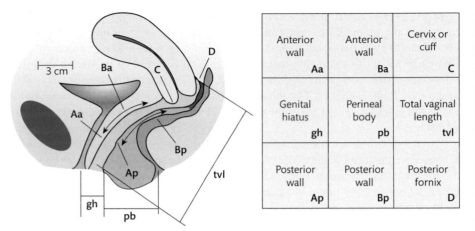

Figure 21.2 Diagram of POP-Q prolapse scoring system.

Reprinted from *American Journal of Obstetrics and Gynecology*, 175:1, Richard C. Bump *et al.*, The standardization of terminology of female pelvic organ prolapse and pelvic floor dysfunction, 10–17. Copyright 1996 with permission from Elsevier.

Point description range of values

Aa Anterior vaginal wall 3 cm proximal to the hymen –3 cm to +3 cm
Ba Most distal position of the remaining upper anterior vaginal wall –3 cm to +tvl
C Most distal edge of cervix or vaginal cuff scar
D Posterior fornix (N/A if post-hysterectomy)
Ap Posterior vaginal wall 3 cm proximal to the hymen –3 cm to +3 cm
Bp Most distal position of the remaining upper posterior vaginal wall –3 cm to +tvl
Genital hiatus (gh) Measured from middle of external urethral meatus to posterior midline hymen
Perineal body (pb) Measured from posterior margin of gh to middle of anal opening
Total vaginal length (tvl) Depth of vagina when point D or C is reduced to normal position

POP-Q Staging Criteria

Stage 0 Aa, Ap, Ba, Bp=−3 cm and C or D ≤ (tvl−2) cm
Stage I Stage 0 criteria not met and leading edge <−1 cm
Stage II Leading edge ≥−1 cm but ≤+1 cm
Stage III Leading edge >+1 cm but < + (tvl−2) cm
Stage IV Leading edge ≥ + (tvl−2) cm

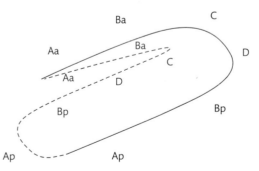

Figure 21.3 Diagram showing prolapse changes described in the study patient (red) compared with the normal anatomical distribution of the POP-Q.

−3 Aa	−8 Ba	−9 C
2 GH	3 PB	10 TVL
−3 Ap	−10 Bp	−10 D

Example of normal POP-Q grading in the absence of prolapse.

−3 Aa	−6 Ba	−6 C
4 GH	2 PB	8 TVL
+2 Ap	0 Bp	No D as no uterus

POP-Q table in the study patient in the absence of the uterus.

Expert comment

The aim of the six-week review is to see the progress in the management of the urinary symptoms, encourage the patient to continue the treatment program and where necessary to increase the dose of anti-muscarinic medication depending on the needs of the patient and the presence of anti-muscarinic side effects. Trials have shown that approximately 50% of patients commenced on the lowest dose of anti-muscarinic therapy have required an increase in dose [18,19]. These were most frequently the patients with the more severe symptoms.

Mrs X was asked to keep a voiding diary over three days. This showed urinary leakage associated with and without urgency, an average of 10 voiding episodes during the day, three episodes at night, and a maximum voided volume (MVV) of 320 ml of urine (Figure 21.4, day 1). She was seen by the continence nurse specialist who started conservative management with bladder training and pelvic floor exercises. The patient was offered antimuscarinic therapy and a plan was made to review her in six weeks in clinic with a new completed bladder diary.

After 3 months on antimuscarinic therapy, the patient returned to clinic with a recently completed bladder diary. This showed seven to eight voiding episodes during day time, between zero and one micturitions at night time, leakage with straining maneuvers, and a MVV of 400 ml of urine (Figure 21.4, day 2). Post void residual volume measured with a bladder scan in clinic showed no significant residual. The severity of her urgency scores showed improvement. In view of the

Day 1				
Time	In	Out	Wet	Urgency
07.00		320	X	E
08.00	Cup of coffee			
09.00	250 ml water	100		B
10.00				
11.00	Cup of coffee	125	X	coughing
12.00		90	X	E
13.00	Cola 500 ml			
14.00		250		B
15.00	Cup of tea	300		C
16.00		200		C
17.00	500 ml water		X	coughing
18.00		300	X	E
19.00	Cup of tea			
20.00		250		B
21.00	Glass of wine 250 ml			
22.00		150		D
23.00	250 ml water			
00.00			X	coughing
01.00		310		D
02.00				
03.00	250 ml water	220		D
04.00				
05.00		200		C
06.00				

Day 2				
Time	In	Out	Wet	Urgency
07.00		390		B
08.00	Cup of coffee			
09.00	and milk with cornflakes			
10.00			X	coughing
11.00	500 ml water			
12.00		300		C
13.00	orange juice			
14.00			X	coughing
15.00	Cup of tea	400		B
16.00				
17.00	250 ml water	250		B
18.00				
19.00	Glass of milk			
20.00		220		B
21.00				
22.00			X	coughing
23.00		380		A
00.00				
01.00				
02.00				
03.00				
04.00				
05.00				
06.00				

A. I felt no need to empty my bladder, but did so for other reasons
B. I could postpone voiding (emptying my bladder) as long as necessary without fear of wetting myself
C. I could postpone voiding for a short while, without fear of wetting myself
D. I could not postpone voiding, but had to rush to the toilet in order not to wet myself
E. I leaked before arriving to the toilet

APPENDIX 1

Figure 21.4 Bladder diary.

❌ **Learning point** Bladder diaries

Bladder diaries (Figure 21.4) are valuable diagnostic tools for the investigation of patients with LUTS. Although electronic versions are available, most are designed in paper format. Patients are required to document their type, time, and volume of fluid intake, and voiding episodes as well as any urinary incontinence episodes associated with or without urinary urgency, or effort, or exertion (such as coughing, sneezing, etc.). As well as describing patterns of dysfunctional voiding, they can also provide clinicians with information regarding compulsive or excessive fluid intake behaviors. They also measure the largest volume(s) of urine voided during a single micturition (Maximal Voided Volume, MVV). This is particularly useful to differentiate between nocturia and nocturnal polyuria, defined as voided volumes at night greater than 20% in the young adult, or 33% in the elderly, of the overall 24-hour urine output [20].

The optimal duration of the bladder diary has not yet been standardized, however studies have shown patient's compliance is reduced with longer diary requirements [21]. In practice, a three-day diary is adequate if it captures days that represent the patient's 'normality', especially if it is completed on days with varied activities.

As well as a being a diagnostic tool, longitudinal diaries can be used to document response to treatment and are an objective measure for clinical research outcome measures.

➕ **Clinical tip** Conservative management of LUTS

- Fluid restriction (daily total fluid intake should be 1500–3000 ml).
- Restrict to 2 litres/day or 24 mls/Kg if frequency is a primary symptom.
- Avoid caffeinated drinks (although avoidance of caffeinated drinks does not improve UI, it does help to improve symptoms such as urgency and frequency).
- Timing of fluids (limit evening fluids if nocturia is troubling).
- Weight loss advice (weight loss > 5% in obese women improves UI).
- Stop smoking.
- Treat constipation.
- Pelvic floor muscle training (PFMT).
- Bladder retraining (especially for OAB).
- Topical oestrogen replacement therapy may be of benefit to the post-menopausal woman [22].

❌ **Learning point** Pelvic floor muscle training (PFMT)

First described by Margaret Morris in 1936 and later popularized by Arnold Kegel [23], who demonstrated that women could improve their stress incontinence through pelvic floor muscle training and exercise. The goal is to teach patients how to enhance urethral closure and bladder-neck support by voluntary coordinated contraction of their pelvic floor muscles.

There is wide variation in PFMT regimes and the optimal regimen has yet to be determined.

In general, good results are achieved using 45–50 PFMT exercises per day. To avoid muscle fatigue, patients are usually advised to spread their exercises in two to three sessions per day.

Accompanying teaching techniques using biofeedback, digital palpation, or electrical stimulation give patients more accurate perception of which muscles to contract.

❝ **Expert comment**

A recent Cochrane systematic review showed that women who did PFMT also reported better continence-specific quality of life, experienced fewer incontinence episodes per day, and less leakage on a short office-based pad test. It concluded that PFMT should be included as first-line conservative management for women with stress, urge, or mixed urinary incontinence. Variations in training regime, and length of treatment require further studies [24].

✅ **Evidence base** Bladder training (BT)

BT is a treatment programme designed to gradually increase a patient's bladder control. Patients are asked to void either according to a fixed voiding schedule, or alternatively, may be encouraged to follow a schedule established by their own bladder diary/voiding chart (habit training).'Timed

(continued)

voiding' is voiding initiated by the patient. Timed and habit voiding are recommended to patients who can void independently. Timed voiding reduces leakage episodes in cognitively intact women. 'Prompted voiding' (voiding initiated by the caregiver), is an alternative in cognitively impaired patients.

- BT alone is as effective in controlling UUI and nocturnal incontinence as anti-muscarinic therapy [25–28].
- The combination of BT and anti-muscarinic drug therapy is more effective than either treatment alone, and is the recommended treatment for OAB [29].
- Two RCTs comparing BT with no intervention found that UI could be improved, but not cured, by timed bladder voiding at intervals of between 2.5 and 4 hours [30].

✦ Expert comment

Conservative management requires significant input from a trained individual, a high degree of motivation from the patient, and time for improvement to take place. The National Institute for Clinical Excellence (NICE) recommended in 2006 that women who present with urinary symptoms for the first time should not be referred for urodynamic investigation before a trial of conservative therapy [31]. In patients presenting with a history of mixed urinary incontinence, it is standard practice to treat OAB symptoms first as these are often harder to treat and could be the underlying cause for the patients stress incontinence. If treatment fails, secondary adverse events develop or the patient has had previous continence surgery, urodynamic assessment is indicated.

Overall, it is estimated that only 60% of patients with a diagnosis of OAB will demonstrate detrusor muscle over-activity during urodynamic investigation [32].

✪ Learning point   Urodynamic testing

This consists of:

- Uroflowmetry (measurement of volume of urine voided and flow rate (ml/second)) in its simplest form is a strain gauge on which is placed a receptacle and as the patient voids, a computer plot of rate of increase in weight of the receptacle over time is measured. The peak flow rate (Qmax) and the appearance of the flow curve is used to assess the presence of voiding dysfunction.

- Standard cystometry

  - Filling cystometry involves the placement of a urethral catheter with either an internal or external pressure transducer. Bladder pressure (pves) is recorded while the bladder is filled naturally or by means of a pump. Normal saline is usually used as the filling medium. An abdominal catheter is used to record abdominal pressure synchronously; this is most commonly inserted rectally (or vaginally) above the anal margin. Urodynamic equipment records vesical and abdominal pressure (pabd) and calculates the detrusor pressure (pdet) from these (pves _ pabd ¼ pdet).
  - Voiding cystometry provides information about voiding patterns and flow rates; however, additional information concerning voiding pressures is obtained with voiding cystometry. This additional information enables more accurate diagnosis of voiding dysfunction.

- Video-urodynamics are the combined measurement of cystometric parameters together with radiographic visualization of the urinary tract. This is usually reserved for more complex cases, and simple cystometry without radiographic imaging is suitable for the majority of patients [38]. Fluoroscopy will allow the visualization of anatomical abnormalities of the lower and possibly the upper urinary tracts, such as the presence of vesico-ureteral reflux, fistulae, bladder diverticulae, urethra hypermobility, and bladder trabeculation.

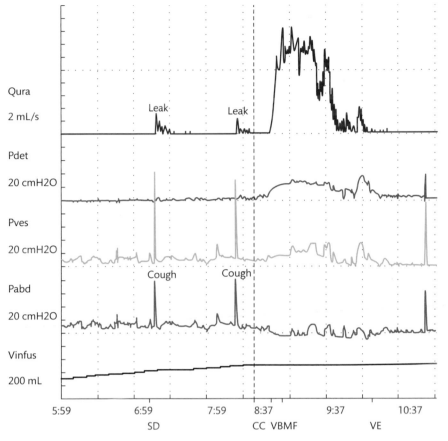

Figure 21.5 Urodynamic stress incontinence. Increasing abdominal pressure (Pabd) during coughing are followed or accompanied by leakage [Qura—urine flow; Pdet—detrusor pressure; Pves—bladder (vesical) pressure; Pabd—abdominal pressure; Vinfus—volume of fluid infused in the bladder.) Note: the test is routinely conducted at full cystometric capacity (full bladder).

Reproduced from Sarris, Bewley, and Agnihotri, *Training in Obstetrics and Gynaecology*, 2009, with permission from Oxford University Press.

significant persistence of her stress urinary incontinence, and her previous continence surgery (Burch colposuspension), she was referred for video-urodynamic assessment. Her video-urodynamic imaging showed both normal bladder capacity and compliance, no detrusor overactivity, moderate urodynamic stress incontinence (USI) (Figure 21.5), and normal pressure flow studies with no post void residual at the end of the investigation.

Videourodynamic studies confirmed the diagnosis of moderate USI (Figure 21.7). There were no involuntary detrusor muscle contractions detected during the filling phase. Following discussion with the patient regarding her surgical options and associated risks, the patient opted for a tension-free vaginal tape obturator (TVT-O) and posterior repair (Figure 21.8). Two days after surgery, the indwelling urethral catheter was removed, the woman voided spontaneously to completion, and was discharged home. At the two months' follow-up visit, the woman was still dry and asymptomatic, thus she was discharged back to her GP.

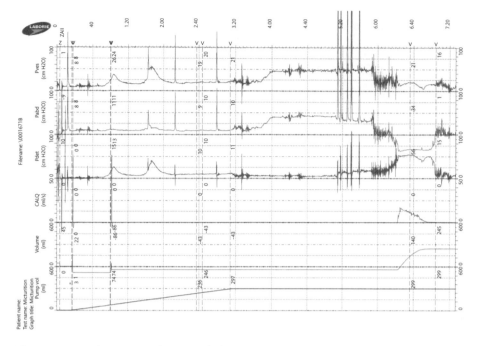

Figure 21.6 Urodynamic trace (cystogram) of a patient with detrusor over-activity characterized by involuntary detrusor contractions (Pdet) during the filling phase which may be defined as systolic or provoked, with subsequent increase in bladder pressure (Pves), and stable abdominal pressure (Pabd).

> ✪ **Learning point** Pharmacotherapy in LUTS
>
> Antimuscarinic (AM) drug therapy (Table 21.2) in combination with bladder retraining and fluid intake advice is the mainstay of treatment for OAB. AMs act by blocking the muscarinic receptors in the bladder wall (both at detrusor and urothelium level) during the storage phase of the micturition cycle. This reduces both muscle contractibility and detrusor sensation. The different antimuscarinic agents available differ in their pharmacokinetic properties (half-life and lipid solubility); pharmacological profiles (receptor affinity and mode of action); and formulation (immediate or extended release, topical, or oral).
>
> Side effects at sites distant from the bladder are a major drawback to successful AM therapy. The most common side effects are dry mouth and constipation. Non-selective antimuscarinic drugs (e.g. oxybutynin) which cross the blood–brain barrier can also have effects on cognitive function, a particular concern in elderly patients who may already have a degree of cognitive impairment. Care must also be exercised when patients have narrow-angle glaucoma.
>
> There are five types of muscarinic receptors. On human detrusor muscle cells, M2 receptors are predominant in number over M3 receptors, however, the M3 receptors are responsible for the normal micturition contraction. The role for the M2 receptors in bladder function has not been fully established but they may play a role in relaxation of the detruror [33]. Newer AM drugs have tried to achieve greater M3 selectivity to reduce unwanted side effects as a result of stimulation of other muscarinic subtypes. Unfortunately, absolute receptor selectivity or bladder selectivity whilst desirable is not possible to achieve. More recent antimuscarinics employ sustained release formulations allowing once-daily dosing which improves patient compliance, and flexible dose escalation allowing drug-dose titration for patients with less responsive symptoms.

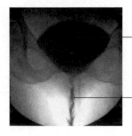

— Full bladder as seen during video-urodynamics using contrast solution

— Loss of contrast solution seen during coughing at maximum cystometric capacity.

Figure 21.7 Voiding cystourethrography showing urodynamic stress incontinence (USI).

Reprinted from *Journal of Urology* 2000; 163:5, 1510–12. Neyssan Tebyani, Percutaneous Needle Bladder Neck Suspension for the Treatment of Stress Urinary Urinary Incontinence in Women: Long-Term Results, Copyright 2000 with permission from Elsevier.

Table 21.2 Common antimuscarinics used in everyday clinical practice

Name	Pharmacokinetic properties	Pharmacological profile	Formulation
Oxybutynin	Tertiary amine muscarinic receptor antagonist	Extensive upper GI and hepatic metabolism	Immediate release form associated with significant side effects, but available as once daily oral form, a gel, and a patch
Solifenacin	Tertiary amine muscarinic receptor antagonist	Terminal half-life 50 hrs with 90% bio-availability. Significant hepatic metabolism	Oral once daily controlled released dosage 5–10 mg
Fesoterodine	Prodrug converted to active metabolite 5-hydroxymethyltoterodine (5-HMT) following ingestion	Metabolized in the liver primarily, but significant renal excretion prior to metabolism and >15% not converted to 5-HMT	Oral once daily 4–8 mg
Darifenacin	Selective M3 receptor antagonist	Absolute bioavailability 90%	Oral once daily controlled release 7.5-15 mg
Trospium	Quarternary ammonium compound with antimuscarinic actions and no selectivity for muscarinic receptor subtypes	Bio-availablity <10%, but no cognitive side effects	Oral twice daily 20 mg

❝ Expert comment

The Fourth International Consultation on Incontinence [34] provides a thorough and up-to-date review of the available AMs and their published data from clinical studies and clinical trials. Ultimately, the choice of agent depends upon local and national guidelines, cost, and personal preference. From a patient perspective, a once-daily formulation with the fewest side effects and greatest efficacy would guide personal choice.

More recently, a once-daily-only beta-3 adrenergic receptor agonist, mirabegron 50 mg, has been released for the treatment of OAB. Several phase III studies [35–37] to-date have demonstrated good safety and efficacy with a relative absence of side effects experienced with antimuscarinic medications due to its different mode of action. Recent studies suggest that a combination of an antimuscarinic and a beta-3 adrenoreceptor agonist may offer superior efficacy with a better side-effect profile than a high-dose antimuscarinic alone. Further studies are awaited.

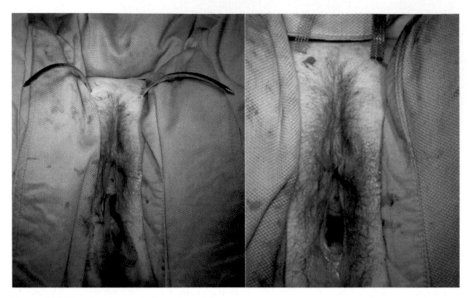

Figure 21.8 Tension-free vaginal tape insertion.

Reproduced from Sarris, Bewley, and Agnihotri, *Training in Obstetrics and Gynaecology*, 2009 with permission from Oxford University Press.

> ⊗ **Learning point** Surgical options for previous failed surgery for USI
>
> Video-urodynamic evaluation is an essential part of the investigation of these patients. The data available on repeat surgery for incontinence are limited and patient numbers are usually too small to draw conclusions from published studies [38]. The success of repeat continence surgery is less than that of primary surgery. The choice of repeat procedure would depend upon the urodynamic diagnosis, the mobility of the urethra, patient factors, and the need for any concomitant pelvic surgery, as well as surgeon's familiarity and confidence.

> ⊗ **Learning point** Tension-free vaginal tapes (TVT)
>
> The mid urethral tension-free vaginal tape was introduced in 1996 and has gained in popularity worldwide since that time [39]. It would now be the normal first-line surgical treatment for urodynamic stress incontinence. The procedure is less invasive, equally efficacious, and less costly than colposuspension.
>
> The tapes can be inserted either retropubically (Figure 21.9), or through the obturator foramina (transobturator, Figure 21.10). In this particular case, Mrs X had undergone a prior colposuspension and therefore it was likely that there would be significant scarring in the retropubic space. A transobturator tape was a more logical choice to avoid adhesions and to minimize the risk of bladder injury. The cure rates of both procedures are similar (Table 21.3).
>
> Other treatment options such as single incision and adjustable slings, bulking agents, or artificial sphincters have more limited indications and variable successful rates.

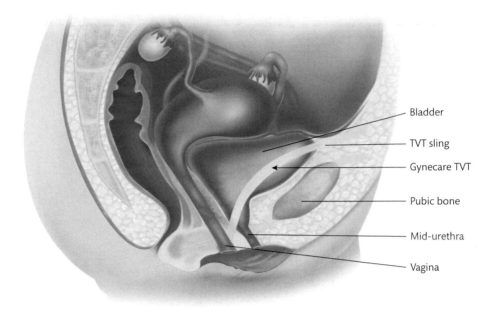

Bladder

TVT sling

Gynecare TVT

Pubic bone

Mid-urethra

Vagina

Figure 21.9 Schematic representation of retropubic insertion of a TVT. Left and right trocars are placed through the endopelvic fascia and along the posterior aspect of the pubic bone until the trocars appear through the suprapubic skin on each side.

Table 21.3 Comparison of outcome after TVT and TVT-O [40–42]

	TVT	TVT-O
Patient reported cure rates	77%	77%
Clinically reported cure rates	85%	85%
Voiding dysfunction	7%	4%
Bladder perforation	5%	0.3%
De-novo urgency	6%	1.7%
Chronic perineal pain	3%	7%

✚ Clinical tip Preparation for a mid urethral tape (MUT) procedure

Women should be adequately counselled preoperatively regarding:

- Possible voiding difficulties
- De novo detrusor over-activity
- Bladder injury
- Tape erosion (uncommon, and can be related to the experience of the operator)
- Most tapes are inserted as a day-case procedure or with an overnight stay
- Commonly performed under spinal anaesthesia/general
- Groin pain if TVT-O is performed
- Re-operation to remove the tape if needed
- Infection
- bleeding
- Future mode of delivery if the family is not completed yet
- Follow-up is usually planned for 6–8 weeks after surgery

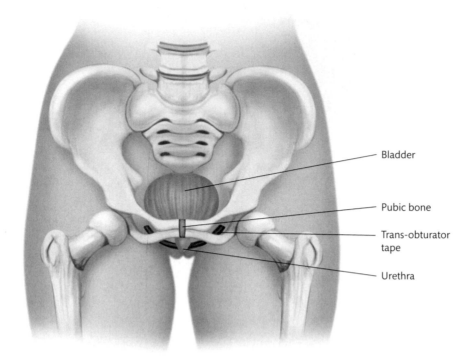

Figure 21.10 Schematic representation of trans-obturator insertion of a TVT-O. Small incisions are placed in the groins (one on each side), and the same small incision is made in the vagina under the urethra, allowing the mesh tape to be placed under the urethra in the correct position without having to pass needles blindly through the retropubic space and the abdominal wall.

Discussion

Lower urinary tract dysfunction including urinary incontinence is common and a significant burden on both individuals and society. Despite the clearly detrimental effect on quality of life, relatively few women seek clinical care for LUTS. In a recent European study [43], it was estimated that only 31 % of affected women had consulted their doctor about their urinary problem. The factors usually associated with seeking help include young age, longstanding duration, and frequency of symptoms, and degree of inconvenience. Willingness to take long-term medication and discussions with other sufferers scored highest as predictors for seeking treatment [44]. Identified barriers for seeking help include urinary symptoms being considered a normal part of ageing or childbirth, or perceiving that medical intervention was unavailable. Consultation rates tend to be higher for urgency, and mixed urinary incontinence compared with stress incontinence, and this may reflect the greater bother that these conditions tend to cause [45].

The overall financial cost of incontinence to the NHS is difficult to calculate. In 1998, the Continence Foundation calculated the figure of £354 million, without including the costs of residential, nursing, or long-term hospital care. In a more recent study by Turner *et al.* [46], it was estimated that the NHS spends £233 million to manage storage symptoms amongst women alone. A study in the United States of America estimated the annual direct cost of UI in America to be $16.3 billion, $12.4 billion for women [47]. However, these studies do not account for the older people who move into residential or nursing homes as a result of their incontinence (incontinence is second only to dementia as an initiating factor for admission to nursing homes). The cost associated with this care (indirect costs) is considerable [48].

Whilst financial costs are significant, the impact on the quality of life for the individual, their families and carers should not be underestimated. Urinary incontinence can affect patients in almost all their daily activities and personal interactions.

The causative mechanisms of stress urinary incontinence are well understood, and the conservative and surgical treatments both logical and effective. From the patient's perspective the introduction of the mid urethral tapes has been hugely advantageous, largely replacing a significantly larger surgical procedure with comparable cure rate and less morbidity.

It is important to remember that all surgical procedures can cause morbidity as well as cure and should only be offered when conservative therapies have failed. Patients must be carefully counselled regarding the common problems encountered during continence surgery generally, in addition to the complications related to the use of tapes specifically. There are currently several large class actions relating to the use of mesh for the treatment of prolapse being fought worldwide, and whilst these do not specifically relate to mid urethral tapes for stress urinary incontinence, the mesh material used is similar. Consequently it is best practice to warn all women regarding the possibility of both pain and tape erosion despite very low incidence of these complications.

A Final Word from the Expert

The treatment of overactive bladder symptoms is less successful than that of stress urinary incontinence. The mechanisms of OAB are multiple and incompletely understood. Appropriate investigations as outlined in the chapter are the key to successful treatment. The importance of simple advice and bladder retraining cannot be overstated. The addition of antimuscarinic drug therapy to these measures allows for even greater treatment effect although the long-term and indeed short-term adherence to AM drug therapy is poor. Newer AM agents with simpler prescribing regimens, and less adverse events have improved treatment efficacy. New drug therapy targeting beta-3 adrenoreceptors may offer an even better treatment option for sufferers. Ultimately, not all patients will improve with current multimodality therapy, or may be unable to tolerate AM agents. When patients fail to tolerate one agent it is sensible to try others. When two or more agents have been used it is safe to conclude that this treatment option has failed and consider other options after thorough investigation of the patient.

For patients who have failed standard treatment for OAB, the options of botulinum toxin injections or neuromodulation are usually the next line when detrusor overactivity has been proven by urodynamic investigations. Both have their advantages and disadvantages, and both are considerably more costly than simpler conservative therapy.

Ultimately for patients, whilst the majority of uncomplicated OAB and stress incontinence can be managed in primary care and by non-specialists, more complex cases should be managed by those with a specialist interest and sub-specialty training.

References

1. Kelleher CJ, Cardozo LD, Khullar V, Salvatore S. A new questionnaire to assess the quality of life of urinary incontinent women. *BJOG* 1997 Dec; 104(12):1374–9

2. Irwin DE, Milsom I, Hunskaar S, Reilly K, Kopp Z, Herschorn S, *et al*. Population-based survey of urinary incontinence, overactive bladder, and other lower urinary tract symptoms in five countries: results of the EPIC study. *Eur Urol* 2006 Dec; 50(6):1306–14; discussion 1314–15. Epub 2006 Oct 2.

3. Haylen BT, de Ridder D, Freeman RM, *et al*. An International Urogynecological Association (IUGA)/International Continence Society (ICS) joint report on the terminology for female pelvic floor dysfunction. *Int Urogynecol J Pelvic Floor Dysfunct* 2010;21:5–26.

4. Ricci JA, Baggish JS, Hunt TL, Stewart WF, Wein A, Herzog AR, Diokno AC. Coping strategies and health care-seeking behavior in a US national sample of adults with symptoms suggestive of overactive bladder. *Clin Ther* 2001 Aug; 23(8):1245–59.

5. Anders K. Coping strategies for women with urinary incontinence. *Best Pract Res Cl Ob* April 2000;14(2):355–61.

6. Diokno AC, Burgio K, Fultz NH, Kinchen KS, Obenchain R, Bump RC. Medical and self-care practices reported by women with urinary incontinence. *Am J Manag Care* 2004 Feb; 10(2 Pt 1):69–78.

7. Peyrat L, Haillot O, Bruyere F, Boutin JM, Bertrand P, Lanson Y. Prevalence and risk factors of urinary incontinence in young and middle-aged women. *BJU Int* 2002 Jan; 89(1):61–6.

8. Burch JC. Urethrovaginal fixation to Cooper's ligament for correction of stress incontinence, cystocele, and prolapse. *Am J Obstet Gynecol* 1961 Feb; 81:281–90.

9. DeLancey JO. Structural support of the urethra as it relates to stress urinary incontinence: the hammock hypothesis. *Am J Obstet Gynecol* 1994 Jun; 170(6): 1713–20

10. Kitchener HC, Dunn G, Lawton V, Reid F, Nelson L, Smith AR; COLPO Study Group. Laparoscopic versus open colposuspension—results of a prospective randomised controlled trial. *BJOG* 2006 Sep; 113(9):1007–13.

11. Dumville JC, Manca A, Kitchener HC, Smith AR, Nelson L, Torgerson DJ; COLPO Study Group Cost-effectiveness analysis of open colposuspension versus laparoscopic colposuspension in the treatment of urodynamic stress incontinence. *BJOG* 2006 Sep; 113(9):1014–22.

12. Bump RC, Mattiasson A, Bø K, Brubaker LP, DeLancey JO, Klarskov P, Shull et al. The standardization of terminology of female pelvic organ prolapse and pelvic floor dysfunction. *Am J Obstet Gynecol* 1996 Jul; 175(1):10–17.

13. Auwad W, Freeman RM, Swift S. Is the pelvic organ prolapse quantification system (POPQ) being used? A survey of members of the International Continence Society (ICS) and the American Urogynecologic Society (AUGS). *Int Urogynecol J Pelvic Floor Dysfunct* 2004 Sep-Oct; 15(5):324–7.

14. Laycock J. Clinical evaluation of the pelvic floor. In:Schussler B, Laycock J, Norton PA, Stanton SL. *Pelvic floor re-education*. London: Springer-Verlag, 2003:42–8.

15. Haylen BT, Law MG, Frazer M, Schulz S. Urine flow rates and residual urine volumes in urogynecology patients. *Int Urogynecol J Pelvic Floor Dysfunct* 1999;10(6):378–83.

16. Costantini E, Mearini E, Pajoncini C, Biscotto S, Bini V, Porena M. Uroflowmetry in female voiding disturbances. *Neurourol Urodyn* 2003;22(6):569–73.

17. Goode PS, Locher JL, Bryant RL, Roth DL, Burgio KL. Measurement of postvoid residual urine with portable transabdominal bladder ultrasound scanner and urethral catheterization. *Int Urogynecol J Pelvic Floor Dysfunct* 2000;11(5):296–300.

18. Cardozo L, Hall T, Ryan J, Ebel Bitoun C, Kausar I, Darekar A, *et al*. Safety and efficacy of flexible-dose fesoterodine in British subjects with overactive bladder: insights into factors

associated with dose escalation. *Int Urogynecol J* 2012 Nov; 23(11):1581–90. doi: 10.1007/s00192–012–1804–1

19. Haab F, Cardozo L, Chapple C, Ridder AM; Solifenacin Study Group. Long-term open-label solifenacin treatment associated with persistence with therapy in patients with overactive bladder syndrome. *Eur Urol* 2005 Mar; 47(3):376–84.

20. van Kerrebroeck P, Abrams P, Chaikin D, Donovan J, Fonda D, Jackson S, *et al*; Standardisation Sub-committee of the International Continence Society. The standardisation of terminology in nocturia: report from the Standardisation Sub-committee of the International Continence Society. *Neurourol Urodyn* 2002;21(2):179–83.

21. Cody JD, Richardson K, Moehrer B, Hextall A, Glazener CM. Oestrogen therapy for urinary incontinence in postmenopausalwomen. *Cochrane Database Syst Rev* 2009 Oct 7;(4):CD001405

22. Larsson G, Victor A. Micturition patterns in a healthy female population, studied with a frequency/volume chart. *Scand J Urol Nephrol Suppl* 1988;114:53–7.

23. Cody JD, Richardson K, Moehrer B, Hextall A, Glazener CM. Oestrogen therapy for urinary incontinence in post-menopausal women. *Cochrane Database Syst Rev* 2009 Oct 7;(4):D001405.

24. Kegel AH, Powell TO. The physiologic treatment of urinary stress incontinence. *J Urol* 1950 May; 63(5):808–14.

25. Dumoulin C, Hay-Smith J. Pelvic floor muscle training versus no treatment, or inactive control treatments, for urinary incontinence in women. *Cochrane Database Syst Rev* 2010 Jan 20;(1) :CD005654

26. Lauti M, Herbison P, Hay-Smith J, Gaye E, Don W. Anticholinergic drugs, bladder retraining and their combination for urge urinary incontinence: a pilot randomised trial. *Int Urogynecol J Pelvic Floor Dysfunct* 2008 Nov; 19(11):1533–43.

27. Mattiasson A, Blaakaer J, Hoye K, et al; Tolterodine Scandinavian Study Group. Simplified bladder training augments the effectiveness of tolterodine in patients with an overactive bladder. *BJU Int* 2003 Jan; 91(1):54–60.

28. Mattiasson A, Masala A, Morton R, et al. Efficacy of simplified bladder training in patients with overactive bladder receiving a solifenacin flexible-dose regimen: results from a randomized study. *BJU Int* 2009 Oct 10.

29. Fitzgerald MP, Lemack G, Wheeler T, Litman HJ. Urinary Incontinence Treatment Network. Nocturia, nocturnal incontinence prevalence, and response to anticholinergic and behavioral therapy. *Int Urogynecol J Pelvic Floor Dysfunct* 2008 Nov; 19(11):1545–50.

30. Burgio KL, Locher JL, Goode PS, Locher JL, Roth DL. Behavioral vs drug treatment for urge urinary incontinence in older women: a randomized controlled trial. *JAMA* 1998 Dec 16;280(23):1995–2000.

31. Blaivas JG. *Techniques of evaluation*. In Yalla SV, McGuire EJ, Elbadawi A, Blaivas JG (eds). *Neurourology and urodynamics, Principles and practice*. New York: MacMillan, 1988:166–74.

32. NICE. Urinary incontinence. The management of urinary incontinence in women London: National Institute for Health and Clinical Excellence, 2006.

33. Al-Ghazo MA, Ghalayini IF, Al-Azab R, Bani Hani O, Matani YS, Haddad Y. Urodynamic Detrusor Overactivity in Patients with Overactive Bladder Symptoms. *Int Neurourol J* 2011 March; 15(1):48–54.

34. Andersson KE. Antimuscarinics for treatment of overactive bladder. *Lancet Neurol* 2004 Jan; 3(1):p 46–53.

35. Abrams P, Andersson KE, Birder L, Brubaker L, Cardozo L, Chapple C, *et al*; Members of Committees; Fourth International Consultation on Incontinence Recommendations of the International Scientific Committee: Evaluation and treatment of urinary incontinence, pelvic organ prolapse, and fecal incontinence. Fourth International Consultation on Incontinence. *Neurourol Urodyn* 2010;29(1):213–40.

36. Nitti V, Herschorn S, Auerbach S, Ayers M, Lee M, Martin N. The selective [beta] 3-adren-oreceptor agonist mirabegron is effective and well tolerated in patients with overactive bladder syndrome. *J Urol* 2011;185:e783–e784

37. Khullar V, Cambronero J, Stroberg P, Angulo J, Boerrigter P, Blauwet M, *et al.* (2011) The efficacy and tolerability of mirabegron in patients with overactive bladder-results from a European-Australian phase III trial. *Eur Urol Suppl* 10:278–9

38. FDA (2012) Summary of safety and efficacy as basis for Advisory Committee briefing document for mirabegron, 5 April 2012. Division of Reproductive and Urologic Products, Office of New Drugs Center for Drug Evaluation and Research of Food and Drug

39. Ashok K, Wang A. Recurrent urinary stress incontinence: an overview. *J Obstet Gynaecol Res* 2010 Jun; 36(3):467–73.

40. Ulmstem U, Henriksson L, Johnson P, Varhos G. An ambulatory surgical procedure under local anesthesia for treatment of female urinary incontinence. *Int Urogynecol J* 1996;7:81–6.

41. Barber MD, Kleeman S, Karram MM, Paraiso MF, Walters MD, Vasavada S, *et al.* Transobturator tape compared with tension-free vaginal tape for the treatment of stress urinary incontinence: a randomized controlled trial. *Obstet Gynecol* 2008 Mar; 111(3):611–21

42. Barber MD, Kleeman, Karram MM, et al. Risk factors associated with failure 1 year after retropubic or transobturator midurethral slings. *Am J Obstet Gynecol* 2008 Dec; 199(6):666.e1–7.

43. Deffieux X, Daher H, Mansoor A, Debodinance P, Muhlstein J, Fernandez H. Transobturator TVT-O versus retropubic TVT: results of a multicenter randomized controlled trial at 24 months follow-up. *Int Urogynecol J* 2010 Nov; 21(11):1337–45.

44. Shaw C, Tansey R, Jackson C, Hyde C, Allan R. Barriers to help seeking in people with urinary symptoms. *Fam Pract* 2001 Feb; 18(1):48–52.

45. Hannestad YS, Rortveit G, Hunskaar S. Help-seeking and associated factors in female urinary incontinence. The Norwegian EPINCONT Study. Epidemiology of Incontinence in the County of Nord-Trøndelag. *Scand J Prim Health Care* 2002 Jun; 20(2):102–7.

46. Shaw C, Gupta RD, Bushnell DM, Assassa RP, Abrams P, Wagg A, *et al.* The extent and severity of urinary incontinence amongst women in UK GP waiting rooms. *Fam Pract* 2006 Oct; 23(5):497–506. Epub 2006 Jul 13.

47. Turner DA, Shaw C, McGrother CW, Dallosso HM, Cooper NJ, and the MRC Incontinence Team. (2004) The cost of clinically significant urinary storage symptoms for community dwelling adults in the UK. *BJU International* 93:1246–52.

48. Irwin DE, Milsom I, Hunskaar S, Reilly K, Kopp Z, Herschorn S, *et al.* Population-based survey of urinary incontinence, overactive bladder, and other lower urinary tract symptoms in five countries: results of the EPIC study. *Eur Urol* 2006 Dec; 50(6):1306–14; discussion 1314–15.

49. Wilson L, Brown J, Shin G, Luc KO, Subak LL. (2001) Annual Direct Cost of Urinary Incontinence. *Obstet Gynaecol* 98:398–406.

22 Post-menopausal bleeding

Josephine Vivian-Taylor

ⓘ Expert Commentary David Luesley

Case history

A 60-year-old woman was referred by her general practitioner to the gynaecology clinic at her local hospital after a single episode of post-menopausal bleeding. She described three days of period-like bleeding. She was otherwise asymptomatic. Her medical history included essential hypertension and type II diabetes. She was sexually active and denied post-coital bleeding. She had no unexplained weight loss, nor abdominal distension. Her last cervical smear three months ago was normal. She had three normal vaginal births, the last being 28 years earlier. She had no previous surgery. Her paternal grandfather and her father were diagnosed with bowel cancer at the ages of 45 and 38 respectively. On examination she had a BMI of 41, there was no peripheral lymphadenopathy, and abdominal examination was unremarkable. Genital examination revealed a normal vulva, vagina, and cervix. Bimanual examination was not possible due to body habitus. A transvaginal ultrasound performed in clinic demonstrated an endometrial thickness of 15 mm (Figure 22.2) and normal ovaries. Direct visualization of the uterine cavity and endometrial sampling were achieved with an outpatient hysteroscopy and pipelle biopsy. At hysteroscopy, the cavity was seen to be lined with friable irregular tissue (Figure 22.3).

> **✪ Learning point** Post-menopausal bleeding (PMB) and the risk of malignancy
>
> - Post-menopausal bleeding is defined as any bleeding from the genital tract after a period of 12 months of amenorrhoea.
> - Whilst predominantly caused by benign conditions such as vaginal or endometrial atrophy, or uterine or cervical polyps, investigation is essential to diagnose or exclude pre-malignant and malignant conditions of the female genital tract.
> - Between 5% and 12% of women who present with post-menopausal bleeding have endometrial cancer, the most common gynaecological malignancy in the developed world [1]. Risk factors for endometrial cancer may be taken into consideration when assessing an individual patient who presents with PMB (Table 22.1).

Table 22.1 Risk factors for development of type I endometrial cancer [16–22]

Risk factors	Relative Risk (RR)/Odd Ratio (OR)
Age	
Oestrogen-only hormone replacement therapy	RR 2.3 (any use) RR 9.5 (10y use)
Obesity	RR 1.59 for each increase in BMI of 5 kg/m2
Type 2 diabetes	RR 2.1
PCOS	RR 2.89
Tamoxifen use	RR 2–4 (2–5y use) 6.9 (≥ 5y use)
Lynch syndrome	40–60% lifetime risk
Protective factors	
Oral contraceptive pill	OR 0.57

❝ Expert comment

This represents a fairly standard presentation of endometrial cancer and illustrates the utility of 'one-stop' clinics allowing all of the key diagnostic data to be collected in a single visit and reassuring the majority of women who do not have endometrial cancer. A high body mass index can hinder accurate clinical assessment. Fortunately, transvaginal ultrasonography can provide some of the missing information which, apart from ovarian assessment and endometrial thickness, should also provide some information on uterine size. Large uteri are considered at higher risk for endometrial cancer than normal-sized uteri, and a laparoscopic approach to surgery might be difficult with a grossly enlarged uterus.

✪ Learning point Endometrial evaluation by ultrasound for postmenopausal bleeding

- The endometrial thickness (ET) is measured via transvaginal ultrasound (TVUS) with the uterus in a sagittal view. It measures the antero-posterior dimension from one basalis layer to the other and is hyperechogenic compared to the myometrium (Figure 22.1).
- An endometrial thickness of ≥ 5 mm in women with post-menopausal bleeding is considered abnormal and warrants further evaluation of the endometrium to exclude endometrial cancer (Figure 22.2). The sensitivity of TVUS at this cut-off is approximately 96% [2,3].
- If the bleeding is persistent, further evaluation of the endometrium is required even if the endometrium appears normal on ultrasound and is < 5 mm [4,5].
- Abnormal endometrial features such as focal lesions, a cystic appearance of the endometrium, and fluid inside the cavity, all warrant further evaluation.
- While the risk of malignancy is lower in asymptomatic women (compared to those presenting with PMB) with an endometrial thickness ≥ 5 mm, the decision to investigate further should be made on a case-by-case basis. The presence of risk factors for endometrial cancer, abnormal features on ultrasound including ET > 11 mm and patient and clinician preferences, will guide practice in this area [4,5]. Screening asymptomatic women to reduce mortality from endometrial cancer, using endometrial thickness, has not been established [6].
- The endometrial thickness cut-off in women on continuous combined HRT is the same as for women on no HRT. This cannot be applied to women on sequential HRT, who require further investigation if they have abnormal vaginal bleeding.

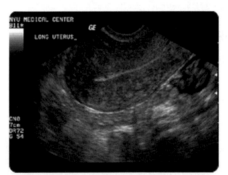

Figure 22.1 Transvaginal ultrasound of a post-menopausal patient. Note: hyperechoic endometrium compared with myometrium.

Reprinted from *American Journal of Obstetrics and Gynecology*, 201:1, Steven R. Goldstein, The role of transvaginal ultrasound or endometrial biopsy in the evaluation of the menopausal endometrium, 5–11 Copyright 2009, with permission from Elsevier.

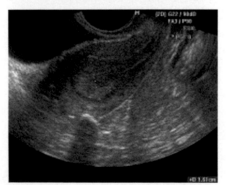

Figure 22.2 Transvaginal ultrasound illustrating thickened endometrium with well-defined outer margins.

Reprinted from *American Journal of Obstetrics and Gynecology*, 201:1, Steven R. Goldstein, The role of transvaginal ultrasound or endometrial biopsy in the evaluation of the menopausal endometrium, 5–11 Copyright 2009, with permission from Elsevier.

➕ **Clinical tip** Endometrial sampling

Office-based endometrial sampling (e.g. Pipelle) is accurate in diagnosing endometrial cancer when an adequate sample is obtained [7,8]. However, this procedure has a failure rate of approximately 8%, and in up to 15% inadequate or insufficient specimen for histopathology is obtained [7]. Additionally, all sampling techniques will miss some endometrial cancers and hyperplasia [5]. Performing a hysteroscopy at the same time as the endometrial biopsy allows identification of focal lesions that may be missed by blind sampling techniques, and provides additional information about the nature of the endometrial cavity when an inadequate or insufficient specimen is obtained [9–11]. Outpatient hysteroscopy and endometrial sampling is as accurate and acceptable to patients as an inpatient procedure [5,12]. If symptoms of post-menopausal bleeding persist, despite a negative hysteroscopy and endometrial histology, a repeat procedure is indicated [5]; in most cases this would be a hysteroscopy, dilatation, and curette under general anaesthetic.

➕ **Clinical tip** Minimizing the risk of uterine perforation at hysteroscopy, dilatation, and curette

- Pre-operative misoprostol.
- Bimanual examination to assess uterine position and straightening of the uterine access with gentle traction with a tenaculum/valsalum on the cervix.
- Use of narrow dilators in cervical stenosis.
- Intracervical vasopressor (avoid in office procedures).
- Dilatation of the external cervical os followed by direct vision with the hysteroscope allows visualization of the internal os and hydrodilation.

❝ **Expert comment**

The need for hysteroscopy in the investigation of PMB is debatable. As demonstrated in this case, the inclusion of routine hysteroscopy may not influence the management decisions. While there are some situations where direct vision of the endometrium is of value, its routine inclusion in the investigation of PMB can increase risk to the patient and health-system costs, and decrease the number of cases that can be seen in any one clinic. Some 'one-stop' PMB clinics prefer to use ultrasound and endometrial sampling, which may be the most cost-effective approach [13].

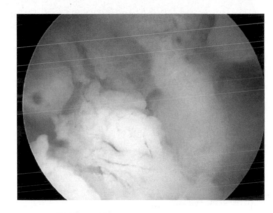

Figure 22.3 Hysteroscopic view of endometrial carcinoma. The uterine cavity is filled with friable, irregular tissue.

Reproduced from Sarris, Bewley, and Agnihotri, *Training in Obstetrics and Gynaecology*, 2009 with permission from Oxford University Press.

The histopathology results demonstrated endometriod endometrial carcinoma grade 3. A pre-operative CT chest and abdomen demonstrated no evidence of metastatic disease and an MRI of the pelvis suggested stage 1A disease with < 50% myometrial invasion and no evidence of lymph node metastases (Figure 22.4).

✪ **Learning point** Histopathology of endometrial cancer [14,15]

Endometrial cancer is classified according to the World Health Organisation and International Society of Gynaecological Pathologists. Type I endometrial cancers endometrioid and type II (non-endometrioid) histologies differ in their pathogenesis, epidemiology and prognosis.

Type I endometrial cancer

- 80% of endometrial cancers are histologically endometrioid which arise from atypical hyperplasia.
- Surrounding endometrium is hyperplastic.

(continued)

- Are oestrogen-receptor-positive tumours and therefore associated with exposure to unopposed oestrogen such as occurs in polycystic ovarian syndrome, obesity, Tamoxifen, and oestrogen-only HRT.
- Occurs in younger women.
- Usually low-grade, less aggressive tumours with a better prognosis.
- Associated with genetic mutations (e.g. Lynch syndrome).

Type II endometrial cancer

- Histological types: serous, clear cell.
- Non-oestrogen-dependent.
- Surrounding endometrium is atrophic.
- Arise in older women.
- High-grade tumours, aggressive with a poorer prognosis.

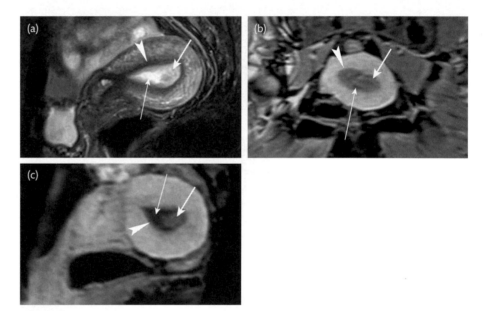

Figure 22.4 MRI scan demonstrating endometrial carcinoma confined to the endometrial cavity, stage IA. (a) Sagittal T2-weighted fat-saturated image of a retroflexed uterus shows an endometrial carcinoma confined to the uterine cavity. The tumor (thick arrow) is slightly lower in signal intensity than the normal endometrium (thin arrow). The low-signal-intensity junctional-zone myometrium (arrowhead) is intact. Dynamic T1-weighted post-contrast images axial (b) and sagittal to uterine body (c) reveal a lobulated enhancing intraendometrial mass (thick arrow) within low-signal-intensity fluid (thin arrow). Fluid and normalenhancingendometrial lining are much better differentiated on the dynamic contrast-enhanced images. Preservation of continuous uninterrupted subendometrial enhancement (arrowhead) is consistentwith a mass confined to the cavity. Surgical pathology confirmed a stage1A tumor confined to the endometrium without myometrial invasion.

Reproduced from Brant and de Lange, *Essentials of Body MRI*, 2012 with permission from Oxford University Press.

✚ **Clinical tip** Benign endometrial cells found incidentally on cervical smear [23]

- Are normal in women < 40 years of age and do not require further investigation if the woman is asymptomatic.
- In women > 40 years of age, they may indicate endometrial pathology. They can also be present when women are receiving oral contraceptives, hormone replacement therapy, or Tamoxifen, or are fitted with an IUCD.
- Menstruating women > 40 years of age who are asymptomatic and have no risk factors for endometrial cancer do not warrant further investigation.
- Post-menopausal women should be investigated for endometrial pathology.

✪ **Learning point** Endometrial cancer and obesity

Obesity (Body Mass Index (BMI) of > 30 kg/m^2) is a risk factor for the development of endometrial cancer. The relative risk of developing endometrial cancer is 1.59 for each increase in BMI of 5 kg/m^2 [21]. It is particularly associated with the development of endometrial cancer in younger women (< 45 years), and prior to menopause [24,25].

The mechanism behind this relationship is multifactorial. The conversion of androstenedione into oestrone, and the aromatization of androgens to oestrodiol in adipose tissue increases oestrogen levels which stimulate proliferation of the endometrium. This proliferation, unopposed by progestins, promotes the development of endometrial hyperplasia and ultimately endometrial cancer. Increased insulin, IGF-1 and leptin levels, and reduced adiponectin levels, are associated with obesity and endometrial cancer, and may also play a role in the mechanisms behind the association [26].

The risk of dying from endometrial cancer is 6.25 times higher in women who are morbidly obese (BMI > 40 kg/m2) [27]. This may relate to ongoing tumour stimulation from the obesity-related factors described, or higher rates of peri-operative morbidity and mortality in obese women undergoing surgical staging for endometrial cancer.

While technically more difficult in obese women, minimally invasive surgical techniques are feasible in this population, with adequate staging, less blood loss, shorter hospital stay, and lower rates of wound infection compared with laparotomy [28,32].

✔ **Evidence base** Pre-operative staging of endometrial cancer

- A meta-analysis of the radiological staging of endometrial cancer found MRI to be more accurate than CT and ultrasound for the assessment of the depth of myometrial invasion. The sensitivity and specificity of MRI for the detection of deep myometrial invasion ranged from 80–100% and 70–100%, respectively. The sensitivity and specificity of MRI in the detection of cervical involvement (stage II disease) ranged from 56–100% and 93–100% respectively [33].
- MRI performs less well (mean sensitivity 72%) when used for the detection of lymph node metastases [34].
- The role of PET/CT for the pre-operative detection of lymph node metastases in endometrial cancer remains controversial. Studies have demonstrated sensitivity and specificity of 60–100% and 98–100% respectively [35–38].
- Intra-operative assessment of the depth of myometrial invasion correlates poorly with final pathology [39].

❝ **Expert comment**

NICE Improving outcomes in gynaecological cancers guidance recommends that women with low-risk endometrial cancer should normally be managed by gynaecological cancer units, and high-risk cancers to be referred to a cancer centre with gynaecological oncologists and medical oncologists in a multidisciplinary team [40]. Other patient factors such as the bariatric challenges posed by this particular patient may also warrant a referral to a cancer centre.

Her case was referred to a gynae-oncologist. After discussion at their Multidisciplinary Team (MDT) meeting, the recommended treatment was a total abdominal hysterectomy (TAH), bilateral salpino-oophorectomy (BSO), and bilateral pelvic lymphadenectomy (BPLND). The gynaecological oncologist was experienced in laparoscopic surgery and proceded to a total laparoscopic hysterectomy bilateral salpingo-oophorectomy and pelvic lymph node dissection. The procedure was uncomplicated.

> ### ⊘ Evidence base Lymphadenectomy in early-stage endometrial cancer
>
> The role of routine pelvic and para-aortic lymph node dissection in the management of early endometrial cancer remains controversial. FIGO surgical staging of endometrial cancer stipulates intra-operative assessment of the pelvic and para-aortic lymph nodes, rather than lymphadenectomy in all cases. Prospective studies have demonstrated the absence of survival benefit from pelvic and para-aortic lymphadenectomy in early endometrial cancer and a major complication rate from lymphadenectomy of 2–6% [41–43].
>
> One of these studies, a large cohort study of 39396 women demonstrated a therapeutic benefit of lymphadenectomy for women with stage 1 grade 3 disease (p < 0.001) and stages II–IV (p < 0.001) [42]. High rates of lymph node involvement and possible therapeutic benefit in high-risk tumours (grade 3, non-endometrioid, stage 1B) has lead some clinicians to advocate lymph node dissection for all but 'low-risk' early endometrial cancer [42,44–46]. Routine lymphadenectomy provides important prognostic information [47], and knowledge of lymph node status may allow a more tailored approach to adjuvant chemoradiotherapy [44].

> ### ◑ Landmark trial Efficacy of systematic pelvic lymphadenectomy in endometrial cancer (ASTEC) [41]
>
> The need for pelvic lymph node dissection remains controversial due to the associated morbidity of this procedure, as well as questions about the therapeutic benefit in early endometrial cancer. A multicentre international randomized control trial (n = 1408 women) found that the pelvic lymphadenectomy conferred no overall, disease-specific, or recurrence-free survival benefit for women with endometrial carcinoma thought pre-operatively to be stage 1. There was no difference in the proportion of women who required post-operative radiotherapy. Critics of the trial suggest that the high proportion of 'low-risk' disease (grade 1 or 2 with < 50% myometrial invasion) could have underestimated the therapeutic benefit of lymphadenectomy in 'high-risk' stage 1 disease. Further study of this high-risk subgroup is required.

> ### ❻ Expert comment
>
> Whether or not a pelvic and or para-aortic lymphadenectomy should be performed at the time of surgical removal of the uterus for all endometrial cancers continues to challenge gynaecological oncologists, and clinical oncologists. Despite a lack of evidence for any benefit (in terms of improved survival), the practice continues and it is not without risk. The lymphoedema that this woman went on to develop is certainly attributable to her surgery.
>
> What do we know? Non-endometrioid histologies are at high risk of nodal metastases and should therefore be treated as such. A proportion of cases will have involved pelvic lymph nodes at the time of first surgical intervention; however, there are no reliable, practical investigations that will definitively identify such cases prior to surgery. There are known risk factors that are associated with an increased incidence of lymph node involvement. These include the grade of tumour and the degree and type of myometrial involvement which can be assessed pre-operatively by endometrial sampling and pre-operative cross-sectional imaging, MRI in particular. These techniques are subject to error.
>
> The next, and most obvious question is, 'Does having knowledge of lymph node status influence outcome?' So far, there are no randomized data showing a survival advantage in low-risk and low-intermediate-risk groups. The ASTEC trial has drawn more than its fair share of criticism but its detractors have yet to provide solid evidence of an advantage associated with lymph node removal. For these reasons, our own cancer centre would not routinely consider pelvic lymphadenectomy in cases deemed at low- or low intermediate risk. Whilst lymph node dissection is considered for type 1 tumours of high and high-intermediate risk, we continue to audit this practice carefully as it can really only be justified if there are effective interventions for those found to have positive nodes.

> **Evidence base** Minimally invasive approaches to the surgical staging of endometrial cancer
>
> The laparoscopic approach to the management of early-stage endometrial cancer is safe and effective. The overall survival, disease-free survival and cancer-related survival did not differ when compared to laparotomy [48]. While operating times were on average longer for laparoscopic approaches, they had less blood loss, shorter hospital stays, and less post-operative complications, when compared to laparotomy [48,49]. About 25% of laparoscopies were converted to laparotomy, usually due to poor visibility [49]. A systematic review looked at the use of robotic surgery in endometrial cancer staging. It found longer operating times compared to laparotomy and laparoscopy but post-op complication rates and transfusion rates similar to laparoscopy [50].

She made a good recovery from surgery and went home on post-operative day 3. The final pathology was confirmed a grade 3 stage 1A endometrioid endometrial cancer (Table 22.2). There was no lymphovascular space invasion (LVSI). The patient was given the options of observation or vault brachytherapy and opted for observation only. Given her strong family history of Lynch syndrome-associated cancers, she was referred to the geneticists. Follow-up was planned at four-month intervals for three years, six monthly for the fourth and fifth years, and yearly thereafter.

> **Expert comment**
>
> It has not, as yet, been possible to demonstrate any benefit in terms of either early detection or, indeed, survival by the application of routine follow-up practices. The risk of relapse is very low in cases such as this, and even if it were to occur, the majority of women will represent with symptoms. By adopting a practice of patient education and patient initiated follow-up a significant amount of outpatient resource can be released for other aspects of patient care.

Table 22.2 FIGO staging and prognosis for endometrial cancer [51]

Stage	Description	5-year survival rate
Stage 1	Tumour confined to the corpus uteri	
1A	Tumour limited to endometrium or invades less than one-half of the myometrium	90%
1B	Tumour invades one-half or more of the myometrium	78%
Stage II	Tumour invades stromal connective tissue of the cervix but does not extend beyond the uterus	74%
Stage III	Local or regional spread of tumour, or both	
IIIA	Tumour involves serosa and/or adenxa, or both	56%
IIIB	Vaginal or parametrial involvement, or both	36%
IIIC1	Positive pelvic nodes	57%
IIIC2	Positive para-aortic nodes with or without positive pelvic nodes	49%
Stage IV	Tumour invades bladder, or bowel mucosa, or distant metastases or all three	
IVA	Tumour invades bladder, or bowel mucosa, or both	22%
IVB	Distant metastases, including intraabdominal metastases, or inguinal lymph nodes, or both	21%

> **Evidence base** Radiotherapy and Chemotherapy in endometrial cancer
>
> The controversy around the need for adjuvant radiotherapy following surgery in stage 1 endometrial cancer is reflected in current treatment guidelines [22,45]. The presence of negative prognostic factors for recurrent disease, which include serous and clear cell histopathology, advanced patient age, grade 3, deep myometrial invasion, presence of lymphovascular space invasion (LVSI) and tumour size, are taken into consideration when planning adjuvant treatment [22,45].
>
> Adjuvant radiotherapy reduces the risk of local regional recurrence in stage 1 endometrial cancer [52,53]. However, studies have failed to demonstrate a reduction in overall survival and cancer-related deaths with the use of adjuvant radiotherapy for low- and intermediate-risk disease. This is attributed to the high rate of successful salvage for isolated vaginal recurrences [52–54]. The PORTEC trial
>
> (continued)

demonstrated a survival rate following isolated vaginal recurrence treated with radiotherapy of 79% at two years and 69% at three years [52]. High-risk stage 1 disease is likely to benefit from adjuvant radiotherapy in terms of cancer related and overall survival [55–57].

Radiotherapy, especially following lymphadenectomy, is associated with both early and late toxicity which can cause significant morbidity or even death. The PORTEC-2 trial [58] compared vaginal brachytherapy (VB) with external beam radiotherapy (EBRT) in early endometrial cancer at risk of recurrence. The rate of gastrointestinal complications was lower in the women receiving VB (12.6%) compared to EBRT (53.8%). There was no difference in the rate of recurrent disease or survival.

Chemotherapy is the recommended as adjuvant treatment of stage III and IV endometrial cancer [45]. It reduces the risk of distant metastases and improves overall survival when compared to no treatment or whole abdominal radiotherapy [59,60]. Further research is underway to establish the role of chemotherapy in early-stage endometrial cancers at increased risk of distant metastases.

⭐ **Learning point** Hereditary non-polyposis colonic cancer (HNPCC) and gynaecological malignancy

HNPCC, otherwise known as Lynch syndrome, is a familial cancer syndrome associated with a lifetime risk of colon and non-colonic malignancies. It carries a lifetime risk of endometrial cancer of 40–60% [22]. It is caused by genetic defects in the mismatch repair genes of MLH1, MSH2, MSH6, PMS2. The inheritance is autosomal dominant with incomplete penetrance and it accounts for approximately 2.3% of endometrial cancers [61]. The Society of Gynaecological Oncology (SGO) has published guidelines for the referral of women for genetic testing, which are based on a personal and family history of endometrial and ovarian cancers and other malignancies associated with Lynch syndrome [61]. Screening of histological specimens for mismatch repair genes is currently not feasible for all endometrial cancers. Women who are known to carry a Lynch syndrome mutation but have never been diagnosed with a gynaecological malignancy should be offered surveillance with TVUS and endometrial sampling from age 30–35 years, and prophylactic surgery at the completion of childbearing [62]. Given the paucity of evidence, further research is required to determine the optimal management of, and screening for Lynch syndrome in women.

✓ **Evidence base** The role of fertility-sparing treatment in early endometrial cancer and complex hyperplasia

The gold standard treatment for early endometrial cancer is surgery +/- adjuvant therapy. Fertility-sparing treatment for women with grade 1, stage 1a endometrial cancer confined to the endometrium remains controversial. Treatments that have been described, include megestrol acetate 80–160 mg BD, medroxyprogesterone acetate 600 mg daily, and levonorgestrol IUS, and GnRH agonist + levonorgestrol IUS [63–65]. Follow-up is with repeat hysteroscopy and endometrial biopsy which are performed at three-monthly intervals. Following a complete response, it is suggested that women actively pursue pregnancy. Hysterectomy is recommended on completion of childbearing.

A systematic review of the literature by Gunderson et al. demonstrated a complete response (CR) rate of 48.2% for medically treated early endometrial cancer and complex endometrial hyperplasia [65]. The median duration to CR was six months, and the risk of recurrence after an initial response was 35.4%. 34.8% of women achieved a pregnancy, either spontaneously or by assisted reproductive techniques. For women with complex hyperplasia, the complete response rates and recurrence rates after an initial response were significantly more favourable. However, pregnancy rates did not differ to those women with endometrial cancer.

Four weeks post-op she reported leakage of a clear fluid from the vagina and was referred back to the gynae-oncologist. On examination, an area of granulation tissue was seen at the vault and there appeared to be urine in the vagina.

> ➕ **Clinical tip** Post-operative urogenital fistulae
>
> - A fistula is a communication between two epithelial surfaces.
> - The risk of fistula formation following gynaecological surgery is increased following ureteric or bladder injury at the time of surgery, and in the setting of malignancy, radical surgery, pelvic infections, and excessive cautery for bleeding intra-operatively.
> - If a urogenital fistula is suspected, the whole urinary tract must be assessed as multiple fistulae may exist.
> - A CT urogram is the radiological modality of choice in the evaluation for ureterogenital fistulae.
> - Cystoscopy is performed to identify a vesico-genital fistula tract. A retrograde pyelogram at the time of cytsocopy may demonstrate a ureterogential fistula close to the trigone.
> - If the patient has a history of pelvic malignancy, a biopsy must be taken to exclude recurrent disease as the cause of fistula formation.

A small vesico-vaginal fistula was diagnosed. It was initially treated conservatively with prolonged catheter drainage for 4 weeks. However, this did not result in closure of the fistula and surgery was required. This procedure was performed vaginally and involved excision of the fistula tract, mobilization of surrounding tissue, and a tension-free closure of each layer. The catheter was removed two weeks post-operatively after cystogram excluded bladder leak. She made a good recovery.

At her six-month follow-up appointment, she reports bilateral swelling of her legs. On examination there was evidence of mild lower extremity lymphoedema. She was referred to the lymphoedema clinic at her local hospital for ongoing management.

> ✖ **Learning point** Lymphoedema following treatment for endometrial cancer
>
> - The risk of lower extremity lymphoedema following pelvic lymph node dissection ranges from 3–38% [66–67].
> - The risk increases with higher numbers of lymph nodes removed, the removal of circumflex iliac nodes to the distal external iliac nodes, and adjuvant radiotherapy [66–67].
> - Whilst it cannot be cured, the management of established lower extremity lymphoedema involves keeping the skin in good condition and reducing the risk of infection, regular exercise and weight control, external compression, and lymphatic drainage (e.g. complex decongestive therapy).
> - Referral to a specialized lymphoedema service is recommended and most countries also have lymphoedema patient-support networks.

At her 12-month follow-up appointment, she reported a three-week history of vaginal bleeding. She was otherwise well. On examination, a lesion was seen at the vaginal vault and a punch biopsy was taken in clinic. The biopsy confirmed the presence of recurrent endometrial cancer. An MRI was performed and demonstrated a 1.5 cm mass at the vaginal vault. A CT/PET scan excluded distant metastases.

> ✖ **Learning point** Vaginal vault recurrence of endometrial cancer
>
> The vaginal vault is a common site of recurrent endometrial cancer. For isolated vaginal recurrence, treatment may be curative. Prior to treatment, it is important to exclude other sites of recurrence. This can be achieved with an integrated positron emission tomography and computed tomography (PET/CT). Survival following vaginal recurrence is better for those who had not received adjuvant radiotherapy [68].
>
> (continued)

Radiotherapy (external beam pelvic radiotherapy +/- brachytherapy) is the first-line treatment for women who were initially treated with surgery alone. The cure rates are lower and complication rates are higher if the woman has had previous radiotherapy to the pelvis or vault [68–69].

Surgery is usually reserved for women who have previously received pelvic radiotherapy or if radiotherapy alone will be insufficient for local control, usually in the setting of large lesions [70]. A partial vaginectomy, or pelvic exenteration, may be required to achieve clear margins. While surgery in this context may be associated with long-term improved survival in carefully selected patients, it is associated with significant mortality and major morbidity [70–71].

She received pelvic radiotherapy and brachytherapy to the vaginal vault. Five years after primary surgery she is disease-free and her lymphoedema is stable.

Discussion

The case highlights a number of dilemmas in endometrial cancer management today. The rising rates of obesity in our community and longer life expectancies are likely to be driving increases in the incidence of endometrial cancer. While survival from endometrial cancer is high, particularly in early-stage disease with favourable histology, optimizing survival outcomes while minimizing the morbidity of treatment remains a challenge.

Screening for early endometrial cancer or endometrial hyperplasia in the general population is not recommended. Disease prevalence is low, most women present with symptoms (abnormal vaginal bleeding) when the disease is at an early stage, and current testing modalities (TV ultrasound and endometrial sampling) have poor sensitivity and specificity in asymptomatic women. With the exception of women with a known-HNPCC mutation, there are insufficient data to support screening of asymptomatic women with risk factors for the development of endometrial cancer, such as those using Tamoxifen, obese women, and those with a history of PCOS. Instead, they should be educated to report any abnormal vaginal discharge, or bleeding to their doctor.

Despite the growing body of evidence that early-stage endometrial cancer can be safely treated with less radical, and thus less morbid approaches, controversy remains and practice differs between individual practitioners and centres. The approach to management which limits the number and morbidity of treatment modalities used, while not compromising disease prognosis, has not been determined for all endometrial cancer cases, particularly those of intermediate grade and prognostic factors. Unlike in the case of breast cancer, where sentinel node biopsy and selective lymph node dissection has become the standard practice, the use of sentinel node detection in the management of endometrial cancer has not been established [72].

A Final Word from the Expert

This case is almost certainly related to background oestrogenic stimulation, but the history does raise the issue of hereditary non-polyposis colonic cancer syndrome (HNPCC) with a strong family history of bowel cancer at an early age. The optimal management of endometrial cancer, in particular the role of routine lymphadenectomy and adjuvant treatments, continues to challenge gynaecological and medical oncologists.

Another area of controversy is the use of Tamoxifen in the management of breast cancer. While it has undoubtedly improved the outcome for post-menopausal women with ER-receptor-positive breast cancer, it is associated with an increased risk of endometrial cancer and hyperplasia and may induce more aggressive tumours if they occur. The IBIS I breast cancer-prevention trial, while not powered to demonstrate an increased risk of endometrial cancer, noted significantly more discontinuation in the Tamoxifen group when compared with placebo, increased endometrial thickness and more gynaecological referrals in the Tamoxifen group [73]. In terms of chemoprevention, this is likely to be important as it impacts on compliance thus partially negating the beneficial effects.

Alternatives to Tamoxifen, such as Raloxifene, are now being increasingly explored that maintain the anti-oestrogenic effect on breast tissue without risk of endometrial stimulation.

References

1. Saso S, Chaterjee J, Georgiou E, Ditri AM, Smith JR, Ghaem-Maghami S. Endometrial cancer. *BMJ* 2011;342: d3954.
2. Smith-Bindman R, Kerlikowske K, Feldstein VA, Subak L, Scheidler J, Segal M, *et al*. Endovaginal ultrasound to exclude endometrial cancer and other endometrial abnormalities. *JAMA* 1998;280(17):1510–17.
3. Timmermans A, Opmeer BC, Khan KS, Bachmann LM, Epstein E, Clark TJ, *et al*. Endometrial thickness measurement for detecting endometrial cancer in women with postmenopausal bleeding: a systematic review and meta-analysis. *Obstet Gynecol* 2010;116(1):160–7.
4. ACOG Committee. ACOG Committee Opinion No. 426: the role of transvaginal ultrasonography in the evaluation of postmenopausal bleeding. *Obstet Gynecol* 2009;113:462–4.
5. Scottish Intercollegiate Guidelines Network. Guideline 61: Investigation of post-menopausal bleeding. 2001.
6. Smith-Bindman R, Weiss E, Feldstein V. How thick is too thick? When endometrial thickness should prompt biopsy in postmenopausal women without vaginal bleeding. *Ultrasound Obstetr Gynecol* 2004;24(5):558–65.
7. Clark TJ, Mann CH, Shah N, Khan KS, Song F, Gupta JK. Accuracy of outpatient endometrial biopsy in the diagnosis of endometrial cancer: a systematic quantitative review. *BJOG* 2003;109(3):313–21.
8. Dijkhuizen F, Mol BWJ, Brölmann HAM, Heintz APM. The accuracy of endometrial sampling in the diagnosis of patients with endometrial carcinoma and hyperplasia. *Cancer* 2000;89(8):1765–72.
9. Epstein E, Ramirez A, Skoog L, Valentin L. Dilatation and curettage fails to detect most focal lesions in the uterine cavity in women with postmenopausal bleeding. *Acta Obstet Gyn Scan* 2002;80(12):1131–6.
10. Gimpelson R, Rappold H. A comparative study between panoramic hysteroscopy with directed biopsies and dilatation and curettage. A review of 276 cases. *Am J Obstetr Gynecol* 1988;158;489–452.
11. Loffer FD. Hysteroscopy with selective endometrial sampling compared with D&C for abnormal uterine bleeding: the value of a negative hysteroscopic view. *Obstet Gynecol* 1989;73:16–20.

12. Tahir M, Bigrigg M, Browning J, Brookes T, Smith PA. A randomised controlled trial comparing transvaginal ultrasound, outpatient hysteroscopy and endometrial biopsy with inpatient hysteroscopy and curettage. *BJOG* 1999;106(12):1259–64.

13. Clark T, Barton P, Coomarasamy A, Gupta J, Khan K. Investigating postmenopausal bleeding for endometrial cancer: cost-effectiveness of initial diagnostic strategies. *BJOG* 2006;113:502–10.

14. Amant F, Moerman P, Neven P, Timmerman D, Van Limbergen E, Vergote I. Endometrial cancer. *Lancet* 2005;366(9484):491–505.

15. Tavassoli FA, Devilee P. Chapter 4: Tumours of the Uterine Corpus. Pathology and genetics of tumours of the breast and female genital organs. Geneva: World Health Organisation, 2003.

16. Bergman L, Beelen ML, Gallee MP, Hollema H, Benraadt J, van Leeuwen FE. Risk and prognosis of endometrial cancer after tamoxifen for breast cancer. *Lancet* 2000;356(9233):881–7.

17. Friberg E, Orsini N, Mantzoros C, Wolk A. Diabetes mellitus and risk of endometrial cancer: a meta-analysis. *Diabetologia* 2007;50(7):1365–74.

18. Gierisch JM, Coeytaux RR, Urrutia RP, Havrilesky LJ, Moorman PG, Lowery WJ, *et al.* Oral Contraceptive Use and Risk of Breast, Cervical, Colorectal, and Endometrial Cancers: A Systematic Review. *Cancer Epidem Biomar* 2013;22:1931–43.

19. Grady D, Gebretsadik T, Kerlikowske K, Ernster V, Petitti D. Hormone replacement therapy and endometrial cancer risk: a meta-analysis. *Obstet Gynecol* 1995;85(2):304–13.

20. Haoula Z, Salman M, Atiomo W. Evaluating the association between endometrial cancer and polycystic ovary syndrome. *Hum Reprod* 2012;27(5):1327–31.

21. Renehan AG, Tyson M, Egger M, Heller RF, Zwahlen M. Body-mass index and incidence of cancer: a systematic review and meta-analysis of prospective observational studies. *Lancet* 2008;371(9612):569–78.

22. Wright JD, Medel NIB, Sehouli J, Fujiwara K, Herzog TJ. Contemporary management of endometrial cancer. *Lancet* 2012 7;379:1352–60.

23. Luesley D, Leeson S, editor. Colposcopy and Programme Management Guidelines for the NHS Cervical Screening Programme 2nd edn. NHS Cancer Screening Programmes, May 2010.

24. Soliman PT, Oh JC, Schmeler KM, Sun CC, Slomovitz BM, Gershenson DM, *et al.* Risk factors for young premenopausal women with endometrial cancer. *Obstet Gynecol* 2005;105(3):575–80.

25. Thomas CC, Wingo PA, Dolan MS, Lee NC, Richardson LC. Endometrial cancer risk among younger, overweight women. *Obstet Gynecol* 2009;114(1):22–7.

26. Fader AN, Arriba LN, Frasure HE, von Gruenigen VE. Endometrial cancer and obesity: epidemiology, biomarkers, prevention and survivorship. *Gynecologic oncology* 2009;114(1):121–7.

27. Calle EE, Rodriguez C, Walker-Thurmond K, Thun MJ. Overweight, obesity, and mortality from cancer in a prospectively studied cohort of US adults. *N Eng J Med* 2003;348(17):1625–38.

28. Eisenhauer EL, Wypych KA, Mehrara BJ, Lawson C, Chi DS, Barakat RR, *et al.* Comparing surgical outcomes in obese women undergoing laparotomy, laparoscopy, or laparotomy with panniculectomy for the staging of uterine malignancy. *Ann Surg Oncol* 2007;14(8):2384–91.

29. Eltabbakh GH, Shamonki MI, Moody JM, Garafano LL, Hysterectomy for obese women with endometrial cancer: laparoscopy or laparotomy? *Gynecol Oncol* 2000;78(3):329–35.

30. Gehrig PA, Cantrell LA, Shafer A, Abaid LN, Mendivil A, Boggess JF. What is the optimal minimally invasive surgical procedure for endometrial cancer staging in the obese and morbidly obese woman? *Gynecol Oncol* 2008;111(1):41–5.

31. Obermair A, Manolitsas T, Leung Y, Hammond I, McCartney A. Total laparoscopic hyster-ectomy versus total abdominal hysterectomy for obese women with endometrial cancer. *Int J Gynecol Cancer* 2005;15(2):319–24.

32. O'Hanlan KA, Dibble SL, Fisher DT. Total laparoscopic hysterectomy for uterine pathol-ogy: impact of body mass index on outcomes. *Gynecol Oncol* 2006;103(3):938–41.

33. Kinkel K, Kaji Y, Kyle KY, Segal MR, Lu Y, Powell CB, *et al*. Radiologic Staging in Patients with Endometrial Cancer: A Meta-analysis. *Radiology* 1999;212(3):711–8.

34. Selman T, Mann C, Zamora J, Khan K. A systematic review of tests for lymph node status in primary endometrial cancer. *BMC Women's Health* 2008;8(1):8.

35. Chao A, Chang TC, Ng KK, Hsueh S, Huang HJ, Chou HH, *et al*. 18 F-FDG PET in the management of endometrial cancer. *Eur J Nuc Med Mol Imaging* 2006;33(1):36–44.

36. Horowitz NS, Dehdashti F, Herzog TJ, Rader JS, Powell MA, Gibb RK, *et al*. Prospective evaluation of FDG-PET for detecting pelvic and para-aortic lymph node metastasis in uterine corpus cancer. *Gynecol Oncol* 2004;95(3):546–51.

37. Park JY, Kim EN, Kim DY, Suh DS, Kim JH, Kim YM, *et al*. Comparison of the validity of magnetic resonance imaging and positron emission tomography/computed tomography in the preoperative evaluation of patients with uterine corpus cancer. *Gynecol Oncol* 2008;108(3):486–92.

38. Suzuki R, Miyagi E, Takahashi N, Sukegawa A, Suzuki A, Koike I, *et al*. Validity of posi-tron emission tomography using fluoro-2-deoxyglucose for the preoperative evaluation of endometrial cancer. *Int J Gynecol Cancer* 2007;17(4):890–6.

39. Case AS, Rocconi RP, StraughnJr JM, Conner M, Novak L, Wang W, *et al*. A prospec-tive blinded evaluation of the accuracy of frozen section for the surgical management of endometrial cancer. *Obstet Gynecol* 2006;108(6):1375–9.

40. Guidance on Commissioning Cancer Services: Improving Outcomes in Gynaecological Cancers. NHS Executive, 1999.

41. Kitchener H, Swart A, Qian Q, Amos C, Parmar M. Efficacy of systematic pelvic lym-phadenectomy in endometrial cancer (MRC ASTEC trial): a randomised study. *Lancet* 2009;373(9658):125–36.

42. Chan JK, Wu H, Cheung MK, Shin JY, Osann K, Kapp DS. The outcomes of 27,063 women with unstaged endometrioid uterine cancer. *Gynecol Oncol* 2007;106(2):282–8.

43. Panici PB, Basile S, Maneschi F, Lissoni AA, Signorelli M, Scambia G, *et al*. Systematic pelvic lymphadenectomy vs no lymphadenectomy in early-stage endometrial carcinoma: randomized clinical trial. *J National Cancer Institute* 2008;100(23):1707–16.

44. Ben-Shachar I, Pavelka J, Cohn DE, Copeland LJ, Ramirez N, Manolitsas T, *et al*. Surgical staging for patients presenting with grade 1 endometrial carcinoma. *Obstet Gynecol* 2005;105(3):487–93.

45. Colombo N, Preti E, Landoni F, Carinelli S, Colombo A, Marini C, *et al*. Endometrial can-cer: ESMO Clinical Practice Guidelines for diagnosis, treatment and follow-up. *Ann Oncol* 2011;22 Suppl 6: vi35–vi9.

46. Creasman WT, Morrow CP, Bundy BN, Homesley HD, Graham JE, Heller PB. Surgical pathologic spread patterns of endometrial cancer: a Gynecologic Oncology Group study. *Cancer* 2011;60(S8):2035–41.

47. May K, Bryant A, Dickinson HO, Kehoe S, Morrison J. Lymphadenectomy for the manage-ment of endometrial cancer. *Cochrane Database Syst Rev* 2010 (1): CD007585.

48. Palomba S, Falbo A, Mocciaro R, Russo T, Zullo F. Laparoscopic treatment for endo-metrial cancer: a meta-analysis of randomized controlled trials (RCTs). *Gynecol Oncol* 2009;112(2):415–21.

49. Walker JL, Piedmonte MR, Spirtos NM, Eisenkop SM, Schlaerth JB, Mannel RS, *et al*. Laparoscopy compared with laparotomy for comprehensive surgical staging of uterine cancer: Gynecologic Oncology Group Study LAP2. *J Clin Oncol* 2009;27(32):5331–6.

50. Gaia G, Holloway RW, Santoro L, Ahmad S, Di Silverio E, Spinillo A. Robotic-assisted hysterectomy for endometrial cancer compared with traditional laparoscopic and laparotomy approaches: a systematic review. *Obstet Gynecol* 2010;116(6):1422–31.

51. Lewin SN, Herzog TJ, Medel NIB, Deutsch I, Burke WM, Sun X, *et al.* Comparative performance of the 2009 international Federation of gynecology and obstetrics' staging system for uterine corpus cancer. *Obstet Gynecol* 2010;116(5):1141–9.

52. Creutzberg CL, van Putten WLJ, Koper PCM, Lybeert MLM, Jobsen JJ, Wárlám-Rodenhuis CC, *et al.* Surgery and postoperative radiotherapy versus surgery alone for patients with stage-1 endometrial carcinoma: multicentre randomised trial. *Lancet* 2000;355(9213):1404–11.

53. Keys HM, Roberts JA, Brunetto VL, Zaino RJ, Spirtos NM, Bloss JD, *et al.* A phase III trial of surgery with or without adjunctive external pelvic radiation therapy in intermediate-risk endometrial adenocarcinoma: a Gynecologic Oncology Group study. *Obstet Gynecol Survey* 2004;92(3):744–51.

54. Brazil K, Sussman J, Whelan T, Brouwers M. Adjuvant external beam radiotherapy in the treatment of endometrial cancer (MRC ASTEC and NCIC CTG EN. 5 randomised trials): pooled trial results, systematic review, and meta-analysis. *Lancet* 2009;373(9658):137–46.

55. Johnson N, Cornes P. Survival and recurrent disease after postoperative radiotherapy for early endometrial cancer: systematic review and meta-analysis. *BJOG* 2007;114(11):1313–20.

56. Kong A, Johnson N, Kitchener HC, Lawrie TA. Adjuvant radiotherapy for stage I endometrial cancer. *Cochrane Database Syst Rev* 2012 (10): DCD003916.

57. Lee CM, Szabo A, Shrieve DC, Macdonald OK, Gaffney DK. Frequency and effect of adjuvant radiation therapy among women with stage I endometrial adenocarcinoma. *JAMA* 2006;295(4):389–97.

58. Nout R, Smit V, Putter H, Jürgenliemk-Schulz I, Jobsen J, Lutgens L, *et al.* Vaginal brachytherapy versus pelvic external beam radiotherapy for patients with endometrial cancer of high-intermediate risk (PORTEC-2): an open-label, non-inferiority, randomised trial. *Lancet* 2010;375(9717):816–23.

59. Johnson N, Bryant A, Miles T, Hogberg T, Cornes P. Adjuvant chemotherapy for endometrial cancer after hysterectomy. *Cochrane Database Syst Rev Cochrane Database Syst Rev* 2011 (10): CD003175.

60. Randall ME, Filiaci VL, Muss H, Spirtos NM, Mannel RS, Fowler J, *et al.* Randomized phase III trial of whole-abdominal irradiation versus doxorubicin and cisplatin chemotherapy in advanced endometrial carcinoma: a Gynecologic Oncology Group Study. *Jf Clin Oncol* 2006;24(1):36–44.

61. Resnick KE, Hampel H, Fishel R, Cohn DE. Current and emerging trends in Lynch syndrome identification in women with endometrial cancer. *Gynecol Oncol* 2009;114(1):128–34.

62. Vasen HFA, Möslein G, Alonso A, Bernstein I, Bertario L, Blanco I, *et al.* Guidelines for the clinical management of Lynch syndrome (hereditary non-polyposis cancer). *J Med Genet* 2007;44(6):353–62.

63. Minig L, Franchi D, Boveri S, Casadio C, Bocciolone L, Sideri M. Progestin intrauterine device and GnRH analogue for uterus-sparing treatment of endometrial precancers and well-differentiated early endometrial carcinoma in young women. *Ann Oncol* 2011;22(3):643–9.

64. Pashov AI, Tskhay VB, Ionouchene SV. The combined GnRH-agonist and intrauterine levonorgestrel-releasing system treatment of complicated atypical hyperplasia and endometrial cancer: a pilot study. *Gynecol Endocrin* 2012;28(7):559–61.

65. Gunderson CC, Fader AN, Carson KA, Bristow RE. Oncologic and Reproductive outcomes with progestin therapy in women with endometrial hyperplasia and grade 1 Adenocarcinoma: A systematic review. *Gynecol Oncol* 2012;125:477–82.

66. Abu-Rustum NR, Alektiar K, Iasonos A, Lev G, Sonoda Y, Aghajanian C, *et al*. The incidence of symptomatic lower-extremity lymphoedema following treatment of uterine corpus malignancies: a 12-year experience at Memorial Sloan-Kettering Cancer Center. *Gynecol Oncol* 2006;103(2):714–18.

67. Todo Y, Yamamoto R, Minobe S, Suzuki Y, Takeshi U, Nakatani M, *et al*. Risk factors for postoperative lower-extremity lymphoedema in endometrial cancer survivors who had treatment including lymphadenectomy. *Gynecol Oncol* 2010;119(1):60–4.

68. Creutzberg CL, van Putten WL, Koper PC, Lybeert ML, Jobsen JJ, Wárlám-Rodenhuis CC, *et al*. Survival after relapse in patients with endometrial cancer: results from a randomized trial. *Obstet Gynecol Survey* 2003;58(8):533. *Gynecol Oncol* 2003;89(2):201-9.

69. Huh W, Straughn Jr J, Mariani A, Podratz K, Havrilesky L, Alvarez Secord A, *et al*. Salvage of isolated vaginal recurrences in women with surgical stage I endometrial cancer: a multiinstitutional experience. *Int J Gynecol Cancer* 2007;17(4):886–9.

70. Del Carmen M, Boruta D, Schorge J. Recurrent endometrial cancer. *Clin Obstet Gynecol* 2011;54:266–77.

71. Barlin JN, Puri I, Bristow RE. Cytoreductive surgery for advanced or recurrent endometrial cancer: a meta-analysis. *Gynecol Oncol* 2010;118(1):14–18.

72. Kang S, Yoo HJ, Hwang JH, Lim M-C., Seo S-S., Park S-Y. Sentinel lymph node biopsy in endometrial cancer: meta-analysis of 26 studies. *Gynecol Oncol* 2011;123:522–7.

73. Cuzick J, Forbes J, Edwards R, Baum M, Cawthorn S, Coates A, *et al*. First results from the International Breast Cancer Intervention Study (IBIS-I): a randomised prevention trial. *Lancet* 2002;360:817–24.

23 Recurrent ovarian cancer

Jayanta Chatterjee, Viren Asher, and
Christina Fotopoulou

Ⓖ Expert Commentary Henry Kitchener
Ⓖ Guest Expert Sarah Blagden

Case history

Mrs M, a 57-year-old post-menopausal healthcare assistant, presented to her general practitioner with a two-month history of worsening spasmodic lower abdominal pain. She had also developed symptoms of urinary urgency and associated incontinence, which were affecting her activities of daily living especially her performance at work. She did not have any bowel symptoms and did not report loss of appetite or weight. There was no family history of cancer. On examination she had a palpable mass in the lower abdomen arising from the pelvis. Her GP referred Mrs M as a matter of urgency to the rapid access clinic (RAC) and ordered a trans-vaginal pelvic ultrasound.

> **✪ Learning point** Presentation of ovarian cancer
> - Ovarian cancer is the second most common gynaecological cancer, the fifth most common cancer in women, and the leading cause of death from gynaecological cancer in the UK.
> - The overall five-year survival rate is less than 40% [1].
> - 80% of cases occur in post-menopausal women over the age of 50 years [1].
> - Whilst most women present with non-specific symptoms, the most frequently reported symptoms of early-stage disease are lower abdominal pain or bloating [2] (Table 23.1).
> - Persistent, new onset, and worsening symptoms (up to 12 months), or ongoing symptoms will help distinguish ovarian cancer from other diagnoses [3].

Table 23.1 Symptoms of ovarian cancer according to disease stage (courtesy CRUK)

	Early Stage	Disease spread beyond the ovary	Late stage disease
Symptoms associated with spread of disease	• Lower abdominal pain • Abdominal bloating or feeling of fullness	• Irregular periods or post-menopausal bleeding • Lower abdominal pain • Back pain • Urinary frequency • Constipation • Dyspareunia • A swollen abdomen • Feeling of fullness or loss of appetite	• Loss of appetite or a feeling of fullness in the abdomen • Nausea/vomiting • Constipation • Tiredness • Shortness of breath • Abdominal distension

Expert comment

Most women will have had symptoms for months before seeking help. Mrs M's symptoms of urinary incontinence and increased frequency are not a classical presentation but may have been caused by pressure arising from a pelvic mass. Clinicians should include ovarian cancer in their differential diagnosis of a post-menopausal woman with non-specific pelvic or abdominal symptoms. Unexplained fatigue, weight loss, or change in bowel habit in women over 50 years-old should also prompt further investigation and consideration of ovarian cancer.

Expert comment

The National Institute for Health Care and Excellence (NICE) guidelines [4] suggest initiating investigations in primary care for any women over 50 years with suspected ovarian malignancy. A CA-125 should have been performed by the GP before referring her to the rapid access clinic.

⭐ Learning Point Risk factors for ovarian malignancy

- **Family history (see Learning Point)**
- **Personal history of cancer:** Women who have had cancer of the breast, uterus, colon, or rectum have a higher risk of ovarian cancer as there is a greater likelihood that they carry the cancer-predisposing genes described [7].
- **Age over 55:** Most women are over the age of 55 when diagnosed with ovarian cancer apart from those with hereditary cancers [1].
- **Nulliparity:** Older nulliparous women have an increased risk of ovarian cancer.
- **Menopausal hormone therapy:** Studies have suggested that post-menopausal women who take oestrogen by itself (oestrogen without progesterone) for 5 or more years have an increased risk of developing ovarian cancer. The overall increased risk was by 30–40% over the usual incidence. This risk is reversed on stopping hormone replacement therapy [8, 9].
- **Obesity:** Women with a BMI of > 30 have an increased risk of developing ovarian cancer [10].

⭐ Learning point Risk of ovarian malignancy and family history

The average woman has a 1.5–2% risk of developing ovarian cancer during her lifetime. For those carrying cancer-predisposing gene mutations, this risk is increased.

A strong family history of specific cancers may indicate the presence of these mutations. Women who have a first-degree relative (i.e. a mother, daughter, or sister) with ovarian or breast cancer have an increased risk of carrying a BRCA mutation which predisposes for the disease. Women with a family history of cancer of the uterus, ovary, colon, or rectum may have an increased risk of carrying a mismatch repair gene mutation (genes MLH1, MSH2, MSH6, or PMS2). This is termed Lynch syndrome or hereditary nonpolyposis colorectal cancer (HNPCC), and carriers have an increased risk of ovarian cancer as well as other cancers.

Heritable mutations in BRCA1 and BRCA2 genes account for approximately 8% to 13% of newly diagnosed ovarian cancer cases. The risk of developing ovarian cancer by the age of 70 in women carrying a BRCA 1 mutation is approximately 35–60% and in women carrying a BRCA 2 mutation the risk is 10–27%. According to the most recent estimates, 55–65% of women who inherit a harmful BRCA1 mutation, and around 45% of women who inherit a harmful BRCA2 mutation, will develop breast cancer by 70 years of age [5, 6]. In comparison, women with Lynch syndrome (Hereditary non-polyposis colorectal cancer (HNPCC/Lynch syndrome), have a 12% risk of developing ovarian cancer and a 60% lifetime risk of both uterine and colon cancer. Similar to BRCA1 and BRCA2, changes in these genes can cause very early-onset cancers, with some of the cancers occurring as early as age 25 [7]. These women and other female members of their family should be counselled about undergoing genetic testing.

At her rapid access clinic appointment, Mrs M underwent a transvaginal ultrasound. This revealed bilateral complex ovarian masses with solid and multi-septate areas arising from her pelvis with a normal postmenopausal uterus and a small amount of ascites (Figure 23.1). These findings needed further clarification and she was referred for an MRI of the pelvis and blood test for tumour markers.

The magnetic resonance imaging (MRI) confirmed bilateral complex masses comprising of a 3.7 × 5 × 5.5 cm predominantly solid lesion on the right ovary, and a 3 × 3 × 5 cm solid and cystic lesion on the left ovary (Figure 23.2). It also showed moderate ascites and an omental cake with a 1.2 cm deposit in the Pouch of Douglas. The uterus was normal in size, and deposits on the Morrison's pouch and diaphragm were also noted with no evidence of lymphadenopathy.

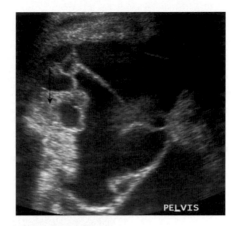

Figure 23.1 Transvaginal ultrasound, showing a complex ovarian cyst with septations and solid areas (arrows).

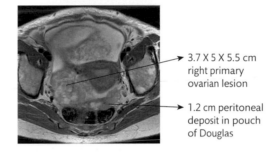

→ 3.7 X 5 X 5.5 cm right primary ovarian lesion

→ 1.2 cm peritoneal deposit in pouch of Douglas

Figure 23.2 Pelvic MRI demonstrating ovarian mass and peritoneal spread.

⊗ **Learning point** Imaging in suspected ovarian malignancy

- Ultrasound examination has a sensitivity of 69% in determining the extent of disease spread [11].
- Recent multivariate logistic regression models have been devised by the IOTA (International Ovarian Tumour Analysis) group to improve discrimination between benign and suspected malignant masses using ultrasound criteria, giving a higher diagnostic sensitivity and specificity [12].
- Magnetic resonance imaging (MRI) has been shown to predict staging correctly in over 80% of cases [13] and is superior to ultrasound in characterizing ovarian morphology and determining malignant features within a cyst such as papillary excrescences, septations, and solid components.

❝ **Expert comment**

Both CT and MRI scan are better than ultrasound in detecting peritoneal disease, disease beneath the diaphragm, and on the liver surface. Both modalities assist in the accurate staging of ovarian cancer [13–15]. MRI scan has been shown to have more sensitivity for detection of lymph node metastasis. The MRI scan in this patient helped to evaluate the extent of Mrs M's disease and informed the decision she should undergo primary debulking surgery, which remains the standard of care. Neither CT nor MRI can accurately assess fine nodule peritoneal cancer deposits, and patients should be made aware that in ovarian cancer there is rarely only 1 peritoneal deposit; rather areas of peritoneum are involved with fine or gross nodular peritoneal disease.

Mrs M's blood results showed that her serum level of tumour marker CA-125 was 885 U/ml (< 35 U/L) and carcinoembryonic antigen (CEA) was < 3 ng/L (3–5 ng/ml). Her haemoglobin was 13.1–g/dl with platelets of 242. Albumin was 46–g/dl, liver function tests were within normal limits, and renal function was also normal. Mrs M was post-menopausal (a score of 3), had two features of malignancy on her TVS (a score of 3), and her Ca125 was 885 U/L. Therefore her RMI score was calculated to be > 250.

❝ Expert commentary

A risk of malignancy (RMI) algorithm has been developed to distinguish between patients with benign and malignant pelvic masses. A RMI of 250 or more has 85% sensitivity and 97% specificity in distinguishing between benign and malignant ovarian masses, with an area under the receiver operating characteristic (ROC) curve of 0.83 [22]. Mrs M had a RMI > 250 and a 75% risk of ovarian cancer, and therefore was best managed in a gynaecological cancer centre [24].

➕ Clinical tip Common serum biomarkers associated with other gynaecological malignancies

- CA19-9 and CEA are mainly raised in bowel neoplasms or in primary or secondary mucinous neoplasms of the ovary.
- CA-153 is a tumour marker elevated in breast cancer.
- AFP is elevated in germ cell tumours of the ovary.
- BHCG levels are used to monitor and diagnose gestational trophoblastic disease.
- Inhibin, Oestradiol (GCT– granulosa cell tumours), and testosterone (Sertoli–Leydig cell tumours) levels are elevated in sex-cord stromal tumours of the ovary.

➕ Clinical tip Calculating risk of malignancy index (RMI) score [11]

The RMI score incorporates a score based on the product of transvaginal (TVS) ultrasound features, menopausal status, and CA-125 level.

$$\text{RMI score} = \text{TVS score} \times \text{menopausal status score} \times \text{CA-125 level.}$$

TVS features	*Score*
1. Multilocular cyst	1—one feature
2. Solid areas in the cyst	3—two to five features
3. Bilateral lesions	
4. Ascites	
5. Metastasis	

Menopausal status	
	1—Pre-menopausal
	3—Post-menopausal

CA-125	
	Level in U/l

✪ Learning point CA-125 A diagnostic biomarker in ovarian cancer

- **CA-125** (cancer antigen 125 or carbohydrate antigen 125), also known as mucin 16 or MUC16, is a protein that in humans is encoded by the MUC16 gene [16].
- To-date, CA-125 is the serum marker that has been most widely studied in the detection of early-stage ovarian cancer (Table 23.3). It was initially used for prognosis to see response following treatment for ovarian cancer.
- Serum CA-125 is elevated in 50% of early-stage and 92% of late-stage ovarian cancers [17].
- The positive predictive value (PPV) of a single CA-125 in early detection of ovarian cancer is 57%. It may not be elevated in non-serous ovarian cancers, such as clear cell and mucinous [18].
- The normal range for CA-125 is < 35 IU/L. CA-125 is raised above the normal range in serous epithelial and endometrioid ovarian cancer.
- CA-125 can be elevated in other cancers such as endometrial, breast, pancreatic, gastrointestinal, and lung cancers.
- CA-125 is also raised in benign gynaecological conditions such as pregnancy, inflammation, endometriosis, menstruation, and pelvic inflammatory disease.
- Various new biomarkers are now being looked at in ovarian cancer. HE4 (human epididymis protein 4) is one of them. The combination of HE4 and CA-125 indicates the risk of ovarian malignancy algorithm (ROMA) index [19].

✪ Learning point Screening for ovarian cancer

- To increase the PPV for screening, CA-125 has been combined with transvaginal ultrasound (TVUS). This strategy has been used in various combinations both sequentially and concurrently to augment the screening process.
- Given the low prevalence of ovarian cancer (16.2/100 000 in UK, 2008) in the general population, an effective and acceptable method of screening must not only have a high sensitivity for detection of early-stage disease (> 75%) but also a very high specificity (99.6%), so that no more than 10 false positive surgical procedures are performed in order to diagnose a single case of ovarian cancer [20].
- There are currently 4 major ovarian cancer screening trials, 2 of which are ongoing, and 2 that have been completed (Table 23.2).
- Routine general population screening for ovarian cancer is not currently recommended [20]. The results of the UKCTOCS Trial are awaited (2015).
- Results from phase I of the UK FOCSS (United Kingdom Familial Ovarian Cancer Screen Study) support the recommendation that women at inherited risk of ovarian cancer who decline RRSO (risk reduction salphingo-oopherectomy) should consider screening (four-monthly CA-125 and annual TVUS) for ovarian cancer from approximately age 35 years. Definitive risk-reducing surgery is recommended no later than in their early 40s [21].

Table 23.2 Findings from major screening trials for ovarian cancer [14]

Screening trial	Years
PLCO (USA)	1993–2001
UKCTOCS (UK)	2001–2005
SCSOCS (Japan)	1985–1999
University of Kentucky (USA)	1987–2011

Study design	Screening test	Numbers screened	Cancers detected	Stage I and II	Stage III and IV	Survival benefit
Randomized Control	TVUSS, CA-125 versus usual care	34 253	212	22%	77%	(-)
Randomized control	TVUSS alone or CA-125 versus usual care	101 279	58	48%	52%	Analysis pending
Randomized control	TVUSS, CA-125 versus usual care	41 688	27	67%	33%	Analysis pending
Population control	Ultrasound	37 293	47	70%	30%	(+)

[a] Trial ongoing. PLCO, The prostate, lung, colorectal and ovarian trial; UKCTOCS, United Kingdom Collaborative Trial of Ovarian cancer Screening; SCSOCS, Shizouka Cohort Study of Ovarian Cancer Screening

Table 23.3 Predictive ability of diagnostic serum markers for ovarian cancer [23]

	Cut-off	SE (%)	SP (%)	PPV	NPV
CA-125	> 35 U/L	82.2	67.3	47.1	91.4
	> 65 U/L	75.6	86.6	66.7	90.9
CA-19-9	> 40 U/ml	35.6	81.1	40	78
CA-15-3	> 32 U/ml	57.1	93.9	75.9	86.7
CEA	> 3 ng/ml (non-smoker) > 5 ng/ml (smoker)	16	93	37	83
AFP (in women < 40)	> 15 ng/ml	85% (germ cell tumours)	20% (in stage I disease)	Poor	Good
B-HCG (in women < 40)	> 5.0 mIU/mL	100% (choriocarcinoma)	10% for germinomatous tumours	Good	Good

PPV—Positive predictive value; NPV—Negative predictive value; SE—Sensitivity; SP—Specificity; CEA—Carcinoembryonic antigen.

Mrs M returned to the rapid access clinic with her husband 2 weeks later for her results. The consultant explained that in light of her RMI, she had a high likelihood of having ovarian cancer. The MRI scan showed that there was evidence the cancer had spread to the rest of her abdomen, and there was some suggestion there were deposits on her diaphragm. The consultant explained that her images and tumour marker results had been reviewed at the gynae-oncology multidisciplinary team meeting (MDT), and the recommendation from the MDT was to offer her primary debulking surgery since she had a good performance status and no comorbidities that prevented radical surgical intervention. Although Mrs M was upset by this news, both she and her husband had already suspected she had cancer. After further discussion, Mrs M was consented for primary debulking surgery and a date arranged for her admission prior to the next available operating list.

> **✪ Learning point** The gynaecological oncology MDT
>
> A typical gynaecological oncology multidisciplinary team is at least composed of a gynaecological oncologist, gynaecological clinical nurse specialist, medical oncologist, clinical oncologist, radiologist, and pathologist. It is recommended that this team meet once a week to discuss the management of gynaecological cancer cases. The MDT observes preset management policies, pathways of referral, and protocols that are agreed by members of the wider cancer network.

Table 23.4 Eastern Cooperative Oncology Group (ECOG) Performance status

Grade	Definition
0	Fully active, able to carry on all pre-disease performance without restriction
1	Restricted in physically strenuous activity but ambulatory and able to carry out work of a light or sedentary nature, e.g. light house work, office work
2	Ambulatory and capable of all self-care but unable to carry out any work activities. Up and about more than 50% of waking hours
3	Capable of only limited self-care, confined to bed or chair more than 50% of waking hours
4	Completely disabled. Cannot carry on any self-care. Totally confined to bed or chair
5	Dead

* As published in Oken MM, Creech RH, Tormey DC, Horton J, Davis TE, McFadden ET, Carbone PP: Toxicity And Response Criteria Of The Eastern Cooperative Oncology Group. *Am J Clin Oncol* 1982;5:649–55.

✪ Learning point Surgical management of ovarian cancer

The current international standard of care for ovarian cancer includes primary debulking surgery that comprises total abdominal hysterectomy (TAH) with bilateral salphingo-oopherectomy (BSO), omentectomy, and removal of disease from affected organs. The initial goals of primary surgery are to diagnose and stage the disease histologically (according to FIGO guidelines), together with complete cytoreduction which will determine the prognosis. Optimal cytoreduction is defined as total macroscopic clearance with no residual disease [34].

Where disease is in *early stage*, pelvic and para-aortic lymph node dissection (systematic LND) may also be performed to help in staging and deciding on adjuvant therapy. In *advanced disease*, where there are other sites of disease involvement, up-front maximal tumour resection is the cornerstone of management (with the aim of achieving complete cytoreduction). Bulky lymph nodes may also be resected. However, in the absence of bulky nodes, systematic LND is not routinely performed as it has no proven prognostic or therapeutic value in advanced disease (the subject of ongoing trials including the Lymphadenectomy in Ovarian Neoplasms (LION) STUDY).

During the pre-operative consent process, it is important that patients are informed that in order to achieve complete tumour resection, surgery may involve resection of part of the bowel and formation of a temporary or permanent stoma, peritoneal stripping in areas with peritoneal carcinosis, with removal of the affected organs if the tumor is more deeply attached (i.e. spleen, stripping of the diaphragm, removal of superficial liver deposits). Appendicectomy is performed if mucinous ovarian neoplasm is suspected arising from the gastrointestinal tract.

This surgical approach requires considerable expertise along with anatomical and practical knowledge of all the abdominal quadrants. The combination of extensive peritonectomy, ascitic and sometimes pleural drainage may necessitate intensive post-operative cardio-pulmonary support for patients in a high-dependency unit with multi-specialty input. Patients should be counselled prior to surgery the morbidity and mortality associated with such procedures based on individual factors such as suspected stage of disease, performance status, and other associated co-morbidities.

⊕ Clinical tip Risk of venous thromboembolism

Patients with ovarian cancer are at increased risk of developing venous thromboembolism (VTE), which is associated with significant morbidity and may complicate further management.

● The risk of developing VTE is highest immediately following surgery and during chemotherapy (15–20%) [30].
● Current NICE guidance [4] recommends use of adapted anti-embolism stockings and prophylactic low molecular weight heparin during admission to hospital.
● For patients with ovarian cancer who have had major pelvic or abdominal surgery, extended post-operative thromboprophylaxsis for 28 days is recommended.

Two weeks later Mrs M was admitted to hospital and underwent a total abdominal hysterectomy, bilateral salpingo-oophrectomy, and supra and infra colic omentectomy. Intra-operatively, the pelvic peritoneum was involved with peritoneal nodules, so an en-bloc resection of uterus, cervix, ovaries, and diseased pelvic peritoneum was performed. A resection of the rectum was not necessary since the Pouch of Douglas peritoneum could be dissected off the rectum. The deposits on the diaphragm were stripped off.

Table 23.5 Impact of residual disease following cytoreduction on survival

Residual disease after cytoreductive surgery	Progression-free Survival (PFS) (risk of disease progression)	Overall survival (OS) (risk of death from all causes)
>1cm	More than twice the risk of disease progression compared to women with only microscopic disease (HR 2.36, 95% CI 2.06–2.71)	Three times the risk of death compared to women with only microscopic disease (HR 3.16, 95% CI 2.26–4.41)
<1cm	Twice the risk of disease progression compared to women with only microscopic disease (HR 1.96, 95% CI 1.72–2.23).	Twice the risk of death compared to women with only microscopic disease (HR 2.20, 95% CI 1.90–2.54)
0cm	Significant and independent 2.3 month increase (95 CI = 0.6-0.4, p = 0.011) in cohort median survival compared to 1.8 month increase (95% CI = 0.6–3.0, $p = 0.004$) in cohort median survival (residual disease ≤ 1 cm) [27].	

Reference: Optimal primary surgical treatment for advanced epithelial ovarian cancer. *Cochrane Review.* Elattar A, Bryant A, Winter-Roach BA, Hatem M, Naik R [35].

Survival impact of complete cytoreduction to no gross residual disease for advanced-stage ovarian cancer: A meta-analyis. Suk-Joon Chang, Melissa Hodeib, Jenny Chang, Robert E. Bristow [36].

> ✪ **Learning point** Neo-adjuvant chemotherapy
>
> Neo-adjuvant chemotherapy as the primary mode of treatment may be considered in certain cases of advanced ovarian cancer:
>
> - In widespread stage IIIC /IV disease where optimal surgical cytoreduction will not be achieved.
> - In patients with significant medical comorbidities with poor performance status.
> - Chemotherapy as primary treatment; may or may not be followed by surgery.
> - Helps identify disease which are chemo-resistant and will not be helped by interval surgery.
> - A recent European study has shown no difference in survival between patients randomised to primary cytoreductive surgery or to neoadjuvant chemotherapy. The study was criticized for low cytoreductive rates and poor median overall survival compared with other studies [37], but it represented real-world practice.

Mrs M had an uneventful post-operative recovery. She had early input with physiotherapy and nutritional support and was discharged on day 5.

Histology showed mixed endometroid and clear cell carcinoma of primary ovarian origin with involvement of omentum, fallopian tube, and mesosalpinx with a histological stage 3c (Table 23.6).

> ⊘ **Evidence base**
>
> A recent Cochrane review highlighted the need for achieving optimal cytoreduction (Table 23.5), and where it is not possible, then aiming for minimal residual disease (< 1 cm). These patients have a better prognosis than those with suboptimal cytoreduction (> 1 cm macroscopic disease) [35] [36].

> ❝ **Expert comment**
>
> In extensive disease spread with diffuse mesenteric or intestinal serosal carcinosis, where a total macroscopic tumor clearance cannot be surgically achieved, there is little point in removing organs like spleen or rectum due to small volume deposits.

> ⊘ **Evidence base** debulking and cytoreduction [32]
>
> - In meta-analysis of 81 studies, the extent of debulking correlated with incremental benefits of survival.
> - Each 10% increase in cytoreduction rates is associated with a 5.5% increase in the duration median survival for the operated cohort.
> - In patient cohorts where surgical cytoreduction was complete in 75%, the median survival was 39 months.
> - In patient cohorts where cytoreduction was complete in less than 75%, the median survival was 22.7 months.

Table 23.6 Staging classification for cancer of the ovary, fallopian tube and peritoneum FIGO Guidelines, 2014

FIGO (2013)	Stage
Descriptor	
I: Tumour confined to ovaries or fallopian tube(s)	I
IA: Tumour limited to one ovary (capsule intact) or fallopian tube; no tumour on ovarian or fallopian tube surface; no malignant cells in the ascites or peritoneal washings	IA
IB: Tumour limited to both ovaries (capsules intact) or fallopian tubes; no tumour on ovarian or fallopian tube surface; no malignant cells in the ascites or peritoneal washings	IB
IC: Tumour limited to one or both ovaries or fallopian tubes, with any of the following	IC
IC1: Surgical spill	IC1
IC2: Capsule ruptured before surgery or tumour on ovarian or fallopian tube surface	IC2
IC3: Malignant cells in the ascites or peritoneal washings	
II: Tumour involves one or both ovaries or fallopian tubes with pelvic extension (below pelvic brim) or primary peritoneal cancer	II
IIA: Extension and/or implants on uterus and/or fallopian tubes and/ or ovaries	IIA
IIB: Extension to other pelvic intraperitoneal tissues	IIB
III: Tumour involves one or both ovaries or fallopian tubes, or primary peritoneal cancer, with cytologically or histologically confirmed spread to the peritoneum outside the pelvis and/or metastasis to the retroperitoneal lymph nodes	III
	IIIA
IIIA1: Positive retroperitoneal lymph nodes only (cytologically or histologically proven)	IIIA1
IIIA1(i) Metastasis up to 10 mm in greatest dimension	IIIA1(i)
IIIA1(ii) Metastasis more than 10 mm in greatest dimension	IIIA1(ii)
IIIA2: Microscopic extrapelvic (above the pelvic brim) peritoneal involvement with or without positive retroperitoneal lymph nodes	IIIA2
IIIB: Macroscopic peritoneal metastasis beyond the pelvis up to 2 cm in greatest dimension, with or without metastasis to the retroperitoneal lymph nodes	IIIB
IIIC: Macroscopic peritoneal metastasis beyond the pelvis more than 2 cm in greatest dimension, with or without metastasis to the retro-peritoneal lymph nodes (includes extension of tumour to capsule of liver and spleen without parenchymal involvement of either organ)	IIIC
IV: Distant metastasis excluding peritoneal metastases	IV
IVA: Pleural effusion with positive cytology	IVA
IVB: Parenchymal metastases and metastases to extra-abdominal organs (including inguinal lymph nodes and lymph nodes outside of the abdominal cavity)	IVB

⊗ **Learning point** Histology and prognosis

- 75% of ovarian cancers are serous adenocarcinoma (SAC), 10% endometrioid and 5–25% clear cell cancers (CCC) [38], and a small proportion have mixed histological disease. 2–4% are mucinous tumours [39].
- Endometrioid adenocarcinoma are associated with better prognosis than the serous type [40], while the CCCs poorly respond to chemotherapeutic agents and recurrence rates are higher [41]. The overall response rate to platinum-based chemotherapy for CCC is significantly lower than that for SAC (11–27% versus 73–81%) [42]. New targeted therapies are warranted.
- Hess et al. [39] demonstrated that advanced-stage (stage 3 and 4) mucinous ovarian cancer have a poorer prognosis than non-mucinous cancer. This is largely related to the platinum resistance of these tumours. Furthermore, the overall survival of patients with non-mucinous tumours, when matched for stage, was 3 times longer than those with mucinous tumours.

> **ⓘ Guest expert comment (medical oncology)**
>
> Patients with advanced disease (stage IC–IV, or stage IA and 1B with adverse histology) will receive post-operative chemotherapy ideally within six to eight weeks of debulking surgery. About 80% of the patients respond to chemotherapy but of those, 75–80% will have tumour recurrence, mostly within 24 months of surgery [43]. Pre-treatment counselling about the short-, medium-, and long-term complications of chemotherapy should be provided by the medical oncologist and clinical nurse specialist (CNS). The information should be supplemented with leaflets, contact numbers for their CNS, and information about support groups.

> **✪ Learning point** Chemotherapy regimes for ovarian cancer.
>
> Standard treatment for epithelial ovarian cancer is six cycles of platinum-based chemotherapy, usually comprising carboplatin and paclitaxel given three-weekly. Although less responsive to platinum-based chemotherapy than serous and endometrioid, the rarer histology ovarian cancers like mucinous and clear cell are generally treated with the same chemotherapy. Various studies are ongoing to evaluate histology-specific regimes.
>
> Patients with stage IA or 1B CCC of the ovary are recommended to have adjuvant chemotherapy as CCC is regarded as a grade 3 tumour. A large retrospective analysis of stage I ovarian CCC showed no statistical differences in survival between patients who had or had not received adjuvant chemotherapy [45]. Furthermore, it demonstrated that peritoneal cytology status and primary-tumour (pT) status were independent prognostic factors for progression free-survival status, implying that adjuvant chemotherapy had little impact upon survival of stage I CCC patients. Therefore, accurate surgical staging with biopsies from all peritoneal surfaces and lymph node dissection (LND) is crucial to determine correct treatment.
>
> Further strategy, such as the addition of molecular targeting agents, could improve survival from ovarian CCC [42], and there is some evidence that anti-angiogenetic agent like avastin could be of some benefit [48].

> **➕ Clinical tip** Assessing response to chemotherapy
>
> A baseline contrast-enhanced CT scan (of chest, abdomen, and pelvis) before the start of chemotherapy helps to compare objective disease response to chemotherapy (with repeat CT scan imaging), following treatment.
>
> Similarly a baseline CA-125 is used as comparative measure of disease response. A static or falling CA-125 indicates stable or responsive disease.

Two weeks after her procedure, Mrs M returned to clinic. She was still experiencing some pain around the wound site but was otherwise well.

Her consultant explained that the procedure had gone well with complete resection of the tumour. After further discussion, Mrs M was subsequently referred to the medical oncologist for adjuvant chemotherapy.

A baseline CT scan performed before starting chemotherapy, three weeks post surgery, showed peritoneal thickening in the right and left paracolic gutters presumed to be inflammatory changes. The CA-125 was within normal limits at 11 U/ml.

Mrs M received six cycles of carboplatin (AUC6) and paclitaxel (175 mg/m^2) given three-weekly. She received prophylactic steroids and anti-emetics to reduce the risk of nausea and vomiting. Mrs M developed alopecia and noticed some tingling in her fingers and toes.

Mrs M and her husband attended a routine follow-up appointment 12 months after completing chemotherapy. She reported that she was feeling better and had returned to work on light duties. Her hair had regrown and the tingling in her fingers and toes was improving. Recently, however, she was feeling tired and had noticed some increased urinary urge and frequency. She underwent a vaginal examination which revealed a mass in the left vaginal fornix. Following this appointment, a CT scan was arranged which demonstrated a left pelvic solid/cystic mass measuring 6.2 × 5.4 cm with no evidence of omental or peritoneal disease (Figure 23.3). Her CA-125 was within normal limits at 23 u/ml.

> **❝ Expert commentary**
>
> The stage and histology of the tumour in this patient are poor prognostic factors with a high chance of future disease recurrence.

> **ⓘ Guest expert comment (medical oncology)**
>
> In the absence of significant disease related symptoms, there appears no detriment to starting chemotherapy up to eight weeks after surgery [51]. This helps the patient to recover from surgery in most cases. Although the optimal time to chemotherapy is unknown, recent research suggests that a delay to starting treatment is associated with worse outcome [52, 53].

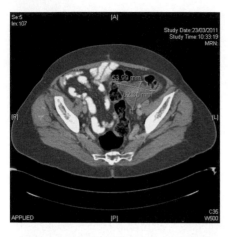

Figure 23.3 A large recurrent left pelvic side-wall cystic mass adherent to sigmoid colon.

> ✚ **Clinical tip** Role of Serum CA-125 in patient follow-up
>
> • Increase in CA-125 to twice the limit of normal has a 85% sensitivity and 91% specificity in detection of disease relapse [56].
> • Rise in CA-125 levels can predate the symptoms and signs by as much as 0–12 months (Median lead time of 63 days) [57]. Therefore the interpretation of rising CA-125 levels should performed with caution.
> • Early treatment based on rising CA-125 alone has shown no survival benefit compared to delayed treatment based on symptoms and clinical evidence of recurrence [58].

> ✪ **Learning point** Side effects of chemotherapeutic agents
>
> • Cisplatin was the first platinum derivative to be used in the treatment of ovarian cancer but was later superceded by carboplatin. Carboplatin is associated with less nephrotoxicity, ototoxicity, neuropathy, and alopecia compared with cisplatin, but has significant hematopoietic toxicity, especially thrombocytopenia.
> • Allergy to carboplatin occurs rarely and is related to cumulative exposure. Reactions typically manifest after a median of eight infusions (54).
> • Paclitaxel is associated with myelosuppression, alopecia, peripheral neuropathy, allergic reactions, and cardiac arrhythmias.

> ❝ **Expert comment**
>
> Within 12 months of completion of chemotherapy, there was recurrent disease evident on Mrs M's CT scan indicating platinum-sensitive recurrence. The CA-125 level remained normal in spite of increase in the mass.

Mrs M's case was discussed at the gynae-oncology multidisciplinary team (MDT) meeting. In view of recurrent mass and the fact that it was a solitary site of recurrence, she was offered surgery to remove the isolated disease.

> ✪ **Learning point** Recurrent Ovarian Cancer (ROC)
>
> • 70–90% of patients diagnosed with advanced ovarian cancer will at some point in time have disease recurrence.
> • Even most patients who go into clinical remission (complete response = CR) after initial therapy will eventually have disease recurrence.
> • The treatment option for recurrent disease depends on the initial outcome of surgical resection, response to chemotherapy, volume and distribution of recurrent tumour, treatment free interval, side effects from initial chemotherapy, and performance status of patient.
> • Secondary cytoreductive surgery, repeat first -line chemotherapy or second-line chemotherapy drugs, are treatment options in recurrent disease.

> ✪ **Learning point** Chemotherapy for recurrent ovarian cancer
>
> Time to recurrence/ relapse after initial therapy is the main determinant for subsequent therapy and expected disease response. The longer the interval between initial complete remission to disease recurrence, the greater will be the sensitivity to the initial chemotherapy.
>
> Recurrence of disease in a patient who has achieved a documented response to initial platinum-based treatment and has been off therapy for more than six months, is defined as *platinum-sensitive disease.*
>
> *Platinum-resistant disease* is defined as disease that has responded to initial chemotherapy but demonstrates recurrence within 6 months following the completion of treatment.
>
> *Refractory ovarian cancer* occurs in patients who have failed to achieve at least a partial response to therapy. This includes patients with either stable disease or actual disease progression during primary therapy, which occurs in approximately 20% of cases. As might be expected, this group has the lowest response rate to second-line therapy.

> ➕ **Clinical tip** RECIST Criteria (Response Evaluation Criteria in Solid Tumours) definitions of response [61]
>
> **Complete response (CR)**—Disappearance of all target lesions.
> **Partial response (PR)**—At least a 30% decrease in the sum of the longest diameter (LD) of target lesions, taking as reference the baseline sum LD.
> **Progressive disease (PD)**—At least 20% increase in the sum of the LD of target lesions, taking the reference the smallest sum LD recorded since the treatment started or appearance of one or more new lesions.
> **Stable disease (SD)**—Neither sufficient shrinkage to qualify for PR nor sufficient increase to qualify for PD, taking as reference the smallest sum LD since the treatment started.

After further discussion, Mrs M agreed to further surgery and was subsequently consented and admitted for a laparotomy. This revealed a fluid-filled cyst, densely adherent to the left pelvic sidewall, and tumour infiltrating the major blood vessel and sigmoid mesentery. There was 2 cm plaque of disease on the rectum that was completely removed with the cyst wall, leaving no macroscopic disease at the end of the procedure.

Subsequent histology revealed fibrovascular connective and ovarian stromal tissue infiltrated with poorly differentiated clear cell adenocarcinoma involving the margins of the capsule.

> 🕙 **Landmark trial** The DESKTOP trial [62]
>
> The DESKTOP I trial proposed a score for the prediction of complete cytoreduction in recurrent ovarian cancer. Resectability was assumed if three factors were present: (1) complete resection at first surgery, (2) good performance status, and (3) absence of ascites. The DESKTOP II trial was planned to verify this hypothesis prospectively in a multicenter setting.
>
> A 75% complete resection rate in 110 prospectively classified patients had to be achieved to confirm a positive predictive value of 2 or higher of 3 with 95% probability.
>
> The rate of complete resection was 76%, thus confirming the validity of this score regarding positive prediction of complete resectability in two or more of three patients. Complication rates were moderate, including second operations in 11% and peri-operative mortality in 0.8%.
>
> This score is the first prospectively validated instrument to positively predict surgical outcome in recurrent ovarian cancer. It may help in the selection of patients who might benefit from secondary cytoreductive surgery and are being enrolled in the recently started randomized prospective DESKTOP III trial investigating the role of surgery in recurrent platinum-sensitive ovarian cancer.

Mrs M was subsequently discussed at the MDT meeting and a decision was made to recommend further chemotherapy to reduce the risk of recurrence. She received further chemotherapy and is currently on clinical follow-up. She was well on her last clinic visit and looking forward to a holiday abroad with her husband.

> 🕙 **Landmark trial** Ovarian Cancer Study Comparing Efficacy and Safety of Chemotherapy and Anti-Angiogenic Therapy in Platinum-Sensitive Recurrent Disease (OCEANS) [63].
>
> This is a randomized, double-blinded, placebo-controlled phase III trial of chemotherapy with or without bevacizumab (BV) in patients with platinum-sensitive recurrent epithelial ovarian, primary peritoneal, or fallopian tube cancer.
>
> Platinum-sensitive ROC patients (recurrence ≥ 6 months after front-line platinum-based therapy) who had measurable disease, were randomly assigned to GC (gemcitabine and carboplatin) plus either BV or placebo (PL) for 6–10 cycles. BV or PL was then continued until disease progression. The primary end-point of this study was to assess progression-free survival (PFS) by RECIST; secondary end-points were objective response rate, duration of response (DOR), overall survival, and safety.
>
> Two patients in the BV arm experienced GI perforation after study treatment discontinuation.
>
> Conclusion: GC plus BV followed by BV until progression, resulted in a statistically significant improvement in PFS compared to the placebo group in platinum-sensitive ROC.

Mrs M will be subsequently followed up jointly between the oncologists and gynae-oncology surgeons. The follow-up visit consists of enquiry about abdominal symptoms with abdominal and vaginal examination to detect recurrence with measurement of CA-125 levels.

> **⊕ Clinical tip** Secondary debulking surgery
>
> Secondary cytoreductive surgery can be offered to these patients who have platinum-sensitive disease to improve their survival, especially if they have disease that is amenable to optimal debulking. The results from DESKTOP III trial are awaited to validate the rationale of secondary cytoreduction in a selected cohort of patients who have recurrent disease [63].

> **❛❛ Expert comment**
>
> There is no optimal interval defined for the regular follow-up of patients after completion of treatment. Most of the patients relapse within the first two years and therefore they are frequently seen during this period. The follow-up protocol greatly varies between different hospitals. The general recommendation is three-monthly follow-up for first two years, and six monthly thereafter. Imaging is not routinely indicated in follow-up of these patients. If needed, CT scan is the modality of choice and is generally performed in symptomatic patients or those where clinical examination reveals an abnormality or those who have rising CA-125 indicating possible recurrence.

Discussion

Mrs M initially presented with disseminated abdominal disease (stage 3c) typically found in 60 % of ovarian cancer patients [1]. Standard treatment comprises surgery to achieve optimal cytoreduction (no residual disease), consistently shown to have better overall survival compared to suboptimal debulking. This patient had mixed clear cell and endometrioid tumour that was completely resected, but following carboplatin and paclitaxel chemotherapy she relapsed. She underwent secondary debulking surgery followed by adjuvant platinum based chemotherapy and she was classified as platinum-sensitive.

A second relapse is almost inevitable and close surveillance during follow-up is required. Many patients, like Mrs M, with high risk of recurrence experience significant psychological morbidity during follow-up. This can be mitigated by close support from specialist nurses and cancer support services.

A multidisciplinary team approach in the management of patients with ovarian cancer has been shown to be a significant factor in improving survival [64]. As well as improving patient survival and quality of life, the centralization of care provided by the multidisciplinary team allows better continuity of care and the development of expertise to deal with rarer cancers. The provision of specialist nurses within multidisciplinary teams can reduce patients' distress, increase satisfaction, and improve information provision [65].

A Final Word from the Expert

This patient had mixed clear cell and endometrioid tumour that had initially completely responded to Carboplatin and paclitaxel chemotherapy but recurred with platinum-sensitive disease in the pelvis. She underwent secondary debulking surgery and this was followed by adjuvant chemotherapy treatment.

The goal of primary surgery in ovarian cancer patients should be to achieve optimal debulking with no residual disease.

Despite complete cytoreduction and chemotherapy, in women with stage 3 disease relapse occurs in the vast majority and following this the prognosis remains very poor. Repeated occurrences of chemotherapy in platinum sensitive patients can prolong survival with good quality of life.

References

1. Office for National Statistics. Survival rates in England, patients diagnosed 2001-2006 followed up to 2007. <http://www.ons.gov.uk/ons/taxonomy/index.html?nscl=Cancer>

2. Mayor S Consensus statement on ovarian cancer aims to settle dispute over symptoms. *BMJ* 2008;337: a2007.

3. Bankhead, CR, Collins C, Stokes-Lampard H, Rose P, Wilson S, Clements A, *et al.* Identifying symptoms of ovarian cancer: a qualitative and quantitative study. *BJOG* 2008:115(8):1008–14.

4. Nice Clinical Guideline 122. Ovarian cancer. April 2011. <http://www.nice.org.uk/guidance/CG122>

5. Chen S, Parmigiani G. Meta-analysis of BRCA1 and BRCA2 penetrance. *Journal of Clinical Oncology* 2007;25(11):1329–33.

6. Howlader N, Noone AM, Krapcho M, Garshell J, Miller D, Altekruse SF, *et al. SEER Cancer Statistics Review, 1975-2010*. Bethesda, MD: National Cancer Institute, 2013.

7. Kehoe SM, Kauff ND. Screening and Prevention of Hereditary Gynecologic cancers. *Seminars in Oncology* 2007;34:406–10.

8. Greiser CM, Greiser EM, Dören M. Menopausal hormone therapy and risk of ovarian cancer: systematic review and meta-analysis. *Hum Reprod Update* 2007;13:453–63.

9. Anderson GL, Judd HL, Kaunitz AM, Barad DH, Beresford SA, Pettinger M, *et al.* Women's Health Initiative Investigators. Effects of oestrogen plus progestin on gynecologic cancers and associated diagnostic procedures: the Women's Health Initiative randomized trial. *JAMA* 2003;290:1739–48.

10. Olsen CM, Nagle CM, Whiteman DC, Ness R, Pearce CL, Pike MC, *et al.* Obesity and risk of ovarian cancer subtypes: evidence from the Ovarian Cancer Association Consortium *Endocr Relat Cancer* 2013;20(2):251–62; doi:10.1530/ERC-12-0395.

11. Davies AP, Jacobs I, Woolas R, Fish A, Oram D The adnexal mass: benign or malignant? Evaluation of a risk of malignancy index. *Br J Obstet Gynaecol* 1993;100(10):927–31.

12. Timmerman D, Ameye L, Fischerova D, Epstein E, Melis GB, Guerriero S, *et al.* Simple ultrasound rules to distinguish between benign and malignant adnexal masses before surgery: prospective validation by IOTA group. *BMJ* 2010;14:341:c6839.

13. Tempany CM, Zou KH, Silverman SG, Brown DL, Kurtz AB, McNeil BJ, *et al.* Staging of advanced ovarian cancer: comparison of imaging modalities-report from the Radiological Diagnostic Oncology Group. *Radiology* 2000;215(3):761–7.

14. Patel VH, Somers S. MR imaging of the female pelvis: current perspectives and review of genital tract congenital anomalies, and benign and malignant diseases. *Crit Rev Diagn Imaging* 1997;38(5):417–99.

15. Kennedy AM, Gilfeather MR, Woodward PJ. *MRI of the female pelvis*. Semin Ultrasound CT MR, 1999. 20(4):214–30.

16. Yin BW, Dnistrian A, Lloyd KO. Ovarian cancer antigen CA125 is encoded by the MUC16 mucin gene. *Int. J. Cancer* 2002;2298(5):737–40.

17. Kobayashi E, Ueda Y, Matsuzaki S, Yokoyama T, Kimura T, Yoshino K, *et al.* Biomarkers for screening, diagnosis and monitoring of ovarian cancer. *Cancer Epidemiology, Biomarkers & Prevention* 2012;21:1902–12

18. Hogdall EVS, Christensen L, Kjaer SK, Blaakaer J, Kjaerbye-Thygesen A, Gayther S, *et al.* CA-125 expression pattern, prognosis and correlation with serum CA-125 in ovarian tumor patients from The Danish 'MALOVA' Ovarian Cancer Study. *Gynecologic Oncology* 2007;104:508–15.

19. Sandri MT, Bottari F, Franchi D, Boveri S, Candiani M, Ronzoni S, *et al.* Comparison of HE4, CA125 and ROMA algorithm in women with a pelvic mass: correlation with pathological outcome. *Gynecol Oncol* 2013 Feb;128(2):233–8.

20. Menon U, Gentry-Maharaj A, Hallett R, Ryan A, Burnell M, Sharma A, *et al.* Sensitivity and specificity of multimodal and ultrasound screening for ovarian cancer, and

stage distribution of detected cancers: results of the prevalence screen of the UK Collaborative Trial of Ovarian Cancer Screening (UKCTOCS). *Lancet Oncology* 2009;10(4):327–40.

21. Rosenthal A. Ovarian cancer screening in the high-risk population-the UK Familial Ovarian Cancer Screening Study (UKFOCSS). *Int J Gynecol Cancer* 2012; Suppl 1

22. Akturk E, Karaca RE, Alanbay I, Dede M, Karaşahin E, Yenen MC, *et al.* Comparison of four malignancy risk indices in detection of malignant ovarian masses. *J Gynecol Oncol* 22;3:177–82.

23. Bosl GJ, Feldman DR, Bajorin DF, Sheinfeld J, Motzer RJ, Rueter VE, *et al.* Cancer of the testis. In:DeVita VT, Hellman S, Rosenberg SA, *et al.* (eds). *Cancer, principles and practice of oncology*, 6th edn. Philadelphia: Lippincott, Williams & Wilkins 2001:1491–518.

24. Junor EJ, Hole DJ, McNulty L, Mason M, Young J. Specialist gynaecologists and survival outcome in ovarian cancer: a Scottish national study of 1866 patients. *Br J Obstet Gynaecol* 1999;106(11):1130–6.

25. Jacobs I, Oram D, Fairbanks J, Turner J, Frost C, Grudzinskas JG. A risk of malignancy index incorporating CA125, ultrasound and menopausal status for the accurate preoperative diagnosis of ovarian cancer. *B J Obstet Gynaecol* 1990;97(10):922–9.

26. Tingulstad S, Hagen B, Skjeldestad FE, Onsrud M, Kiserud T, Halvorsen T, *et al.* Evaluation of a risk of malignancy index based on serum CA125, ultrasound findings and menopausal status in the pre-operative diagnosis of pelvic masses. *Br J Obstet Gynaecol* 1996;103(8):826–31.

27. Morgante G, la Marca A, Ditto A, De Leo V. Comparison of two malignancy risk indices based on serum CA125, ultrasound score and menopausal status in the diagnosis of ovarian masses. *Br J Obstet Gynaecol* 1999;106(6):524–7.

28. Aslam N, Tailor A, Lawton F, Carr J, Savvas M, Jurkovic D. Prospective evaluation of three different models for the pre-operative diagnosis of ovarian cancer. *BJOG* 2000;107(11):1347–53.

29. Tailor A, Jurkovic D, Bourne TH, Collins WP, Campbell S. Sonographic prediction of malignancy in adnexal masses using multivariate logistic regression analysis. *Ultrasound Obstet Gynecol* 1997;10(1):41–7.

30. Agnelli G, Verso M. Management of venous thromboembolism in patients with cancer. *J Thromb Haemost* 2011;9(Suppl 1):316–24.

31. Jelovac D, Armstrong DK. Recent progress in the diagnosis and treatment of ovarian cancer. *CA Cancer J Clin* 2011;61(3):183–203.

32. Bristow RE, Tomacruz RS, Armstrong DK, Trimble EL, Montz FJ. Survival effect of maximal cytoreductive surgery for advanced ovarian carcinoma during the platinum era: a meta-analysis. *J Clin Oncol* 2002;20(5):1248–59.

33. Oken MM, Creech RH, Tormey DC, Horton J, Davis TE, McFadden ET, Carbone PP. Toxicity And Response Criteria Of The Eastern Cooperative Oncology Group. *Am J Clin Oncol* 1982;5:649–55.

34. Stuart GC, Kitchener H, Bacon M, duBois A, Friedlander M, Ledermann J, *et al.* 2010 Gynecologic Cancer InterGroup (GCIG) consensus statement on clinical trials in ovarian cancer: report from the Fourth Ovarian Cancer Consensus Conference. *Int J Gynecol Cancer* 2011;21(4):750–5.

35. Elattar A, Bryant A, Winter-Roach BA, Hatem M, Naik R. Optimal primary surgical treatment for advanced epithelial ovarian cancer. *Cochrane Database Syst Rev* 2011(8):CD007565.

36. Chang S-J., Hodeib M, Chang J, Bristow RE. Survival impact of complete cytoreduction to no fross residual disease for advanced-stage ovarain cancer: A meta-analyis. *Gynecol Oncol* 2013;130;493–8.

37. Vergote I, Tropé CG, Amant F, Kristensen GB, Ehlen T, Johnson N, *et al.* Neoadjuvant chemotherapy or primary surgery in stage IIIC or IV ovarian cancer. *N Engl J Med* 2010;363;943–53.

38. Anglesio MS, Carey MS, Köbel M, Mackay H, Huntsman DG; Vancouver Ovarian Clear Cell Symposium Speakers Clear cell carcinoma of the ovary: a report from the first Ovarian Clear Cell Symposium, 24 June 24 2010. *Gynecol Oncol* 2011;121(2):407–15.

39. Hess V, A'Hern R, Nasiri N, King DM, Blake PR, Barton DP, *et al.* Mucinous epithelial ovarian cancer: a seperate entity requiring specific treatment. *J Clin Oncol* 2004;22:1040–4.

40. Storey DJ, Rush R, Stewart M, Rye T, Al-Nafussi A, Williams AR, *et al.* Endometrioid epithelial ovarian cancer : 20 years of prospectively collected data from a single center. *Cancer* 2008;112(10):2211–20.

41. Behbakht K, Randall TC, Benjamin I, Morgan MA, King S, Rubin SC. Clinical characteristics of clear cell carcinoma of the ovary. *Gynecol Oncol* 1998;70(2):255–8.

42. Itamochi H, Kigawa J, Terakawa N. Mechanisms of chemoresistance and poor prognosis in ovarian clear cell carcinoma. *Cancer Science* 2008;99(4):653–8.

43. Ushijima K. Treatment of recurrent ovarian cancer—at first relapse. *J Oncol* 2010, Article ID 497429, 7 pages doi:10.1155/2010/497429

44. Takakura S, Takano M, Takahashi F, Saito T, Aoki D, Inaba N, *et al.* Randomized Phase II trial of Paclitaxel plus Carboplatin Therapy versus Irinotecan plus Cisplatin Therapy as First-Line Chemotherapy for Clear Cell Adenocarcinoma of the Ovary. A JGOG study. *Int J Gynecol Cancer* 2010;20:240–7.

45. Takano M, Kikuchi Y, Yaegashi N, Suzuki M, Tsuda H, Sagae S, *et al.* Adjuvant chemotherapy with irinotecan hydrochloride and cisplatin for clear cell carcinoma of the ovary. *Oncol Rep* 2006;16:1301–6.

46. <http://public.ukcrn.org.uk/search/StudyDetail.aspx?StudyID=5275>

47. Alexandre J, Ray-Coquard I, Selle F, Floquet A, Cottu P, Weber B, *et al.* Mucinous advanced epithelial ovarian carcinoma: clinical presentation and sensitivity to platinum-paclitaxel-based chemotherapy, the GINECO experience. *Ann Oncol* 2010 Dec;21(12):2377–81.

48. Hall M, Gourley C, McNeish I, Ledermann J, Gore M, Jayson G, *et al.* Targeted antivascular therapies for ovarian cancer: current evidence. *British Journal of Cancer* 2013;108:250–58.

49. van der Burg MEL, Boere IA, Berns PM. Dose-dense therapy is of benefit in primary treatment of ovarian cancer: contra. *Annals of Oncology* 2011;22(Supplement 8): viii33–viii39.

50. Gonzalez-Martin A, Gladieff L, Tholander B, Stroyakovsky D, Gore M, Scambia G, *et al.* Efficacy and safety results from OCTAVIA, a single-arm phase II study evaluating frontline bevacizumab, carboplatin and weekly paclitaxel for ovarian cancer. *Eur J Cancer* 2013, Sep 2. pii: S0959-8049(13) 00757-0. doi:10.1016/j.ejca.2013.08.002

51. Rosa DD, Clamp A, Mullamitha S, Ton NC, Lau S, Byrd L, *et al.* The interval from surgery to chemotherapy in the treatment of advanced epithelial ovarian carcinoma. *Eur J Surg Oncol* 2006;32(5):588–91.

52. Mahner S.Eulenburg C, Staehle A, Wegscheider K, Reuss A, Pujade-Lauraine E, *et al.* Prognostic impact of the time interval between surgery and chemotherapy in advanced ovarian cancer: analysis of prospective randomised phase III trials. *Eur J Cancer* 2013 Jan;49(1):142–9.

53. Hofstetter G.Concin N, Braicu I, Chekerov R, Sehouli J, Cadron I, *et al.* The time interval from surgery to start of chemotherapy significantly impacts prognosis in patients with advanced serous ovarian carcinoma—Analysis of patient data in the prospective OVCAD study. *Gynecol Oncol* 2013;131(1):15–20.

54. du Bois A, Quinn M, Thigpen T, Vermorken J, Avall-Lundqvist E, Bookman M, *et al.* 2004 consensus statements on the management of ovarian cancer: final document of the 3rd International Gynecologic Cancer Intergroup Ovarian Cancer Consensus Conference (GCIG OCCC 2004). *Ann Oncol* 2005;16(Suppl 8): viii7–viii12.

55. Markman M, Kennedy A, Webster K, Elson P, Peterson G, Kulp B, *et al.* Clinical features of hypersensitivity reactions to carboplatin. *J Clin Oncol* 1999 Apr;17(4):1141.

56. Gu P, Pan LL, Wu SQ, Sun L, Huang G. CA 125, PET alone, PET-CT, CT and MRI in diagnosing recurrent ovarian carcinoma: a systematic review and meta-analysis. *Eur J Radiol* 2009;71(1):164–74.

57. Vergote I, Rustin GJ, Eisenhauer EA, Kristensen GB, Pujade-Lauraine E, Pamar MK, *et al.* Re: new guidelines to evaluate the response to treatment in solid tumors [ovarian cancer]. Gynecologic Cancer Intergroup. *J Natl Cancer Inst* 2000;92(18):1534–5.

58. Rustin GJ, van der Burg ME, Griffin CL, Guthrie D, Lamont A, Jayson GC, *et al.* Early versus delayed treatment of relapsed ovarian cancer (MRC OV05/EORTC 55955): a randomised trial. *Lancet* 2010;376(9747):1155–63.

59. Chi DS, McCaughty K, Diaz JP, Huh J, Schwabenbauer S, Hummer AJ, *et al.* Guidelines and selection criteria for secondary cytoreductive surgery in patients with recurrent, platinum-sensitive epithelial ovarian carcinoma. *Cancer* 2006;106(9):1933–9.

60. Markman M, Bookman MA. Second-Line Treatment of Ovarian Cancer. *The Oncologist* 2000;5:26–35.

61. Eisenhauer EA, Therasse P, Bogaerts J, Schwartz LH, Sargent D, Ford R, *et al.* New response evaluation criteria in solid tumours: revised RECIST guideline (version 1.1). *Eur J Cancer* 2009;45(2):228–47.

62. Harter P, Sehouli J, Reuss A, Hasenburg A, Scambia G, Cibula D, *et al.* Prospective validation study of a predictive score for operability of recurrent ovarian cancer: the Multicenter Intergroup Study DESKTOP II. *Int J Gynecol Cancer* 2011 Feb;21(2):289–95.

63. Aghajanian C, Blank SV, Goff BA, Judson PL, Teneriello MG, Husain A, *et al.* OCEANS: a randomized, double-blind, placebo-controlled phase III trial of chemotherapy with or without bevacizumab in patients with platinum-sensitive recurrent epithelial ovarian, primary peritoneal, or fallopian tube cancer. *J Clin Oncol* 2012 Jun 10;30(17):2039–45.

64. Junor EJ, Hole DJ, Gillis CR. Management of ovarian cancer: referral to a multidisciplinary team matters. *Br J Cancer* 1994;70(2):363–70.

65. NHS Executive. *Improving outcomes in gynaecological cancer: the manual.* 1999: NHS Executive.

66. Van der Burg MEL, van Lent M, Buyse M, Kobierska A, Colombo N, Favallie G, *et al.* The Effect of Debulking Surgery after Induction Chemotherapy on the Prognosis in Advanced Epithelial Ovarian Cancer. Gynecological Cancer Cooperative Group of the European Organization for Research and Treatment of Cancer. *N Engl J Med* 1995;332:629–34.

24 Cervical cancer

Jayanta Chatterjee,
Kavitha Madhuri Thumuluru,
and Pubudu Pathiraja

✪ **Expert Commentary** Sean Kehoe and Christina Fotopoulou

Case history

A 25-year-old nulliparous woman attended her GP practice following an invitation for her first cervical smear test. She had no other significant gynaecological history of note with regular menstrual cycles every 28 days, lasting for five days. She did not report any inter-menstrual or post-coital bleeding. She had been in a steady relationship for five years using condoms for contraception. She was otherwise fit and well.

Two weeks later, she received a letter informing her that her cervical smear showed 'severe dyskaryosis', and that an urgent referral for colposcopy had been made on her behalf, which she attended the following week.

At colposcopy, it was noted that she had 'dense acetowhite changes at the squamocolumnar junction with widespread coarse punctuation and raised irregular mosaics with umbilication and irregular pollarded vasculature' suggestive of early invasive cancer'.

Due to the highly suspicious nature of the colposcopy findings, a large loop excisional biopsy of the transformation zone (LLETZ) was performed under general anaesthesia. The patient underwent an uneventful primary conisation without any complications. Macroscopic dimensions of the excised cervical tissue were 25 × 15 × 20 mm.

> ✪ **Learning point** Cervical cancer epidemiology
>
> Worldwide, cervical cancer remains the fourth most common malignancy in women. Over 80 % of these cases are found in developing countries. In 2012, there were 528 000 new cases diagnosed worldwide, accounting for 7 % of all cancer related deaths in women [1].
>
> In the UK, there were 972 deaths due to cervical cancer in 2011, accounting for 1 % of all female cancer deaths. Five-year relative survival rates for cervical cancer have increased from 52 % in England and Wales during 1971–1975 to 66.6 % in England during 2005–2009 [2–5].
>
> Cervical cancer accounts for 2 % of new cancer diagnoses in females in the UK. The age specific incidence rates show two peaks, the first in women aged 30–34 (at 21 per 100 000 women), and the second in women aged 80–84 (at 13 per 100 000 women). The earlier peak is related to increased sexual activity amongst girls in their late teens/early twenties [6,7], giving rise to an increase in human papilloma virus (HPV) infections, a necessary cause of cervical cancer [8]. There has also been an increasing incidence of high-grade CIN in younger women over the last twenty years [9–10]. The second smaller peak is due to increasing cancer incidence with age. In the UK between 2008 and 2010, an average of 20 % of cervical cancer cases were diagnosed in women aged 65 years and over [11–14].
>
> Histologically, over 80 % of cases are squamous cell carcinoma. Adenocarcinoma comprises approximately 10 % of cases. Rarer variants include adenosquamous, clear cell/mucinous adenocarcinoma, and neuroendocrine histology.

❝ Expert comment

Pre-invasive cervical disease with HPV infection is rare in older women but is not unusual in women under the age of 25 years where in most cases spontaneous regression of the lesions occur [15–17]. Hence one reason for the re-evaluation of screening in this population, as unnecessary interventions, is not without morbidity. The morbidity would not only entail that associated with the surgical procedure itself, but also other sequelae, in particular, the association between treatment and premature labour in subsequent pregnancies. Cervical cancer is extremely rare in women under the age of 25, with just 2.6 cases per 100 000 women [18]. Therefore, the harms of screening women under the age of 25 are currently thought to outweigh the benefits. Further epidemiological studies need to be undertaken to assess the impact of lower age of first sexual contact and higher promiscuity rate in relation to exposure to the HPV virus, so guidelines can be adjusted accordingly.

✪ Learning point Cervical screening

Cervical cancer is considered largely preventable through screening and subsequent treatment of precancerous lesions. The UK NHS cervical screening programme [19], set up in 1988, is an example of a national screening programme, aimed at reducing the incidence and mortality from cervical cancer. Cervical cancer screening is done by taking cervical smears which are analysed using the recently introduced liquid-based cytology (LBC) method, to reduce the false positive ratio [19] (Figures 24.1 and 24.2).

The program screened about 3.57 million women between the ages of 25 and 64 in England alone in 2012–2013, with coverage of 78.3 %. Screening and treatment of cervical abnormalities in England costs £175 million a year [20]. A total of 167 394 referrals to colposcopy were reported in 2012–2013, an increase of 13.2 per cent from 2011–2012 (147 889 referrals). The large increase in referrals is likely to be partly due to the roll-out of HPV testing.

All women between the ages of 25 and 64 are invited for cervical screening. Screening interval depends on age:

25 yrs: first invitation

25–49 yrs: 3-yearly

50–64 yrs: 5-yearly

65+: only those women with no smears since the age 50 or with recent abnormal smears [21].

Cervical screening can prevent nearly half of all cervical cancers in women in their 30s, and more than 75 % of cervical cancers in older women in their 50s and 60s, provided they attend screening regularly [21].

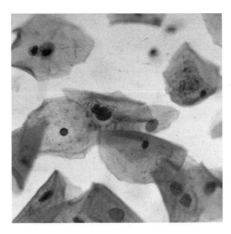

Figure 24.1 Normal smear (cytology picture). Normal squamous cells from the cervix with regular and small nuclei.

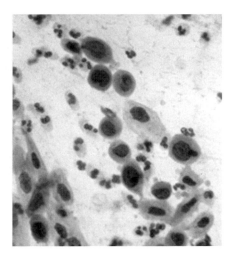

Figure 24.2 Severe dyskaryosis (cytology picture); in comparison, the dyskaryotic nuclei here show hyperchromasia, irregular outlines, and abnormal chromatin pattern.

Figures 24.1 and 24.2 courtesy Miss Maria Kyrgiou, Consultant in Gynaecological Oncology, Imperial Hospitals NHS Academic Trust.

⊕ **Clinical tip** Symptoms of cervical cancer

Although cervical cancer may be asymptomatic and a dyskaryotic smear may be the first abnormal finding, the commonest symptoms are listed:

- Inter-menstrual bleeding.
- Post-coital bleeding.
- Post-menopausal bleeding.
- Unpleasant vaginal discharge.
- Dyspareunia.
- Rarely haematuria or backache (advanced disease).

⊕ **Clinical tip** Urgent referral

- Referrals for colposcopy from primary care for women with high index of suspicion for malignancy on screening should be made via the two-week rule (TWR) to the gynaecological oncology team.
- Screening is not appropriate for women who have symptoms and conducting a cervical screening test may delay the proper diagnostic process in such cases. If the woman is symptomatic, such as experiencing bleeding between periods or after sex, she needs to consult her GP immediately.

ᴳ Expert comment

The National Institute of Health and Care Excellence (NICE) has recently evaluated two new adjunctive colposcopy techniques in evaluating the uterine cervix—DySIS and the Niris Imaging systems. DySIS comprises a digital video colposcope and dynamic spectral imaging technology that are used in combination with each other during clinical examination. The Niris Imaging System uses optical coherence tomography as an adjunct to a standard colposcope.

NICE has recommended that the DySIS is cost-effective and should be considered when NHS organizations are planning to buy colposcopy equipment. However, there is insufficient evidence to work out if the Niris Imaging system provides value for money [22].

❂ Learning point Human papilloma virus (HPV)

It is now known that HPV infection is associated with most cervical cancers [23]. Persistent exposure to HPV DNA is a pivotal element in the development of cervical malignancies. Exposure to high-risk HPV (HR HPV) infection, type 16 and 18, has shown to cause about 70% of all cervical cancers [8,24, 25]. The World Health Organisation (WHO) International Association for Research on Cancer (IARC) identifies 13 types of HPV strains as oncogenic. These high-risk types of HPV are: 16, 18, 31, 33, 35, 39, 45, 51, 52, 56, 58, 59, and 68; all have been shown to directly cause cervical cancer [26].

Risk factors for HPV infection include: number of sexual partners, a relatively recent new sexual relationship, and a history of previous miscarriage [28]. Among HPV-positive women, early age at first coitus, long duration of the most recent sexual relationship, and cigarette smoking are associated with development of CIN 3 [27].

HR HPV testing has recently been introduced in the National Cervical Screening Programme, both as a primary triaging investigation for low-grade and borderline abnormality as well as a test of cure following treatment for high-grade cervical dyskaryosis [28] (Figure 24.3). Whilst the ARTISTIC (A Randomised Trial of HPV Testing in Primary Cervical Screening, n = 25 000) trial has shown that routine HPV testing did not add significantly to the effectiveness of liquid-based cytology (LBC) screening [29], primary HPV triaging has a higher negative predictive value for dyskaryosis, which could potentially facilitate longer screening intervals.

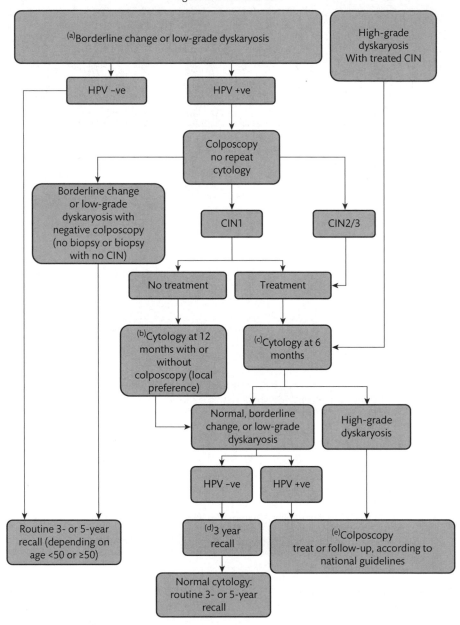

Figure 24.3 An example of an HPV testing and test of cure protocol [30].

HPV triage and text of cure in the cervical screening programme in England, reproduced from Gov.UK (31) under the Open Government License v2.0.

➕ **Clinical tip**

Adenocarcinomas are more commonly associated with HPV types 18 and 45 principally rather than type 16, which is the commonest HPV type for SCC of the cervix with lymphovascular space invasion (LVSI).

> ❝ **Expert comment**
>
> Vaccination against HPV has been rolled out in many countries in recent years, although to affect the global aspect of this disease a major focus has to be on targeting developing countries.
>
> HPV vaccination was introduced in the UK in September 2008 and is presently being offered to schoolgirls aged 12–13 using the quadrivalent vaccine (Gardasil) which protects against HPV types 6, 11 as well as high risk HPV16 and 18.
>
> Research indicates that the HPV vaccine could prevent up to two-thirds of cervical cancers in women under the age of 30 by 2025 but only if uptake of the HPV vaccination is at 80% [31]. To-date, the UK has achieved this level each year in the national HPV immunization programme.

> ✪ **Learning point** Risk factors for cervical cancer
>
> - Smoking has been associated with an increased risk of squamous cell carcinoma (SCC). A recent study by Parkin *et al.* suggested 7% of cases in 2010 were associated with smoking [32]. A recent meta-analysis suggests a 50% increased risk of SCC in current smokers [33].
> - Low socio-economic status has also shown to be a risk factor, with the risk multiplying by almost three in most deprived areas [34–36].
> - A meta-analysis found risk of invasive cervical cancer in current users of combined oral contraceptives (OC) increases by 7% for each year of use. The risk increase for five years of use is approximately 40%. The risk increase is temporary, and the risk returns to the level of someone who had never used the pill after 10 years of stopping use [37]. As with smoking, the direct cause and effect from COCs on cervical cancer is complicated by confounding sexual behaviour.
> - Women with HIV/AIDS have a six-times increased risk of developing cervical cancer, and women who have undergone organ transplant have twice or more the risk, strongly suggesting that immunosuppression plays an important role [38].

> ➕ **Clinical tip** Advice for patients after cervical treatment
>
> Prior to any excisional cervical treatment, the patient should be advised that:
>
> - The risk of preterm labour in treated patients is more than doubled when compared to the untreated group (Chapter 8).
> - This risk is the greatest in women who undergo cold knife conisation, followed by excisional treatment and least in women who have ablative treatment.
> - The depth and size of cone biopsy also has an impact on this risk. Cone biopsies measuring less than 10 mm carry less risk [39,40].
> - Patients should be advised not to wear tampons and refrain from sexual intercourse for 4 weeks after treatment.
> - Bleeding (secondary haemorrhage) post-procedure complicates 2–5% of cases.

The LLETZ histology confirmed a grade 3 adenocarcinoma of the cervix (15 mm in width and 3 mm in depth, extending to the lateral margins without LVSI and incompletely excised). Her case was discussed at the multidisciplinary team (MDT) meeting and an examination under anaesthetic (EUA) was recommended for staging purposes. Imaging in the form of magnetic resonance imaging (MRI) of the abdomen and pelvis was also arranged, along with CT scan of the chest.

EUA along with cystoscopy and sigmoidoscopy was undertaken. On examination, the vulva and vagina appeared normal. The cervix showed evidence of recent loop biopsy and normal non-infected granulation tissue was seen. The cervix appeared to be of normal size and shape and mobility. The uterus felt anteverted, normal sized, and mobile with no palpable adnexal masses. On per vaginal and per rectal

> ➕ **Clinical tip** Histological specimen examination
>
> Important prognostic factors to take into consideration are:
>
> - Size of specimen (influences stage), including width and depth of invasion.
> - Is excision complete, are margins clear.
> - Grade of tumour.
> - Histological subtype.
> - Presence of lymphovascular space invasion (LVSI).

examination, both parametrium felt regular and normal. Saline cystoscopy showed a normal bladder and sigmoidoscopy a normal rectum and sigmoid. The cervical cancer was clinically staged as FIGO stage 1B1.

> ✪ **Learning point** Cervical cancer staging
>
> The International Federation of Gynaecology and Obstetrics (FIGO) staging of cervical cancer is clinical, based on findings at EUA performed by an experienced clinician (Table 24.1). Due to the high incidence of this disease in the developing world, it is not dependent on lymph node status or imaging (MRI, CT scan), as this resource is not uniformly available worldwide [41]. Chest X-ray and intravenous pyelography are widely available and are taken into account for metastatic disease in the developing world. CT and MRI define lymph node status according to size, and hence may not accurately detect normal-sized nodal metastases [42].
>
> **Table 24.1 FIGO staging [43]**
>
> | Stage | |
> |---|---|
> | I | The carcinoma is strictly confined to the cervix (extension to the corpus would be disregarded). |
> | IA | Invasive carcinoma, which can be diagnosed only by microscopy with deepest invasion ≤5 mm and largest extension ≥7 mm. |
> | IA1 | Measured stromal invasion of ≤3.0 mm in depth and extension of ≤7.0 mm. |
> | IA2 | Measured stromal invasion of >3.0 mm and not >5.0 mm with an extension of not >7.0 mm. |
> | IB | Clinically visible lesions limited to the cervix uteri or preclinical cancers greater than stage IA.[b] |
> | IB1 | Clinically visible lesion ≤4.0 cm in greatest dimension. |
> | IB2 | Clinically visible lesion >4.0 cm in greatest dimension. |
> | II | Cervical carcinoma invades beyond the uterus but not to the pelvic wall or to the lower third of the vagina. |
> | IIA | Without parametrial invasion. |
> | IIA1 | Clinically visible lesion ≤4.0 cm in greatest dimension. |
> | IIA2 | Clinically visible lesion >4.0 cm in greatest dimension. |
> | IIB | With obvious parametrial invasion. |
> | III | The tumour extends to the pelvic wall and/or involves lower third of the vagina and/or causes hydronephrosis or nonfunctioning kidney.[c] |
> | IIIA | Tumor involves lower third of the vagina with no extension to the pelvic wall. |
> | IIIB | Extension to the pelvic wall and/or hydronephrosis or nonfunctioning kidney. |
> | IV | The carcinoma has extended beyond the true pelvis or has involved (biopsy proven) the mucosa of the bladder or rectum. A bullous edema, as such, does not permit a case to be allotted to stage IV. |
> | IVA | Spread of the growth to adjacent organs. |
> | IVB | Spread to distant organs. |
>
> [a]Adapted from FIGO Committee on Gynecologic Oncology [43]
> [b] All macroscopically visible lesions—even with superficial invasion—are allotted to stage IB carcinomas. Invasion is limited to a measured stromal invasion with a maximal depth of 5 mm and a horizontal extension of not >7 mm. Depth of invasion should not be >5 mm taken from the base of the epithelium of the original tissue—superficial or glandular. The depth of invasion should always be reported in mm, even in those cases with 'early (minimal) stromal invasion' (~1 mm).
> The involvement of vascular/lymphatic spaces should not change the stage allotment.
> [c]On rectal examination, there is no cancer-free space between the tumour and the pelvic wall. All cases with hydronephrosis or nonfunctioning kidney are included, unless they are known to be the result of another cause.

> ➕ **Clinical tip** Examination under anaesthetic
>
> Assessment parameters include:
>
> - Size of cervical tumour and extent.
> - Is the tumour extending down into the vagina?
> - Are the parametria-free on both sides or involved by tumour on PV and PR examination.
> - Is there extension into the pelvic side-wall?
> - On cystoscopy: is there obvious bladder involvement or there is oedema/bulging of the bladder mucosa or fistulation?
> - On sigmoidoscopy: is there involvement of the rectal mucosa or fistulation?

Her MRI scan was reviewed at the MDT meeting and this confirmed a small residual central tumour limited to the cervix (Figure 24.4). The scan also revealed slightly enlarged bilateral pelvic (iliac) nodes, which were suspicious for disease metastases by size criteria. A whole body PET/CT scan was requested to confirm this.

The PET/CT showed FDG avid uptake area in the pelvis with no uptake in any lymph nodes (Figure 24.5).

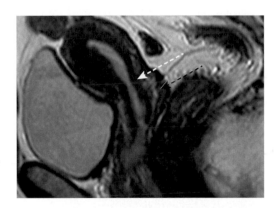

Figure 24.4 An exophytic mass arising from the anterior lip of the cervix and presence of deep cervical stromal invasion with stage IB1 invasive adenocarcinoma of the uterine cervix. Sagittal image show a tumour (T) within 5mm of the internal os. The orange arrow is the tumour showing deep stromal invasion and the green arrow is the internal os.

Image courtesy of *Radiology*.

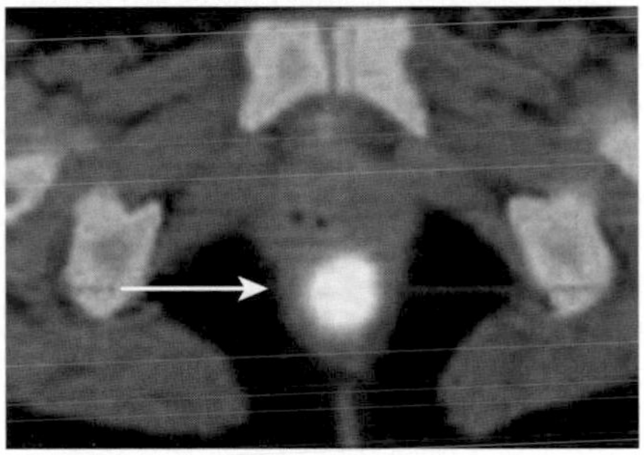

Figure 24.5 The PET/CT shows FDG avid uptake area in the pelvis (tumour, white arrow). No other uptake is seen higher up in the lateral part of pelvis, thus suggesting the iliac nodes to be negative.

❝ Expert comment

The MRI finding of enlarged iliac nodes may represent inflammatory change secondary to the recent LLETZ; the PET scan was requested to confirm this.

❝ Expert comment

If the lymph nodes had been positive, radical surgery would not be recommended.

❝ Expert comment

In resource-rich countries, more than one type of imaging is often undertaken to determine volume of disease and extent of spread. PET/CT combines images from both positron emission tomography (PET) as well as X-ray CT, and hence images from both the devices are available sequentially in the same patient at the same session and superimposed. The principle relies on a radiotracer like FDG (fluorodeoxyglucose) being able to trace glucose metabolism concentrated in hypermetabolic (cancerous) areas as well as areas of micrometastases, and the images of the PET demonstrate cellular activity which are then superimposed on the anatomical CT scan. There are studies currently underway to establish the sensitivity and specificity of PET/CT scans in cervical cancer in detecting metastatic disease. A recent prospective study with histopathological results as a reference found that combined PET and CT may be useful for detecting smaller nodal metastases [44].

Following discussion at MDT, the patient was reviewed in clinic and she reiterated the need to preserve her fertility if at all possible. The MDT recommended a fertility-sparing surgery of radical trachelectomy and pelvic lymphadenectomy, but this would be recommended only if the pelvic nodes were negative for disease. This was considered to be a viable option as the tumour was less than 2 cm and the lymph nodes were negative on PET CT.

✪ Learning point Radical trachelectomy [45]

Eligibility criteria

- FIGO stage IA1 with lymph-vascular space involvement (LVSI), or
- Stage IA2/IB1 histological subtypes: squamous, adenosquamous, adenocarcinoma.
- No evidence (clinical or radiological) to suspect extra-pelvic spread or lymph node metastases.
- Lesion diameter > 2 cm.
- Desire to preserve fertility.
- No diagnosis or indication to suspect infertility.
- Favourable age (relating to fertility outcomes).

Procedure

A fertility-preserving operation, known as 'radical trachelectomy', was coined in 1994 in a seminal paper by the late Daniel Dargent, who described a new technique suitable for exophytic tumours of stages IA–IIA. This procedure preserves the uterine body while removing the cervix, parametrium, and upper one-third of the vagina. Formation of a neocervix and application of a permanent cervical cerclage is also a part of the procedure.

Types of radical trachelectomy that are now recognized are: vaginal (VRT), abdominal (ART), and more recently laparoscopic (LART)/robotic abdominal radical trachelectomy (RART).

Abdominal radical trachelectomy (ART) is a safer option with regards to bulky, exophytic or > 2-cm diameter tumours, as the extent and location of tumours this size and shape requires an increased thoroughness of parametrial, sacro-uterine, vesico-cervical, and pelvic lymphatic tissue resection, which is not possible with VRT, where the approach limits the parametrial resection to tissue in the medial half of the broad ligament. VRT has certain advantages over ART, mainly a shorter hospital stay and post-operative recovery, and possibly less bladder and bowel dysfunction.

✪ Learning point Principles of treatment and management of cervical cancer

Treatment of cervical cancer is determined by stage with surgery being offered for early-stage disease and chemo-radiotherapy (CRT) for advanced-stage disease as shown in the schematic below.

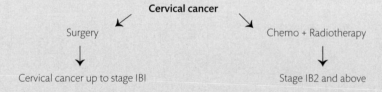

The principles of surgical treatment are excision of the central tumour and assessment of nodal disease. Volume of tumour (not only the size) is a determinant of operability [48].

For central disease (tumour confined to the cervix), depending on tumour volume and stage, either conservative simple excision or radical excision with or without fertility-sparing options is recommended.

(continued)

A stage-wise treatment option is described:

Stage Ia1 disease

- FIGO Ia1 cervical cancer (depth of invasion > 3 mm and width > 7 mm) may be managed conservatively.

Options available in the absence of lymph vascular space involvement (LVSI) include:

- Conization with adequate margins in women wishing to preserve fertility, or
- Simple hysterectomy if no desire to preserve fertility.

In the presence of LVSI, options are:

- Conisation and laparoscopic/open pelvic lymphadenectomy (the risk of nodal involvement with LVSI is less than 1% [49]).
- Radical trachelectomy with PLND for fertility conservation, or
- Modified radical hysterectomy with PLND.

Stage Ia2 disease

- Women with stage Ia2 (depth 3–5 mm and width > 7 mm) are informed of a nodal risk of 7%. In the absence of LVSI, they may be managed conservatively as for stage Ia1 with conisation and laparoscopic pelvic lymphadenectomy.
- If LVSI has been noted, then:
  –Radical trachelectomy with PLND for fertility conservation, or
  –Radical hysterectomy with PLND.

Stage IB–IIA cervical cancer

- Worldwide, no standard management exists for the management of stage IB–IIA cervical cancer.
- Most patients are offered either radical surgery or radical CRT.
- Although both options are considered to be equally effective, morbidity from surgery alone is considerably less. Combination treatment has been shown to have the highest toxicity.
- Treatment decisions depend on patient age, comorbidities, and tumour stage and treatment options available locally. Standard treatment for stage IBI is radical hysterectomy with PLND. In small volume tumours (> 2 cm) radical trachelectomy with PLND may be entertained if there is a desire to preserve fertility.

Stage IB2 –IV

- For locally advanced cervical cancer, radiotherapy has always played a major role.
- Standard treatment includes external beam radiotherapy plus brachytherapy with appropriate dosing of the central tumour and pelvic side wall boost.
- The addition of chemotherapy has significantly improved survival (67% versus 41%) [50].

---

⑥ Expert comment Neoadjuvant chemotherapy (NACT) in locally advanced cervical cancer

Concurrent chemoradiotherapy (CCRT) is the standard care for locally advanced cervical cancer and achieves a 6% improvement in five-year survival when compared to radiotherapy alone. A greater advantage in survival is noted when adjuvant chemotherapy is given after CCRT. In a similar clinical situation when NACT is followed by radical hysterectomy, a meta-analysis of five randomized clinical trials has shown this combination to significantly improve survival when compared to radiotherapy alone [51].

Benedetti-Panici et al. [52] showed survival benefit for NACT arm versus radiotherapy arm was significant for stage IB2–IIB patients but not for stage III disease. NACT is also sometimes considered in special situations in patients diagnosed with cervical cancer in pregnancy who decline surgical option due to the risk of miscarriage and premature labour [53].

❝ Expert comment

In cervical adenocarcinomas, the risk of metastasis is </= 8% and consideration should be given to performing a bilateral salpingo-oopherectomy at the same time if fertility-sparing treatment is not being considered [57].

✪ Learning point Prognostic factors in cervical cancer treatment

In addition to the FIGO stage of disease, the outcome following surgery is associated with a variety of prognostic factors such as:

- Larger tumour size.
- Presence or absence of LVSI.
- Nodal status.
- Deep stromal invasion.
- Close margins (less than 3 mm) or positive surgical resection margins.

Patients with early-stage disease have an intermediate risk of recurrence if any two of the aforementioned factors are present. A RCT evaluating 277 women with stage IB disease (radiotherapy versus 'no further treatment') and at least 2 risk factors showed that adjuvant radiotherapy decreased the rate of recurrence and improved disease-free survival. However, the two groups showed no overall difference in survival [54]. Therefore, despite the positive findings, options regarding adjuvant radiotherapy for surgical patients with selected risk factors remain debatable.

Studies by Landoni *et al.* [55] demonstrated that morbidity following radical surgery and radical radiotherapy is significantly greater. Treatment efficacy is similar for both in early-stage disease, and where possible, patient is triaged into either surgery or CRT.

In order to reduce morbidity from combination treatment, Daniel Dargent in 1987 pioneered laparoscopic pelvic lymphadenopathy, and subsequently proposed a 'two-stage technique' for the surgical management of cervical cancer [56]. In the first instance, a laparoscopic pelvic lymphadenectomy is performed, and if the nodes are histologically negative, then surgery in the form of either simple/radical hysterectomy can be undertaken. If fertility-sparing treatment is being considered, then radical trachelectomy may be considered.

❝ Expert comment

In 1958, McCall *et al.* described the technique of ovarian transposition (oopheropexy) as a way of preserving ovarian function in women receiving radiotherapy by surgically moving the ovaries out of the pelvic brim, outside of the radiotherapy field, while preserving their blood supply, and used to be performed by open surgery. This technique does not prevent loss of fertility and is purely to avoid premature, radiation induced, menopause. Results, however, are variable as devascularization of ovarian pedicles may occur due to tethering of vessels [58]. Today, it is undertaken by minimal access approach with improved results due to improved visualization offered by laparoscopic/robotic approach.

✪ Learning point Standard surgical management in operable cervical cancer

Radical hysterectomy is usually performed by open approach (laparotomy) [59]. However, minimal access surgery (laparoscopic, robotic) is preferred in centres with facilities and expertise due to significant reduction in short- to medium-term morbidity (although intra-operative morbidity is higher), and reduced blood loss from improved visualization at surgery [60].

A radical hysterectomy (Wertheims) involves removal of the cervix and corpus uteri along with the parametria and upper third of the vagina with clear margins.

The patient was keen to conserve fertility and underwent a laparoscopic abdominal radical trachelectomy (LART) and pelvic lymphadenectomy (Figure 24.6). The histology from the frozen section done at the time of the surgery confirmed that all the nodes were free of disease. The procedure was completed uneventfully and she was discharged on second post-operative day.

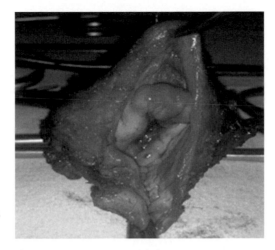

Figure 24.6 Specimen following a laparoscopic abdominal radical trachelectomy showing the cervix, parametria, and upper third of the vagina for FIGO IB1 cervical adenocarcinoma.

Courtesy of Mr Alan Farthing and Miss Maria Kyrgiou, Consultants in Gynaecological Oncology, Imperial Hospitals NHS Academic Trust, West London Gynaecological Cancer Centre.

⊕ Clinical tip Complications of radical surgical management

When discussing surgical management options, appropriate counselling should be offered. For fertility-sparing surgery, the risk of recurrence, risk of premature delivery, and second-trimester miscarriage of the order of 25% should be explained [61]. Besides the common side effects following a hysterectomy, radical surgery carries the risk of being associated with voiding dysfunction with an incidence of 0.4-3.7% for ureteric and bladder injuries. Fistula rates for both vesico-vaginal as well as utero-vaginal range from 0.9-2% [62].

⊘ Learning point Survival according to stage [63]

The chances of living for at least five years after being diagnosed with cervical cancer are:

- **Stage 1**–80–99%
- **Stage 2**–60–90%
- **Stage 3**–30–50%
- **Stage 4**–20%

In the UK, just fewer than 1000 women die from cervical cancer every year.

❝ Expert comment

Minimal access surgery offers the ability to undertake nerve-sparing techniques which are associated with less post-operative morbidity. Robotic surgery has vastly improved this and the advantages to both the surgeon and the patient are shown in Table 24.2.

Table 24.2 Advantages of robotic surgery

Benefits to patients	Benefits to surgeon
Reduced blood loss	Camera positioned by surgeon
Reduced blood transfusion	No camera shake or tremor
Reduced post-operative pain	3D HD image
Reduced hospital stay	Consistently good image avoids time wastage
Reduced risk of post-op complications	Operating time reduced
Fertility-sparing options	Better appreciation of anatomy
Nerve-sparing radical surgery feasible	Accuracy of surgery delivery
MAS available to more people	Reduced blood loss improves vision
Faster return to normal activities	Ergonomics

Her histology was discussed at the MDT meeting. The trachelectomy specimen showed CIN3 with clear margins and did not contain any residual cancer. Routine follow-up was recommended.

⊕ Clinical tip Follow-up after surgery

- Post Trachelectomy patients are usually followed up with three- to four-monthly clinical examinations for the first two years, and six-monthly vagino-isthmic smears. After the initial two years, annual follow-up is carried out up to 10 years with smears and clinical examination and or colposcopy.
- There is no recommended way of following up these patients, and surveillance for recurrence varies according to the experience at the local treatment centre
- Follow-up after radical hysterectomy for surgical management of early cervical cancer is usually by colposcopy and or vault smear as per the protocol of the treatment centre. The follow up is usually carried on up to 10 years. Clinical assessment for recurrence in these patients is done by recto-vaginal assessment and nodal examination (mainly supraclavicular).

> **⊘ Evidence base** Clinical trials in cervical cancer
>
> There are several ongoing clinical trials in cervical cancer:
>
> - The surgical trials include study on sentinel nodes and various techniques for surgical staging.
> - *CIRCCa* (Cediranib in Recurrent Cervical Cancer) is a trial of carboplatin–paclitaxel plus cediranib versus carboplatin–paclitaxel plus placebo in metastatic/recurrent cervical cancer. This study looks at which chemotherapy combination helps in improving survival in recurrent/metastatic cervical cancer.
> - A study looking at ways of increasing the number of young women who take up the offer of cervical screening (*STRATEGIC*) is presently ongoing in the UK.
> - A study comparing MRI scan with PET–CT scan for cervical and womb cancer (*MAPPING*) in presently recruiting patients. This study looks at DW MRI scan or a PET–CT scan may be better than a standard MRI scan in accurately diagnosing lymph node metastases. The researchers will also look at two different radioactive tracers used for the PET–CT scan.
> - A trial of chemotherapy before chemoradiation for cervical cancer (*INTERLACE*) is also recruiting participants. This study looks at improving survival for locally advanced cervical cancer using any of these strategies.

Discussion

Cervical cancer continues to impact women's health with more than half a million new cases being diagnosed each year worldwide. The majority of these are diagnosed in developing countries. Since the introduction of a national cervical screening programme in the UK, there has been a significant reduction in mortality and improvement in survival from early detection of cervical cancer and treatment of cervical pre-cancerous lesions. However, there has been a steady increase in the diagnosis of cervical cancer in young women (< 35 years) over the last decade and cervical cancer is now the most common cancer diagnosed in women in this age group. Pre-cancerous changes or very early-stage disease, as in the described clinical scenario, are usually asymptomatic and diagnosed by cervical smear. This case illustrates the importance of regular attendance for smears.

Grade of tumour, depth, and width of invasion, and presence or absence of lymphovascular space invasion, are prognostic factors that are taken into account before deciding on management. The impact of clinical staging when compared to surgical staging on survival is similar [64]. The treatment for early-stage cervical cancer is by surgery. The mode of surgery depends on the expertise, skills, and protocols followed at the treatment centre. In this case, an abdominal trachelectomy and pelvic lymph node dissection was performed as a fertility-preserving procedure. Adequate counselling about the impact of such surgery on survival, recurrence, and successful pregnancy needs to be fully explored with the patient. The significant risk of preterm labour following abdominal trachelectomy is addressed by referring these patients very early on in their subsequent pregnancy to dedicated preterm labour/high-risk obstetric clinics. There is presently ongoing research into sentinel node biopsy for stage IA2–IB disease, and whether pelvic lymph node dissection can be omitted in patients with a sentinel node negative result. The prognosis for this woman is very good due to early detection and adequate treatment for her cancer, and at the same time preserving her fertility.

A Final Word from the Expert

The presence of HPV is a major factor in the development of cervical cancer. However most women will be exposed to HPV infection during their lifetime, but only few will get cervical cancer. Nevertheless the elimination of high-risk HPV through a vaccination programme will reduce cervical cancer by about 70%. Equally, HPV presence can be used to facilitate the triage of patients with abnormal smears, and indeed eventually may replace the cervical smear as a screening tool. In resource-poor countries, a simpler and affordable screening programme and universal access to cheaper vaccination may be the most effective way of dealing with this disease.

References

1. Ferlay J, Soerjomataram I, Ervik M, Dikshit R, Eser S, Mathers C, *et al*. GLOBOCAN 2012 v1.0, Cancer Incidence and Mortality Worldwide: IARC CancerBase No. 11 [Internet]. Lyon, France: International Agency for Research on Cancer; 2013. <http://globocan.iarc.fr>

2. Office for National Statistics (ONS). Cancer survival in England: Patients diagnosed 2005-2009 and followed up to 2010. London: ONS; 2011.

3. Coleman MP, Babb P, Damiecki P, Grosclaude P, Honjo S, Jones J, *et al*. Cancer Survival Trends in England and Wales, 1971–1995: Deprivation and NHS Region. Series SMPS No. 61 London: ONS, 1999.

4. Office for National Statistics (ONS). Cancer Survival: England and Wales, 1991–2001, twenty major cancers by age group. London: ONS, 2005.

5. Rachet B, Maringe C, Nur U, Coleman MP, Babb P, Damiecki P, *et al*. Population-based cancer survival trends in England and Wales up to 2007. *Lancet Oncol* 2009;10:351–69. (Age-standardized figures were provided by the author on request.)

6. Foley G, Alston R, Geraci M, Brabin L, Kitchener H, Birch J, *et al*. Increasing rates of cervical cancer in young women in England: an analysis of national data 1982–2006. *Br J Cancer* 2011;105(1):177–84.

7. Tripp J, Viner R. Sexual health, contraception, and teenage pregnancy. *BMJ* 2005;330(7491):590–3.

8. Bosch FX, Lorincz A, Muñoz N, Meijer CJ, Shah KJ. The causal relation between human papillomavirus and cervical cancer. *J Clin Pathol* 2002;55(4):244–65.

9. <http://www.cancerscreening.nhs.uk/cervical>

10. HSIC–Health and Social Care Information Centre –Cervical Screening Program England 2012–2013.

11. Data were provided by the Office for National Statistics on request, June 2012. Similar data can be found here: <http://www.ons.gov.uk/ons/search/index.html?newquery=cancer+registrations>

12. Data were provided by ISD Scotland on request, April 2012. Similar data can be found here: <http://www.isdscotland.org/Health-Topics/Cancer/Publications/index.asp>

13. Data were provided by the Welsh Cancer Intelligence and Surveillance Unit on request, April 2012. Similar data can be found at: <http://www.wales.nhs.uk/sites3/page.cfm?orgid=242pid=59080>

14. Data were provided by the Northern Ireland Cancer Registry on request, October 2012. Similar data can be found at: <http://www.qub.ac.uk/research-centres/nicr/CancerData/OnlineStatistics>/

15. Sasieni P, Castañón A, Cuzick J. Effectiveness of cervical screening with age: population based case-control study of prospectively recorded data. *BMJ* 2009;339. doi: 10.1136/bmj.b 2968.

16. Nobbenhuis MA, Helmerhorst TJ, van den Brule AJ, Rozendaal L, Voorhorst FJ, Bezemer PD, *et al.* Cytological regression and clearance of high-risk human papillomavirus in women with an abnormal cervical smear. *Lancet* 2001;358(9295):1782–3.

17. Castle PE, Schiffman M, Wheeler CM, Solomon D. Evidence for frequent regression of cervical intraepithelial neoplasia-grade 2. *Obstet Gynecol* 2009;113(1):18–25.

18. Cancer Statistics Registrations, England (Series MB1) No. 40, 2009. Office for National Statistics.

19. <http://www.cancerscreening.nhs.uk/cervical>

20. HSIC–Health and Social Care Information Centre –Cervical Screening Program England 2012–2013.

21. Sasieni P, Adams J, Cuzick J. Benefit of cervical screening at different ages: evidence from the UK audit of screening histories. *Br J Cancer* 2003 Jul 7;89(1):88–93

22. <http://guidance.nice.org.uk/DG4>

23 Walboomers JMM, Meijer C. Do HPV-negative cervical carcinomas exist? [Editorial]. *Journal Pathology* 1997;181:253–4.

24. Bosch FX, Burchell AN, Schiffman M, Giuliano AR, de Sanjose S, Bruni L, *et al.* Epidemiology and natural history of human papillomavirus infections and type-specific implications in cervical neoplasia. *Vaccine* 2008. 26(10), K1–16.

25. Parkin DM. Cancers attributable to infection in the UK in 2010. *Br J Cancer* 2011;105(S2):S49–S56.

26. Szarewski A. 2012. Cervarix: a bivalent vaccine against HPV types 16 and 18, with cross-protection against other high-risk HPV types. *Expert Rev Vaccines* 2012;11(6):645–57.

27. Deacon JM, Evans CD, Yule R, Desai M, Binns W, Taylor C, *et al.* Sexual behaviour and smoking as determinants of cervical HPV infection and of CIN 3 among those infected. A case-control study nested within the Manchester cohort. *Br J Cancer* 2000;83:1565–72.

28. Kelly RS, Patnick J, Kitchener HC, Moss SM; NHSCSP HPV Special Interest Group. HPV Testing as a triage for borderline or mild dyskaryosis on cervical cytology: results from the sentinel sites studies, *Br J Cancer* (2011);105:983–8.

29. Kitchener HC, Almonte M, Gilham C, Dowie R, Stoykova B, Sargent A, Roberts C, Desai M, Peto J, on behalf of the ARTISTIC Trial Study Group ARTISTIC: a randomised trial of human papillomavirus (HPV) testing in primary cervical screening. *Health Technol Assess* 2009;13(51):1–150.

30. <http://www.cancerscreening.nhs.uk/cervical/hpv-triage-test-flowchart.pdf>

31. Cuzick J, Castanon A, Sasieni P. 2010. Predicted impact of vaccination against human papillomavirus 16/18 on cancer incidence and cervical abnormalities in women aged 20-29 in the UK. *Br J Cancer* 102, 933–9.

32. Parkin DM. Tobacco-attributable cancer burden in the UK in 2010. *Br J Cancer* 2011;105(S2):S6–S13.

33. International Collaboration of Epidemiological Studies of Cervical Cancer. Comparison of risk factors for invasive squamous cell carcinoma and adenocarcinoma of the cervix: collaborative reanalysis of individual data on 8,097 women with squamous cell carcinoma and 1,374 women with adenocarcinoma from 12 epidemiological studies. *Int J Cancer* 2007;120(4):885–91.

34. Quinn M, Babb P, Brock A, Kirby L, Jones J. Cancer Trends in England & Wales 1950–1999. Vol. SMPS No. 66 London: ONS, 2001.

35. Harris V, Sandridge AL, Black RJ, Brewster DH, Gould A. Cancer Registration Statistics: Scotland 1986–1995. 1998, Edinburgh: ISD Scotland Publications.

36. Brown J, Harding S, Bethune A. Incidence of Health of the nation cancers by social class. *Popul Trends* 1997 Winter; 90:40-7, 49-77.

37. Appleby P, Beral V, Berrington de González A, Colin D, Franceschi S, Goodhill A, *et al.* Cervical cancer and hormonal contraceptives: collaborative reanalysis of individual data for 16,573 women with cervical cancer and 35,509 women without cervical cancer from 24 epidemiological studies. *Lancet* 2007;370(9599):1609–21.

38. Grulich AE, van Leeuwen MT, Falster MO, Vajdic CM. Incidence of cancers in people with HIV/AIDS compared with immunosuppressed transplant recipients: a meta-analysis. *Lancet* 2007;370(9581):59–67.

39. Kyrgiou M, Koliopoulos G, Martin-Hirsch P, Arbyn M, Prendiville W, Paraskevaidis E. Obstetric outcomes after conservative treatment for intra-epithelial or early invasive cervical lesions: a systematic review and meta-analysis of the literature. *Lancet* 2006;367:489–98.

40. Arbyn M, Kyrgiou M, Simoens C, Raifu AO, Koliopoulos G, Martin-Hirsch P, *et al.* Perinatal mortality and other severe adverse pregnancy outcomes associated with treatment of cervical intraepithelial neoplasia: a meta-analysis. *BMJ* 2008;337:a1284.

41. Elkas J, Farias-Eisner R. Cancer of the uterine cervix. *Curr Opin Obstet Gynecol* 1998;10:47–50.

42. Hricak H, Gatsonis C, Chi DS, Amendola MA, Brandt K, Schwartz LH, *et al.* Role of imaging in pretreatment evaluation of early invasive cervical cancer: results of the intergroup study American College of Radiology Imaging Network 6651-Gynecologic Oncology Group 183. *J Clin Oncol* 2005;23:9329–37.

43. Pecorelli S. Revised FIGO staging for carcinoma of the vulva, cervix, and endometrium. *Int J Gynaecol Obstet* 2009;105(2):103–4.

44. Sironi, S, Buda A, Picchio M, Perego P, Moreni R, Pellegrino A, *et al.* Lymph node metastasis in patients with clinical early-stage cervical cancer: detection with integrated FDG PET/CT. *Radiology* 2005;238:272–9.

45. Saso S, Ghaem-Maghami S, Chatterjee J, Naji O, Farthing A, Mason P, *et al.* Abdominal radical trachelectomy in West London. *BJOG* 2012;119:187–93.

46. Saso S, Chatterjee J, Smith JR. Radical trachelectomy: need for a randomized controlled trial? *Acta Obstet Gynecol Scand* 2012; Jun 91(6):758.

47. Plante M, Renaud MC, Roy M. Radical vaginal trachelectomy: a fertility-preserving option for young women with early stage cervical cancer. *Gynecol Oncol* 2005;99(3 Suppl 1): S143–6.

48. Soutter WP, Hanoch J, D'Arcy T, Dina R, McIndoe GA, deSouza NM. Pre-treatment tumour volume measurement on high-resolution magnetic resonance imaging as a predictor of survival in cervical cancer. *BJOG* July 2004;111:741–7.

49. Bekkers RLM, Keyser KGG, Bulten J, Hanselaar AGJM, Schijf CPT, Boonstra H, *et al.* The value of loop electrosurgical conization in the treatment of Stage IA1 microinvasive carcinoma of the uterine cervix. *Int J Gynecol Cancer* 2002;12:485–9.

50. Al-Mansour Z, Verschraegen C. Locally advanced cervical cancer: what is the standard of care? *Current Opinion in Oncology* 2010;22:503–12.

51. González-Martín A, González-Cortijo L, Carballo N, Garcia JF, Lapuente F, Rojo A, *et al.* The current role of neoadjuvant chemotherapy in the management of cervical carcinoma. *Gynecol Oncol* 2008;110:S36–S40.

52. Benedetti-Panici P, Greggi S, Colombo A, Amoroso M, Smaniotto D, Giannarelli D, *et al.* Neoadjuvant chemotherapy and radical surgery versus exclusive radiotherapy in locally advanced squamous cell cervical cancer: results from the Italian multicenter randomized study. *J Clin Oncol* 2002:20:179–88.

53. Dawood R, Instone M, Kehoe S. Neo-adjuvant chemotherapy for cervical cancer in pregnancy: a case report and literature review. *Eur J Obstet Gynecol Reprod Biol* 2013;171:205–8.

54. Rotman M, Sedlis A, Piedmonte MR, Bundy B, Lentz SS, Muderspach LI, *et al.* A phase III randomized trial of postoperative pelvic irradiation in stage IB cervical carcinoma with poor prognostic features: follow-up of a gynecologic oncology group study. *Int J Radiat Oncol Biol Phys* 2006;65:169–76.

55. Landoni F, Maneo A, Colombo A, Placa F, Milani R, Perego P, Favini, *et al.* Randomised study of radical surgery versus radiotherapy for stage Ib-IIa cervical cancer. *Lancet* 1997;350:535–40.

56. Dargent D, Enria R. Laparoscopic assessment of the sentinel lymph nodes in early cervical cancer. Technique-preliminary results and future developments. *Crit Rev Oncol Hematol* 2003;48:305–10.

57. Landoni F, Zanagnolo V, Lovato-Diaz L, Maneo A, Rossi R, Gadducci A, Cosio S, *et al.* Ovarian metastases in early-stage cervical cancer (IA2-IIA): a multicenter retrospective study of 1965 patients (a Cooperative Task Force study). *Int J Gynecol Cancer* 2007 May-Jun; 17(3):623–8.

58. Hwang JH, Yoo HJ, Park SH, Lim MC, Seo SS, Kang S, *et al.* Association between the location of transposed ovary and ovarian function in patients with uterine cervical cancer treated with (postoperative or primary) pelvic radiotherapy. *Fertil Steril* 2012 Jun; 97(6):1387–93.e1–2.

59. Papacharalabous E, Tailor A, Madhuri TK, Giannopoulos T, Butler-Manuel SA. Early experience of laparoscopically-assisted radical vaginal hysterectomy (Coelio-Schauta) versus abdominal radical hysterectomy for early-stage cervical cancer. *Gynaecological Surgery* 2009;2:97–100.

60. Nezhat FR, Datta MS, Liu C, Chuang L, Zakashansky K. Robotic radical hysterectomy versus total laparoscopic radical hysterectomy with pelvic lymphadenectomy for treatment of early cervical cancer. 2008 *JSLS* Jul–Sep; 12(3):227–37.

61. Shepherd JH, Mould T, Oram DH. Radical trachelectomy in early stage carcinoma of the cervix: outcome as judged by recurrence and fertility rates. *BJOG* 2001 Aug; 108(8):88–5.

62. Likic IS, Kadija S, Ladjevic NG, Stefanovic A, Jeremic K, Petkovic S, *et al.* Analysis of urologic complications after radical hysterectomy. *Am J Obstet Gynecol* 2008 Dec; 199(6):644.e1–3.

63. Waggoner SE. Cervical cancer. *Lancet* 2003;361:2217–25.

64. Lai CH, Huang KG, Hong JH, Lee CL, Chou HH, Chang TC, *et al.* Randomized trial of surgical staging (extraperitoneal or laparoscopic) versus clinical staging in locally advanced cervical cancer. *Gynecol Oncol* 2003;89:160–7.

INDEX